Cardiac Rehabilitation

CONTEMPORARY CARDIOLOGY

CHRISTOPHER P. CANNON, MD
SERIES EDITOR

CARDIAC REHABILITATION

Edited by

WILLIAM E. KRAUS, MD, FACC, FACSM

Professor of Medicine,
Medical Director,
Cardiac Rehabilitation,
Duke University Medical Center,
Durham, NC

and

STEVEN J. KETEYIAN, PHD, FACSM

Director, Preventive Cardiology,
Division of Cardiovascular Medicine,
Henry Ford Hospital,
Detroit, MI

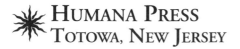

HUMANA PRESS
TOTOWA, NEW JERSEY

Production Editor: Tracy Catanese

Cover design by Patricia F. Cleary

For additional copies, pricing for bulk purchases, and/or information about other Humana titles, contact Humana at the above address or at any of the following numbers: Tel.: 973-256-1699; Fax: 973-256-8341, E-mail: orders@humanapr.com; or visit our Website: www.humanapress.com

This publication is printed on acid-free paper. ∞

ANSI Z39.48-1984 (American National Standards Institute) Permanence of Paper for Printed Library Materials.

Photocopy Authorization Policy:

Printed in the United States of America. 10 9 8 7 6 5 4 3 2 1

eISBN 978-1-59745-491-9

Library of Congress Control Number: 2007928909

Acknowledgements

This volume is dedicated to Andrew G. Wallace, who as Division Chief of Duke Cardiology pioneered cardiac rehabilitation nationally and at Duke in the late 1970s, shepherding it through the early days of coverage by national insurance carriers; and to Frederick R. Cobb, who spent the last 15 years of his abruptly shortened but distinguished career dedicated to the secondary cardiovascular prevention principles that underlie modern cardiac rehabilitation. Finally, this volume is also dedicated to Sidney Goldstein, who, as Chief of Cardiovascular Medicine at Henry Ford Hospital, both appreciated and advanced the use of randomized clinical trials to evaluate a variety of secondary prevention strategies in patients with heart disease; treatment strategies that included risk factor management and exercise training.

PREFACE

The era of cardiac rehabilitation in the United States dates back at least thirty years, when Herman Hellerstein at Case Western Reserve, Andy Wallace at Duke and Ken Cooper in Dallas envisioned that a comprehensive lifestyle approach to the rehabilitation and prevention of patients having had a cardiac event would potentially yield great benefits for the individual patient and the health care system. Until that time, the thought of vigorous exercise in the cardiac patient soon after an event was close to anathema. One of us (WEK) was introduced to Herman Hellerstein in Cleveland in the late 1960's, when his father sought medical opinion from him for a cardiac condition. WEK was introduced to Andy Wallace in 1979 by which time the latter had started a multidisciplinary, geographically regional cardiac rehabilitation program at Duke based upon consultations with Hellerstein and Cooper. By then, cardiac rehabilitation was progressing beyond the vision of exercise only, and since then the concept of cardiac rehabilitation has grown into the comprehensive multidisciplinary program that we know today and that we attempt to describe in this volume.

The practice of cardiac rehabilitation has grown and metamorphosed in the last thirty years in parallel with the growth and metamorphosis of the practice of cardiovascular medicine. During the formative stages of cardiac rehabilitation, the use of coronary care units was in its infancy. The coronary artery bypass operation was less than ten years old. The LIMA bypass had not been invented. There were no statins and the use of angiotensin converting enzyme inhibitors was just beginning. And of course, angioplasty was just a twinkle in the eye of forward looking pioneers in cardiovascular medicine. Thus, the modern practice of both cardiac rehabilitation and cardiovascular medicine represent new realities that are ever evolving. As an example, just last year, in 2006, the Center for Medicare and Medicaid Services (CMS), approved three new indications for cardiac rehabilitation reimbursement (Percutaneous Coronary Intervention-PCI, cardiac transplantation and valvular surgery) to accompany the previous three indications of chronic stable angina, post bypass and post myocardial infarction. More importantly and significantly, CMS recognized cardiac rehabilitation as the truly multidisciplinary program that it is – beyond just exercise therapy for the cardiac patient. And, as this text is in development, the American Association of Cardiovascular and Pulmonary Rehabilitation, the American Heart Association and the American College of Cardiology are combining efforts to publish the first set of performance measures for referral to and delivery of Cardiac Rehabilitation.

To reflect this new reality, we are pleased to have developed this volume. However, this text is not meant as a comprehensive compendium of the history and medical literature supporting the medical practice of cardiac rehabilitation. Rather, such overviews are available in other texts and in Cochrane reviews. Rather, we have specifically designed this as a practical manual for those newly introduced to the specialty, such as ancillary health personnel or cardiology fellows, or for established cardiologists wishing to begin a program in their practice or assuming the role as Medical Director of established programs. We trust that it will serve this purpose well. The text is divided into several sections.

After an Introduction and Overview by the editors (Kraus and Keteyian) and a brief introduction to Exercise Principles, we delve into the essential components of a comprehensive cardiac rehabilitation program. In a section devoted to nutrition, Gene Erb and Julie Pruitt discuss the use of contemporary diets in cardiac rehabilitation and Joh Ehrman discusses the approach to obesity.

Assessment of psychological state and supporting behavior and lifestyle change, whether in nutrition, exercise, smoking cessation or stress and anger management is an essential component of a comprehensive cardiac rehabilitation program. In a section on behavioral aspects of cardiac rehabilitation, Krista Barbour discusses the approaches to depression, and Ruth Quillian-Wolever the approach to stress management. Readiness for Change theory, or the Transtheoretical Model is used a basis for behavior change in multiple venues and Charlotte Collins presents this paradigm for treatment. Last in this section, Jennifer Davis presents the essential approach to smoking cessation.

Exercise Testing is used for prognostication, diagnosis and assessment of exercise capacity and therapeutic progress in the cardiac rehabilitation setting. In this section Bill Kraus presents the basis and uses of exercise testing and Clinton Brawner presents the essential of performing and interpreting the exercise stress test. Dan Bensimhon describes the indications, performance standards and interpretation of the cardiopulmonary exercise test and Vera Bittner does the same for the six minute walk test.

Medical therapy is a mainstay of the comprehensive cardiac rehabilitation program. Treating to goal has become a standard of cardiac post event and prevention programs. As the medical therapy for cardiac often cannot be optimized during their hospital admission, the outpatient cardiac rehabilitation setting when one patient can be seen up to 36 times over the course of three months has become an optimal setting to titrate medical therapies to goal. In this section, Christie Ballantyne and Ryan Neal describe treating lipids to goal in the cardiac rehabilitation setting. Neil Gordon does the same for diabetes mellitus and hypertension.

In a section unto its own, John Schaier and Steven Keteyian describe the various Cardiac Populations for which cardiac rehabilitation is typically prescribed and the vagaries of exercise therapy in these settings. Coronary artery disease is a disease that often presents in the setting of other co-morbid conditions that may require significant modifications of the standard therapeutic approaches. In this section on exercise and co-morbidities, Dalynn Badenhop addresses hypertension and Jennifer Green offers what one needs to know about diabetes mellitus. Neil Macintyre, a well known expert in pulmonary rehabilitation, addresses the needs of the pulmonary patient with cardiac disease. Chris Womack discusses the special needs of the patient in cardiac rehabilitation that has peripheral artery disease. Kim Huffman discusses the issues associated with the cardiac rehabilitation patient with associated arthritis and Dan Forman discusses the challenges and approaches for the elderly patient.

One of the particularly satisfying part of being involved in cardiac rehabilitation is the programmatic advances that have taken place over the course of the last thirty years. When cardiac rehabilitation first started, there was no reimbursement for services. Now, the Program and Medical Directors require broad knowledge regarding several dimensions about running a program, including how to handle referrals, the physicians role, and billing and reimbursement. In this Programmatic section we address these issues. Linda Hall discusses soliciting and handling programmatic referrals. Phil Ades addresses the physician Medical Director's role. Bill Kraus presents an innovative way to provide programmatic assessment and treatment of risk in the cardiac rehabilitation and associated clinic setting. Greg Lawson presents the various staffing models and Pat Comoss discusses billing and reimbursement.

We are pleased to present to you, the interested reader, what we hope will be a useful and thorough overview of the component elements of state of the art cardiac rehabilitation. We trust that the new initiate to cardiac rehabilitation will find useful information. To facilitate communication and quick reference, many of the chapters have highlighted summary tables of important information. We hope that even seasoned veterans will find some innovative hints on how to improve their programs. And we welcome feedback from the reader on how we can make this effort better as we all participate in the coming future evolution of cardiac rehabilitation in the 21st century.

William E. Kraus, MD
Durham
Steven J. Keteyian, PHD
Detroit

CONTENTS

CONTRIBUTORS

PHIL A. ADES, MD • University of Vermont, College of Medicine, Burlington, VT

DALYNN T. BADENHOP, PHD • University of Toledo Medical Center, Toledo, OH

CHRISTIE BALLANTYNE • Director, Center for Cardiovascular, Disease Prevention, Methodist DeBakey Heart Center, Houston, TX 77030

KRISTA A. BARBOUR, PHD • Clinical Associate, Medical Psychiatry, P.O. Box 3119, Duke University Medical Center, Durham, NC 27710

DANIEL BENSIMHON, MD • Associate in Medicine, 3912 Hazel Ln., Greensboro, NC 27408

VERA BITTNER, MD • Professor of Medicine, University of Alabama at Birmingham, Birmingham, AL

CLINTON A. BRAWNER, MS • Henry Ford Hospital, ACSM Registered Clinical Exercise Physiologist Detroit, MI

MEGHAN L. BUTRYN

PAUL CHASE

CHARLOTTE A. COLLINS, PHD • One Hoppin Street, Providence, RI 02903

PATRICIA McCALL COMOSS, RN • Nursing Enrichment Consultants, Harrisburg, PA

JENNIFER DAVIS, MS • Clinical Psychologist, P.O. Box 3022, Duke Center for Living, Duke University Medical Center, Durham, NC 27710

JONATHAN K. EHRMAN • Henry Ford Hospital, Detroit, MI

GENE ERB, JR • Clinical Dietician, P.O. Box 3487, Duke University Medical Center, Durham, NC 27710

DANIEL E. FORMAN, MD • Brigham and Women's Hospital, Boston, MA

NEIL F. GORDON, MD, PHD • INTERVENT USA, Inc., 340 Eisenhower Drive, 1400 Central Park, Suite 17, Savannah, GA 31406

JENNIFER B. GREEN, MD • Assistant Clinical Professor, Division of Endocrinology, Metabolism and Nutrition, Department of Medicine, P.O. Box 3222, Duke University Medical Center, Durham, NC 27710

LINDA K. HALL, PHD • Hattiesburg, MS

KIM M. HUFFMAN, MD, PHD • P.O. Box 3327, Duke University Medical Center, Durham, NC 27710

ERNESTINE G. JENNINGS

JAVIER JURADO • University of Toledo Medical Center, Toledo, OH

STEVEN J. KETEYIAN, PHD • Henry Ford Hospital, Detroit, MI

WILLIAM E. KRAUS, MD, • Professor of Medicine, Medical Director, Cardiac Rehabilitation, Duke University Medical Center, Durham, NC 27710

GREGORY J. LAWSON, MS • Providence Everett Medical Center, Everett, WA

NEIL MacINTYRE, MD • Professor, Department of Medicine, Division of Pulmonary Medicine, P.O. Box 3911, Duke University Medical Center, Durham, NC 27710

RYAN NEAL • Professor of Medicine and Pediatrics, Baylor College of Medicine, 6565 Fannin St. MS A601, Houston, TX 77030

JULIE PRUITT • ActivHealth Coordinator, P.O. Box 3022, Duke University Medical Center, Duke Center for Living, Durham, NC 27710

JOHN R. SCHAIRER, DO • Henry Ford Hospital, Detroit, MI

RUTH Q. WOLEVER, PHD • Assistant Clinical Professor, Medical Psychiatry, Duke Center for Integrative Medicine, P.O. Box 3022, Duke University Medical Center, Durham, NC 27710

CHRISTOPHER J. WOMACK, PHD • Department of Kinesiology, Harrisonburg, VA

1 Introduction

William E. Kraus, MD,
and Steven J. Keteyian, PhD

Although the field of contemporary cardiac rehabilitation has a relatively short (25 years) history in terms of its contribution to evidence-based care for patients with cardiovascular disease, it stands as a subspecialty deserving of a textbook devoted to helping clinicians better understand how best to provide secondary preventive care to patients recovering from a cardiac-related event. In addition, cardiac rehabilitation is undergoing great change. Specifically, to reflect the importance of targeted initiatives in the management of risk factors, changes in program scope have broadened to shift the emphasis away from cardiac rehabilitation from serving as program devoted only to instituting exercise therapy to one that embraces a comprehensive secondary preventive strategy addressing the multiple medical, exercise, nutritional, and behavioral factors that place a patient at increased risk of a subsequent cardiac event.

Consistent with this change in program scope, third party payers – such as Medicare – now recognize the importance of comprehensive secondary prevention. In fact, the new national coverage decision policy from Medicare specifies that rehabilitation should not be solely an exercise program but rather one that is multidisciplinary and aimed at reducing subsequent cardiovascular disease risk through intensive risk factor management and institution of therapeutic lifestyle changes.

For the physician and allied health professional interested in the secondary prevention of cardiovascular disease, a good summary of the secondary prevention goals and treatment guidelines can be found in a recent American Heart Association/American College of Cardiology (AHA/ACC) paper on this topic *(1)*. Table 1 in this introductory chapter provides a summary of these goals. In addition, the American Association of Cardiovascular and Pulmonary Rehabilitation (AACVPR) also has been a long-standing proponent of the multidisciplinary programmatic concept, such that cardiac rehabilitation programs address the broad scope of cardiovascular disease and its risk-related morbidities (diabetes, hypertension, dyslipidemias, metabolic syndrome, psychosocial stress, and smoking behavior) through both medical and multicomponent lifestyle interventions *(2)*. In fact, both the ACC and the AACVPR, along with the American

From: *Contemporary Cardiology: Cardiac Rehabilitation*
Edited by: W. E. Kraus and S. J. Keteyian © Humana Press Inc., Totowa, NJ

Table 1
Summary of the American Heart Association/American College of Cardiology
Goals for Secondary Prevention in Patients with Coronary and other
Atherosclerotic Vascular Disease *(1)*

Risk factor or therapy	Goal
Smoking	Complete cessation. No exposure to environmental tobacco smoke.
Blood pressure	< 140/90 or < 130/80 mmHg if patient has diabetes or chronic kidney disease
Lipid management	Low density lipoprotein cholesterol < 100 mg/dL; if triglycerides are ≥ 200 mg/dL then non-high density lipoprotein cholesterol should be < 130 mg/dL
Physical activity	30 minutes, 7 days per week (minimum 5 days per week)
Weight management	Body mass index, 18.5–24.9 kg/m^2
	Waist circumference, men < 40 inches and women < 35 inches
Diabetes management	Hemoglobin A_{1c} < 7%
Antiplatelet agents/anticoagulants	See full paper for treatment recommendations *(1)*
Renin-angiotensin-aldosterone system blockers	See full paper for treatment recommendations *(1)*
Beta-adrenergic blockers	See full paper for treatment recommendations *(1)*
Influenza vaccination	Patients with cardiovascular disease should be vaccinated

College of Sports Medicine (ACSM), the American Hospital Association, and other organizations and individuals, were instrumental in providing the scientific evidence and opinion comment that led to the most recent changes in Medicare's national coverage policy *(3)*. A summary of these changes are outlined in Table 2. As is evident, Medicare now expects rehabilitation programs to extend service provision beyond exercise only by using an interdisciplinary team approach to promote recovery from a cardiac event and reduce the risk of subsequent events. To facilitate this thinking, this volume strives to provide background evidence and helpful guidance in many of these multidisciplinary elements for the new practitioner to cardiac rehabilitation, whether this be an established medical practitioner starting a program for the first time, the cardiac fellow being exposed to the discipline as part of training, or one of the myriad of ancillary programmatic practitioners joining an established program or assisting in the creation of a new one.

The timing is right for a textbook that provides the cardiac rehabilitation practitioner with both the theoretical and the practical aspects of working in the cardiac

Table 2
Summary of Important Changes in Medicare National Coverage Decision Policy
from 1982 to March 2006 and from March 2006 (3)

	1982–March 2006	As of March 26, 2006
Program components	Stipulated exercise only	Medical evaluation, risk factor modification, exercise, and education
Program duration	36 visits in 12 weeks	36 visits in 18 weeks (following review, up to 72 visits in 36 weeks)
ECG rhythm strips	Required	Clinician-determined need for ECG monitoring
Level of physician supervision	Proximal to exercise area	Hospital premises (within 250 yards for separate buildings on campus). Off hospital campus then present and immediately available
"Incident to" physician	Unclear	Can vary based on setting of the services provided; however, ordering physician, primary care physician, or program medical director should all suffice as long as there is documentation in the medical record of interactions between the physician and rehabilitation staff concerning patient status.
Indications	STEMI, NSTEMI, CABG, and stable angina	NTEMI, STEMI, CABG, angina, PTCA, coronary stenting, heart valve surgery, and cardiac transplant

CABG, coronary artery bypass graft surgery; NSTEMI, non-ST segment elevation myocardial infarction; PTCA, percutaneous transluminal coronary angioplasty; and STEMI, ST segment elevation myocardial infarction.

rehabilitation setting. This volume addresses all aspects of cardiology-related secondary prevention including

- medical, exercise, and nutritional management of hypertension, diabetes, and lipid abnormalities;
- behavioral strategies to facilitate smoking cessation, proper nutrition, stress management, and effective weight management;
- exercise testing and training principles, with an emphasis on patients with various cardiovascular disease;

- potential comorbidities that complicate programmatic components, such as diabetes, pulmonary disease, and arthritides;
- program implementation issues such as staffing requirements and models, optimizing insurance reimbursement, program promotion, and expanding program scope to include disease management; and
- special topics such as exercise and rehabilitation in older patients and the role and responsibilities of the medical director in cardiac rehabilitation.

There are two other important changes of note in Medicare coverage guidelines for cardiac rehabilitation. They are the expansion of program duration from 36 visits in 12 weeks to 36 visits is 18 weeks and the policy to leave to the on-site clinicians and local fiscal personnel to what extent electrocardiogram (ECG) monitoring is indicated for selected patients. Concerning the former, rehabilitation staff now have the ability to implement and complete treatment plans over a period of time that better accommodates interruptions in patient attendance because of commonly experienced complicating medical, family, and social reasons. Additionally, the Medicare national coverage decision policy now allows programs to extend a patient's program duration to 72 visits in 36 weeks, should it be clinically indicated. Examples of criteria that might warrant continued rehabilitation beyond 36 visits include

- an exercise training work rate while in rehabilitation of less than four METs (metabolic equivalent);
- stable but reoccurring angina at a low (less than three METs) work rate during rehabilitation or activities of daily living;
- use of prophylactic sublingual nitroglycerine to exercise symptom free during rehabilitation; and
- in the absence of supervision by trained rehabilitation professionals, patient is at high risk of non-compliance to proper nutritional and physical activity habits.

Concerning ECG telemetry monitoring, the Medicare national coverage decision policy no longer mandates that all patients must undergo such monitoring. The decision as to which patients should receive ECG monitoring and which patients should not is now based on the clinical characteristics and responses as observed by the staff working in the program. One reason that Medicare no longer requires ECG telemetry monitoring on all patients is the substantive body of research published in the 1990s, which showed that such monitoring rarely detects a previously unknown, asymptomatic problem that leads to a change in the patient care plan, either within the cardiac rehabilitation setting or within the overall cardiology patient care plan *(4)*. Examples of criteria to consider when trying to determine which patients might benefit from partial-program or full-program telemetry monitoring include

- patients who did not have a graded exercise test prior to starting rehabilitation, especially those with stable angina or recovering from a recent myocardial infarction;
- patients with a history of myocardial infarction complicated by cardiogenic shock or heart failure or left ventricular dysfunction with or without heart failure;
- patients who demonstrated exercise-induced ischemia, atrial fibrillation, or a ventricular arrhythmia appearing or increasing during their precardiac rehabilitation stress test;
- survivor of sudden cardiac death; and
- patients who are unable to self-monitor heart rate because of physical or mental impairment.

Clearly, these are exciting times for professionals working in the field of cardiac rehabilitation and secondary prevention. However, although much is known about how patients respond to and benefit from regular exercise and therapeutic lifestyle changes, more work is needed relative to improving long-term compliance to known beneficial lifestyle and medical therapies, improving referral rates of eligible patients to secondary prevention programs, and improving retention of patients who are referred to and begin participation in cardiac rehabilitation. And despite cardiac rehabilitation representing a Class 1B guideline therapy for most patients with cardiovascular disease, gender, age, and race discrepancies persist in terms of program access and utilization. Like other therapies available to patients with cardiovascular disease, cardiac rehabilitation has a bright future for serving as a cost-effective strategy that improves mood, restores functional capacity, lessens or alleviates symptoms, and lowers the risk of and occurrence of subsequent clinical cardiovascular events, with all of the attendant social, economic, and medical benefits that ensue from its successes. The authors of this volume are pleased and eager to share the full and bright vista of cardiac rehabilitation with readers.

REFERENCES

1. Smith SC, Allen J, Blair SN, Bonow RO, Brass LM, Fonarow GC, Grundy SM, Hiratzka L, Jones D, Krumholz HM, Mosca L, Pasternak RC, Pearson T, Pfeffer MA, Taubert KA. AHA/ACC Guidelines for Secondary Prevention for Patients with Coronary or Other Atherosclerotic Vascular Disease: 2006 Update. *J Am Coll Cardiol.* 2006;47:2130–2139. doi:10.1016/j.jacc.2006.04.026.
2. Williams MA, Balady GJ, Carlson JJ, Comoss P, Humphrey R, Lounsbury PF, Roitman JL, Southard DR. *Guidelines for Cardiac Rehabilitation and Secondary Prevention Programs*, 4th ed. Champaign, IL: Human Kinetics Publishers; 2004.
3. Centers for Medicare and Medicaid Services. Medicare Coverage Database. Decision Memo for Cardiac Rehabilitation Programs (CAG-00089R). Available at https://www.cms.hhs.gov/mcd/viewdecisionmemo.asp?id=164, accessed on November 4, 2006.
4. Keteyian SJ, Mellet PA, Fedel FJ, McGowan CM, Stein PD. Electrocardiographic Monitoring During Cardiac Rehabilitation. *Chest.* 1995;107:1242–1246.

2 Principles for Prescribing Exercise in Cardiovascular Disease

Steven J. Keteyian, PhD

INTRODUCTION

The practice of prescribing exercise in sedentary healthy people, in patients with clinically manifest disease, and even in high-performance athletes is more similar than you might think. Despite any obvious differences in performance level among these three groups or concerns you may have about exercise-related complications being more likely to occur in one group versus another, there are two basic tenets that apply to everyone when establishing an exercise training program. These are *specificity of training* (e.g., mode or type of training) and *progressive overload* (i.e., intensity, duration, and frequency of training) *(1)*.

SPECIFICITY OF TRAINING

To develop the predominate energy pathway or organ system(s) (e.g., cardiorespiratory) of interest, the organ system or systems needed to perform the activity must first be identified, and then an individualized exercise plan that meets the specific needs of the patient must be crafted. For example, following a myocardial infarction, performance of a muscular task at work or at home that requires repetitive lifting can be made easier by developing muscle strength, muscle endurance, and neuromuscular coordination through resistance training. Conversely, to improve cardiorespiratory function for the purposes of risk factor management, general fitness, or as a secondary

From: *Contemporary Cardiology: Cardiac Rehabilitation*
Edited by: W. E. Kraus and S. J. Keteyian © Humana Press Inc., Totowa, NJ

preventive strategy requires engaging in exercises that stress oxygen transport (cardiac output) and utilization (peripheral blood flow and muscle function). Whether the person wishes to chop wood, shovel dirt, walk in the park, swim laps, or lift weights, the training program that is established must be specific to develop the primary organ system(s) that are responsible for the task of interest.

PROGRESSIVE OVERLOAD

Although the concept of overload training applies to both aerobic training and resistance training, let us begin our discussion by first focusing on aerobic or cardiorespiratory training programs. To accomplish this, it is necessary to introduce three important training principles: *intensity, duration*, and *frequency* of exercise. Ultimately, these principles must be adjusted to provide a sufficient "overload" stimulus on the organ system and energy pathways of interest to induce the corresponding adaptations that lead to desired outcomes, such as improvements in daily function, risk factors, or exercise capacity.

Intensity

Of the above three principles, intensity of effort requires the most consideration. The two methods that are typically used to guide intensity in patients with clinically manifest disease are heart rate and ratings of perceived exertion.

The relationship between heart rate and exercise intensity (i.e., power output or peak oxygen consumption, VO_2) is generally quite linear in healthy people and those with cardiovascular disease (Figure 1); therefore, it is appropriate to train an individual at a target rate or within a target heart rate range that will elicit the necessary overload

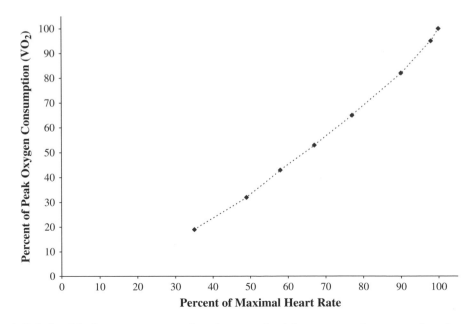

Fig. 1. Relationship between percent of peak or maximal heart rate and percent of peak oxygen consumption.

stimulus on the cardiorespiratory system. The two common formulas for determining a heart rate-based training intensity are the straight percent of peak heart rate method and the heart rate reserve method.

Using both heart rate-based formulas, in Table 1, we describe computed training heart rate ranges for two patients, one taking a beta-adrenergic blocking agent and the other not on beta-blockade. Typically, training intensities set at 60–85% (or 90%) of peak heart rate or 50–80% of heart rate reserve are sufficient to produce the organ system overload stimulus needed to improve aerobic performance. Also, note that in Table 1, regardless of the method used to determine target heart rate training range, the upper limit of the range is quite similar for both patients. However, because the heart rate reserve method accounts for the difference between peak and resting (sitting) heart rates, the lower limit of the target range is usually higher when using the heart rate reserve method, regardless of beta-blockade therapy. This observation is consistent with what occurs in healthy people and in patients with cardiovascular disease and is the main reason why the heart rate reserve method is preferred over the percent of peak heart rate approach.

In some people, time does not permit the teaching of pulse taking, whereas in others with certain clinical conditions (e.g., atrial fibrillation and diabetes), pulse taking is rendered less accurate. In these instances, we can use a scale named after the individual who developed it, the Borg Rating of Perceived Exertion (RPE) scale (2). This scale (Table 2) has been tested in various healthy and patient populations and represents a valid means to guide exercise intensity because of its coexisting linear relationship to both heart rate and VO_2 during exercise testing and training. It involves asking the patient to rate their over-all (not just legs or breathing) body exertion or fatigue, using a scale of 6–20. A value of 6 corresponds to sitting in a chair, and a value of 20 is described as all-out maximal effort to exhaustion.

Table 1

Examples of Heart Rate-Based Training Intensities in a 62-Year-Old Patient both Taking and not Taking a Beta-Adrenergic Blocking Agent

	Measured peak heart rate (beats • min^{-1})	Resting heart rate (beats • min^{-1})	Exercise training heart rate range (beats • min^{-1})	
			Lower limit	Upper limit
No Beta Blockade				
HRR	150	70	110	134
Percent of peak HR	150	NA	90	128
On beta-blockade				
HRR	126	52	89	111
Percent of peak HR	126	NA	76	107

Heart rate reserve (HRR) method is computed as: (peak HR − resting HR) × 0.50 + resting HR = lower limit and (peak HR − resting HR) × 0.8 + resting HR = upper limit. % peak HR method is computed as: peak HR × 0.60 = lower limit and peak HR × 0.85 = upper limit. HR, heart rate and NA, not applicable.

Table 2
The Borg Rating of Perceived
Exertion Scale *(2)*

6	
7	Very, very light
8	
9	Very light
10	
11	Fairly light
12	
13	Somewhat light
14	
15	Hard
16	
17	Very hard
18	
19	Very, very hard
20	

Relative to exercise training intensity, an RPE of 11–12 is equivalent to light to moderate work and a heart rate approximating 50–60% of peak. Training within an RPE range of 12–14 is common among patients with stable cardiovascular disease, in that it is both safe and sufficient to induce improvement in peak VO_2 and health.

Frequency and Duration

Duration can refer to both the length of a single training bout (number of minutes or hours) and how long the patient has been training over-all (months vs. years). Generally, the more frequent the program (5 days per week vs. 2 days per week) and the longer the over-all program, the greater the improvement in exercise capacity or function. For example, a 24-week exercise training study in our laboratory involving patients with chronic heart failure initially showed an improvement of 14% in peak VO_2 at week 12 and a further increase to 16% at week 24 *(3)*.

The recommended frequency for most patients with cardiovascular disease is 3–5 days per week *(4)*. We also know that, assuming training intensity is unchanged, duration and frequency of training can, to a certain extent, be traded off. If, for some reason, a patient's training frequency during a week is decreased from 6 to 3 or 2 days, then total duration per training session should be increased to ensure that the total overload stimulus (minimal of exercise/session × sessions/week) that is accomplished for that week is similar to that of a 6-day per week training regimen. Table 3 summarizes a typical training regimen for improving aerobic or cardiorespiratory fitness (see also chapter 15 for any unique or disease-specific changes or considerations that may be needed when developing an exercise prescription).

Table 3
General Training Guidelines for Improving Health
and Aerobic Fitness

Training factor	Guidelines*
Intensity	60–85% of peak HR
	50–80% of HRR
Frequency	4–6 days/week
Sessions/day	One
Duration	≥ 8 weeks
Duration/Session	≥ 30 min/session

*Target goal is $150\,Kcal \bullet day^{-1}$ ($1000\,Kcal \bullet wk^{-1}$).
HR, heart rate and HRR, heart rate reserve.

RESISTANCE TRAINING

The above discussion concerning specificity of training and progressive overload focused on activities that involve the entire body during an aerobic-type activity. Increasingly common among patients with cardiovascular disease or risk factors is the use of weight training or resistance training. Such training often improves one's muscular strength and endurance and allows patients to more easily engage in activities of daily living, manage risk factors, reduce incidence of falls, and lessen frailty. One difference between developing fitness using resistance training versus an aerobic-type regimen is that the former involves a regional or joint-specific activity to focus on a singe muscle or muscle group, whereas the latter usually represents a gross motor activity that involves many major muscle groups to improve cardiorespiratory function. As a result of these differences, the concepts of intensity, duration, and frequency of activity take on slightly different meanings.

An important point to keep in mind when discussing/recommending resistance training to patients with cardiovascular disease is that the load should be modified. Specifically, among healthy people and athletes, maximal strength gains are best achieved by an overload program that incorporates (a) higher intensities (more weight), (b) more sets, and (c) fewer repetitions. Additionally, gains in muscular endurance are also derived from this type of training, as well as from a regimen that incorporates moderate intensity lifts completed in sets that incorporate more repetitions.

In patients with clinically manifest disease, a sufficient overload can be accomplished by using a moderate-intensity (weight), more-repetition model. Therefore, as most patients can benefit from gains in muscle strength and endurance, it is prudent to use a lower-weight, fewer-set, and higher-repetition training model – for example, two sets of 8–12 repetitions at 50–70% of 1 repetition maximum (RM). Although some controversy exists relative to whether or not there is more benefit if a patient weight trains 3 versus 2 (or one) days per week, there is little evidence that substantial gains can be realized among patients performing resistance exercise more than 3 days per week. For the patient who has never engaged in weight lifting before or has been away from it for several years, it is prudent to limit training frequency to two times per week and progress to three per week after demonstrating no problems at the initial level.

FEATURE BOX...PROPER TECHNIQUE
AND RESISTANCE TRAINING

Any discussion about resistance training would be incomplete without the mention of the necessary steps one must take to minimize injury and increase the effectiveness while training. General recommendations include the following *(5)*:

- All lifts should be conducted throughout the full range of motion.
- Breathe out (exhaling) during the lift phase and breathe in (inhaling) during the recovery phase.
- Never arch the back during any lifting.
- Always control the recovery phase of the lift, instead of allowing the weights to "crash" down in preparation for the next repetition.
- Be sure that patients always train with a partner.
- Review with patients the signs and symptoms of excessive fatigue (e.g., higher than usual heart rate at rest or during training, general weakness, and unsteady lift technique) that can occur during training, especially within the first three weeks for patients starting a weight lifting program. Instruct patients to curtail the remainder of training during a session should excessive fatigue be present.
- Clinical exercise staff familiar with resistance training should conduct an initial orientation with each patient concerning the various lifts they will be doing, as well as be available for regular re-evaluations and assistance during training sessions.

Establishing the correct weight or load to lift per repetition can be accomplished in patients with cardiovascular disease using an approach that assumes that for each time a weight is lifted, the percent RM is reduced by 2.5% *(5)*. Thus, a load lifted only once represents 100% of 1 RM, whereas the lifting of a weight five repetitions, without the ability to lift it a sixth repetition, represents 90% of the 1 RM (i.e., a reduction of 2.5% for each successful lift beyond 1, so that $4 \times 2.5\% = 10\%$ and $100 - 10\% = 90\%$). From this, the 1 RM can be estimated from the following equation:

$$\frac{\text{weight lifted}}{[1.0 - (\text{the number of lifts} \times 0.025)]} = 1\text{RM}$$

Among patients with clinically manifest disease, the indirect 1-RM method is believed to reduce even further the already very small risk of an abnormal response occurring during resistance training, such as an orthopedic injury, a hypertensive response, left ventricular dysfunction, or arrhythmia.

Flexibility

Although not mentioned earlier, there is a third component to consider when developing a patient's total fitness, beyond cardiorespiratory or muscle strength/endurance. This third component of fitness pertains to muscle and joint flexibility and is important because it can help restore the normal pattern of movement, reduce pain due to injury or disease, improve function during routine activities of daily living, and maintain functional independence. Joint flexibility is influenced by variables such as the distensibility of the joint capsule, adequate warm-up, muscle viscosity, and any pain due to an acute or chronic injury. And just as no single exercise can induce total body strength or endurance, no single exercise yields total body flexibility. In other words, flexibility is a joint-specific and muscle group-specific type of fitness.

Improving flexibility is usually accomplished through static or passive (versus dynamic) stretching exercises. This approach to stretching involves gently lengthening a muscle group to the point of resistance or mild discomfort (no pain), holding it in that lengthened position for a period of time, and then relaxing. Each time the muscle is stretched it should be held for 30–60 s. This entire process is repeated two or three more times for the same muscle group, before moving on to the next. As with resistance training, patients should be instructed to avoid breath holding while stretching.

In almost every instance, the benefits of mild passive stretching outweigh any risks; however, it is important to point out that the potential for injury due to "over-stretching," although extremely rare, does exist. This is especially true among patients who present with an already unstable or hypermobile joint. Stretching is contraindicated at a fracture site, and caution is advised in patients with osteoporosis.

CONCLUSION

For most patients with cardiovascular disease, the above training principles will apply for the purposes of developing cardiorespiratory fitness or muscles strength or endurance. However, because of the sometimes unique pathophysiology of each disorder, certain modifications or adjustments in the usual training guidelines may be needed *(4,5)*. These considerations are described in chapter 15, for several of the more common cardiovascular diseases.

REFERENCES

1. Foss ML, Keteyian SJ. *Fox's Physiological Basis for Exercise and Sport*. New York: McGraw Hill; 1998.
2. Borg G. Subjective Effort in Relation to Physical Performance and Working Capacity. In Psychology: From Research to Practice, HJ Pick, JE Singer, A Steinschneider and H Stevenson (eds). New York: Plenum; 1978, 333–361.
3. Keteyian SJ, Levine AB, Brawner CA, Kataoka T, Rogers FJ, Schairer JR, Stein PD and Levine TB. Exercise Training in Patients with Heart Failure. *Ann Int Med*. 1996;124:1051–1057.
4. American College of Sports Medicine. *Guidelines for Exercise Testing and Prescription*, 7th ed. Philadelphia, PA: Lippincott Williams & Wilkins; 2005, pp. 133–183.
5. Ehrman JK, Gordon PM, Visich PS, Keteyian SJ. *Clinical Exercise Physiology*. Champaign: Human Kinetics; 2003, pp. 103–128.

3 Nutrition in Cardiac Rehabilitation

Gene Erb, Jr, and Julie Pruitt

CONTENTS

INTRODUCTION

Healthy nutrition plays an essential role in improving the cardiovascular risk profile following a cardiac event. Recognizing the impact that healthy dietary behaviors can have on recovery, the American Heart Association stated that "...nutritional counseling should be provided to all participants in cardiac rehabilitation" *(1)*. Research has shown that the combination of regular exercise and healthy nutrition together significantly slows the progression of coronary heart disease *(2)*. Increasing fruit and vegetable intake and managing fat in the diet are also critical in the management of other heart disease risk factors such as hypertension, type 2 diabetes mellitus, and dyslipidemias of many varieties.

National guidelines published by the American Association of Cardiovascular and Pulmonary Rehabilitation (AACVPR) *(3)* specifically require assessment of and targeted intervention on the nutrition status of all cardiac rehabilitation participants. The methods and tools used to achieve these requirements vary from program to program. The size of the program, additional state regulatory requirements, program resources, and other considerations will all influence the choice of tools and methods employed by each program. One element essential for all programs to include, regardless of size or

From: *Contemporary Cardiology: Cardiac Rehabilitation*
Edited by: W. E. Kraus and S. J. Keteyian © Humana Press Inc., Totowa, NJ

resources, is personalization of information for each participant. Personalization begins with an individualized look at the participant's nutritional status. Once an assessment is complete, each participant should have access to appropriate nutrition education. The nutrition therapy portion of a cardiac rehabilitation program should culminate with healthy personalized recommendations. On the basis of the structure of the program, these services may be provided through individual consultation with program staff or through interactive classroom instruction.

Core Components of Nutritional Counseling in Cardiac Rehabilitation

Evaluation – Assess caloric and nutrient intake, assess eating habits, and assess target areas for intervention.
Intervention – Develop individualized diet plan aimed at general heart healthy recommendations and specific risk reduction strategies; counsel participant and family; incorporate behavior change and compliance strategies.
Expected outcomes – Participant understanding of basic dietary principles, plan to address eating behavior problems, and adherence to diet.

Adapted from Balady 2000 *(4)*

DIETARY INTAKE AND THE MANAGEMENT OF HEART DISEASE

Extensive research has been conducted on many different individual nutritional components and the impact they have on coronary heart disease and the associated risk factors. Hu and Willett completed a review of 147 original investigations and reviews of major dietary factors. They identified increased intake of fruits, vegetables, and whole grains, substitution of non-hydrogenated unsaturated fats for saturated and *trans*-fats, and increased intake of omega-3 fatty acids as the major effective dietary strategies for preventing coronary heart disease *(5)*. Additionally, incorporation of low-fat dairy products on a daily basis helps to control blood pressure and may possibly assist in weight management *(6,7)*. Structuring cardiac rehabilitation nutrition education around these principles will support the goal of secondary prevention in participants.

FRUITS AND VEGETABLES

Numerous studies have demonstrated that diets rich in fruits and vegetables are correlated with the prevention of coronary heart disease and associated risk factors *(5)*. In a large epidemiologic study, a significant inverse correlation between risk of coronary heart disease and intake of fruits and vegetables was noted. Every 1 serving-per-day increase in intake was correlated with a 4% decrease in risk. Individuals in the highest quintile of intake (9.15–10.15 servings/day) had a 20% lower relative risk of developing coronary heart disease than individuals in the lowest quintile of intake (2.54–2.93 servings/day). Especially beneficial were leafy green vegetables and Vitamin C-rich fruits and vegetables (Joshipura) *(20)*. In the landmark Dietary Approaches to Stop Hypertension (DASH) trials, increased consumption of fruits and vegetables in the setting of additional healthy food behaviors led to markedly decreased blood pressure levels *(6)*. The beneficial effects of including fruits and vegetables in the diet are thought to come, in part, from the provision of potassium, fiber, phytochemicals, and the displacement of unhealthier food choices.

Counseling participants with regard to the inclusion of additional fruits and vegetables in their diets must include several key elements. First, emphasize the importance of serving the fruits and vegetables in a healthy and an appealing manner. People often offset the benefit gained from the inclusion of fruits and vegetables in the diet by adding copious amounts of fats and sugars during food preparation. Second, starchy vegetables such as corn, potatoes, peas, and beans are included in the *starch* food group and not in the *vegetable* food group. Starchy vegetables, as the name implies, have carbohydrate and calorie contents similar to other starches. When developing a meal plan, treating them as such is necessary, especially when blood glucose management is a factor in meal composition. Non-starchy vegetables are very low in calories and can be consumed liberally, even in the setting of weight management. Finally, encourage the selection of whole fruits and vegetables whether they are fresh, frozen, or canned in their own juice or light syrup over juices. Whole fruits and vegetables provide the extra benefit of fiber and increased satiety. In general overconsumption of calories from fruit rarely occurs and only when a participant consumes more than the recommended amount of juice or dried fruit—less satisfying foods. Increasing the consumption of healthily prepared fruits and vegetables may be a new experience for many cardiac rehabilitation participants. Increasing their self-efficacy through education and counseling to establish these new habits is critical in their eventual success.

DIETARY FATS

There is undeniable evidence that diets high in saturated and *trans*-fats are significant contributors to the risk of coronary heart disease, whereas inclusion of healthy monounsaturated and polyunsaturated fats reduces risk. Differences in total fat intake, with the exception of difficult-to-adhere-to very low-fat diets (< 10% of total calories from fat), do not significantly influence coronary heart disease risk; only substitution of saturated and *trans*-fats with monounsaturated and polyunsaturated fats significantly impacts risk (8–10). In the Women's Health Initiative Study, an 8.3% reduction in total fat intake (2.9% from saturated fat, 0.6% *trans*-fats, 3.3% monounsaturated fats, 1.5% polyunsaturated fats) did not result in significant impact on coronary heart disease risk (9). However, the replacement of 5% of energy from saturated fat and 8.2% of energy from *trans*-fat with monounsaturated and polyunsaturated fats was associated with a 42 and 53% lower risk of coronary heart disease, respectively, in the Nurses' Health Study (10). Targeted reductions and substitutions of fat subtypes are critical to improving a person's cardiac risk profile.

In addition to replacing unhealthy fats in the diet with healthy fats, inclusion of omega-3 fats in the diet provides substantial benefit. Inclusion of approximately eight or more servings of omega-3 fatty acid-rich fish each month reduced sudden cardiac death by 50% compared with consumption of less than one serving of omega-3 fatty acid-rich fish each month (11). Plant-based sources of omega-3 fatty acids have also been indicated in the secondary prevention of coronary heart disease (11). It is important to encourage participants to increase omega-3 fatty acids in their diet by including two 3-ounce servings of low-contaminate fatty fish each week and plant-based sources such as flaxseed, English walnuts, and canola oil.

Fish Advisory

Some fatty fish such as shark, swordfish, king mackerel, and tilefish have higher mercury content. Limit your consumption of these fish to no more than 7 ounces per week. Consumption of fish with lower mercury contamination such as tuna, red snapper, and orange roughy should be limited to no more than 14 ounces per week. Woman of childbearing age, pregnant woman, and children should avoid fish with high mercury contamination altogether, and limit lower mercury fish to not more than 12 ounces per week.

American Heart Association *(12)*

Managing the balance of fat in the diet through the replacement of unhealthy saturated and *trans*-fats with healthy omega-3, monounsaturated and polyunsaturated fats can represent a significant lifestyle change for many cardiac rehabilitation participants. This will likely be a shift away from many of the comfort foods that are ingrained in their home environment. Acknowledging the difficulty of these changes can be helpful as the participant begins to set goals for change. Smaller, more attainable goals lead to early success and increased self-efficacy. Work with the participant to identify one or two specific areas for change and target efforts there. For example, someone who is not eating any fish may choose to include one serving of fish rich in omega-3 fats once a week. A second goal may be substituting canola or olive oil for shortening when cooking. Both of these actions can considerably improve the participant's diet without an overwhelming, unnecessary, and expensive pantry overhaul, the sheer magnitude of which could cause a total resistance to all change.

Saturated fat	*Trans*-fat
• Usually solid at room temperature	• Results from hydrogenating unsaturated fats
• Sources include animal-based products such as meats and plant-based hydrogenated vegetable oils (shortening)	• Major sources include fast foods, baked goods, and stick margarine

Polyunsaturated fat	Monounsaturated fat	Omega-3 fat
• Usually liquid at room temperature	• Usually liquid at room temperature	• Marine sources include fatty fish such as salmon, herring, sardines, and mackerel
• Sources include corn oil, safflower oil, cotton seed oil, and soy bean oil	• Sources include olive oil, avocado, canola oil, and most nuts	• Plant-based sources include walnuts and flaxseed

DAIRY PRODUCTS

Dairy products may play a role in managing blood pressure and weight. Adding low-fat dairy products such as milk and yogurt to a diet rich in fruits and vegetables compounds the diet's ability to reduce cardiac risk. In the setting of weight maintenance, the DASH-feeding studies noted that addition of two to three servings of low-fat dairy products to the basic diet more than doubled the reduction in blood pressure achieved by subjects using this dietary approach *(6)*. While these positive effects on blood pressure have been well-documented, newer research demonstrates the potential for even more risk-reduction benefits through dietary changes.

Recent studies support the role of calcium and low-fat dairy products in weight and body fat mass management. Including dairy (i.e., three servings of yogurt per day) in the setting of energy restriction improved total body fat loss and trunk fat loss by 61 and 81%, respectively *(7)*. If energy intake is held constant and suboptimal calcium intake is increased through the inclusion of three servings of dairy per day, body fat mass decreases (−5.4%), especially in the trunk region (−4.6%), while body weight remains stable *(7)*. A recent randomized control trial compared increased calcium through supplementation and inclusion of dairy products. While individuals taking calcium supplements experienced improvement over the control group in weight, total body fat, and trunk fat loss, individuals in the dairy group had substantially greater losses *(7)*.

These smaller trials indicate that provision of dairy products in the diet is beneficial in the management of weight and body fat, however more extensive research is needed. Virtually all cardiac rehabilitation participants can benefit from the inclusion of two to three servings of dairy products in their daily diet. Primarily, these servings should come from low-fat milk and yogurt. Owing to their higher fat content and lower calcium content, cheese and butter are considered when determining daily fat intake, rather than as dairy servings.

WHOLE GRAINS AND STARCHES

In the past several years, starches have received volumes of negative press, with some fad diet creators suggesting virtual elimination of starches from the diet. However, starches are critical components of a healthy diet, as they provide essential nutrients and serve as an important energy source. Starches also serve an integral function in satiation. The distinction to be made is in the type of starch that is recommended for inclusion in the diet. While refined grains are stripped of their nutrients and are often included in popular high-fat products, whole grains provide a bounty of nutrients, phytochemicals, and fiber.

Inclusion of whole grains and cereal fiber in the diet also decreases risk of disease. In the Iowa Women's Health study, Jacobs et al. *(13)* found a clear inverse relationship between intake of whole grains and risk of heart disease. Individuals in the highest quintile of intake (3.2 servings per day) had a 30% lower relative risk of heart disease than individuals in the lowest quintile of intake (0.2 servings per day) *(13)*. Similarly, results from the Nurse's Health Study also demonstrated a 34% lower risk of heart disease in women in the highest quintile of fiber intake. The decreased risk was only significant for dietary fiber from cereal grains and not for fiber from fruits and vegetables *(14)*.

Introduction or increasing whole grain products in the diet can be structured in a stepwise manner with the goal of at least half of all starch servings in the diet provided by whole grain products. It is productive to have the participant begin to examine the starch products currently consumed and identify areas for change. Initial increases may come from mixing whole grain breakfast cereals with favorite refined grain cereals or from purchasing whole grain pastas. Eventually, the participant can continue to transition to additional whole grain products as the palate and gastrointestinal tract adjusts.

ADDITIONAL DIETARY COMPONENTS

Stanols and Sterols

Plant stanols and sterols are organic compounds found naturally in vegetable oils, cereals, fruits, and vegetables. Additionally, they now are added to products such as margarines and orange juice. Owing to their cholesterol-like structure, these compounds interfere with the absorption of cholesterol and cholesterol-building blocks in the digestive tract. The net effect of this lowered absorption is a 6–15% reduction in low-density lipoprotein (LDL) cholesterol (NCEP). The Third Report of the National Cholesterol Education Program Expert Panel of Detection, Evaluation, and Treatment of High Blood Cholesterol in Adults (Adult Treatment Panel III) recommends consuming 2 g of plant stanol and sterol esters per day as a therapeutic option for managing LDL cholesterol *(15)*. To achieve an optimal intake level, inclusion of fortified products is necessary as the amount of stanols and sterols occurring naturally in foods is minimal.

Alcohol

While alcohol intake and a reduction in cardiac events has been widely publicized in the popular media and supported by several research studies, encouraging the addition of alcohol in the diet of a cardiac rehabilitation participant is not recommended. The addictive nature and adverse consequences of over-consuming alcohol do not outweigh the potential benefits. Also, it is becoming clear that many of the studies that found a potential benefit of moderate alcohol consumption, perhaps overestimated the benefits by incorrectly including reformed high-volume alcoholic consumers in the abstinence group. While the proper role of alcohol in the diet and for risk reduction is being investigated, the American Heart Association recommends limiting intake to not more than one drink per day for women and two drinks per day for men *(16)*.

Sodium

Numerous studies have shown that reducing intake of dietary sodium can have a significant effect on lowering blood pressure. In the DASH-sodium trial, subjects were maintained on sodium intakes of approximately 3300 mg/day, 2400 mg/day, and 1500 mg/day in a cross-over design. Blood pressure was significantly reduced with each incremental drop in sodium intake (Sacks) *(21)*. While sodium intake at the lowest level showed the greatest overall effect, maintaining this level of intake is difficult at best. Therefore, the American Heart Association recommends consuming no more than 2400 mg of sodium per day *(16)*. To remain under the recommended level of intake, it is important to counsel cardiac rehabilitation participants to steer clear from high sodium-canned meats, soups and vegetables, and salty snacks, and to avoid adding salt when cooking or at the table.

ALTERNATIVE DIETARY PATTERNS

One of the most significant ways that cardiac risk can be reduced is through achieving and maintaining a healthy body weight. As a result, cardiac rehabilitation participants often solicit advice about initiating one of the numerous popular diets for weight loss. For this reason, health professionals need to be aware of two key points emerging from research in this field. Several studies have noted that weight loss is not significantly different after 12 months in subjects following any one of several popular diets (17–19). In a randomized clinical trial comparing a low-carbohydrate, high-protein, high-fat diet to a low-calorie, high-carbohydrate, low-fat diet, greater improvement of some cardiac risk factors [triglycerides and high-density lipoprotein (HDL)] was experienced on the low-carbohydrate diet (17). Changes in other risk factors (LDL, blood pressure, and insulin sensitivity), however, were not significantly different between the groups or, as demonstrated by meta-analysis, were found to be unfavorable on a low-carbohydrate diet (17,19). When discussing alternative popular diets with participants, it is important to examine restrictions set forth by the popular diet that limit the consumption of the proven beneficial foods (fruits, vegetables, low-fat dairy products, and whole grains). The long-term health ramifications and safety of excluding or limiting these foods is, as of yet, unknown.

CALORIES AND DIETARY PATTERN

Practical implementation of a healthy diet pattern begins with laying a foundation of appropriate caloric intake. The following tool was developed by dietitians at the Duke Center for Living and Duke Cardiac Rehabilitation program. Extrapolated from the Harris Benedict equation, it is a user-friendly tool requiring minimal calculations to approximate caloric intake. Once an appropriate calorie level is identified, one should determine the recommended contributions from each dietary component. A healthy cardiac diet allows for an estimated 25–30% of total calories from fat—mainly from healthy monounsaturated and polyunsaturated fats by limiting unhealthy saturated fat to 7% of total calories. A quick reference for total fat and saturated fat gram allowance for varying calorie levels is provided. One can select the calorie level closest to the participant's calculated needs, erring on the side of less versus more calories in the diet.

Determining Your Daily Calorie Allowance

Step 1: Write current weight_____ (lbs) then multiply by 10 = _____

Step 2: Choose one from Steps a – e below. (It is important not to have a calorie level < 1200 without evaluation by a registered dietitian.)

    a. If you want to tone up your body, maintain weight or lose less than 10 lbs, then add 500.
    b. If you want to lose 10–25 lbs, then add 0. _____
    c. If you want to lose greater than 25 lbs, subtract 500.
    d. If you weigh 350 lbs or more, subtract 1000.
    e. If you want to gain weight, add 1000.

Step 3: Add the calories from steps 1 and 2.
    This is your estimated calorie needs per day _____calories per day

Above calorie levels are based on person engaging in approximately 30 min of exercise 3–5 days/week.

Daily Fat Gram Budget Chart

Calorie needs	Maximum daily total fat gram budget	Maximum daily saturated fat gram budget
1300	40	10
1400	43	11
1600	48	12
1800	51	14
2000	58	16
2200	66	17
2400	73	19
2600	79	20
2800	87	22
3000	95	23

Taking into account the calories from fat and the recommendations for following a diet pattern rich in fruits, vegetables, low-fat dairy products, and whole grains, the following are suggested meal plans for healthy living. The first plan includes provisions for participants who consume beef, poultry, seafood, eggs, and cheese, while the second is specifically designed for lacto-ovo vegetarians (individuals who do not consume animal products with the exception of eggs, cheese, and dairy products). One should begin by finding the caloric level that most closely matches the participant's recommended caloric intake.

SUGGESTED MEAL PLANS FOR HEALTHY EATING

Chart 1 is a Plan for Individuals Who Eat Beef, Poultry, Seafood, Eggs, and Cheese

Chart 1	1300	1400	1600	1800	2000	2200	2400	2600	2800	3000
Fat grams	≤ 43	≤ 45	≤ 52	≤ 58	≤ 64	≤ 70	≤ 78	≤ 84	≤ 90	≤ 98
Starch*	4	4	5	5	6	7	7	8	9	10
Fruit	2	3	4	4	5	5	5	6	7	7
Vegetable	3+	4+	4+	5+	5+	6+	6+	6+	7+	7+
Dairy	2	2	2	2	2	2	3	3	3	3
M&P**	3	3	4	6	6	8	8	8	8	9

Chart 2 is a Plan for Individuals Who are Lacto-Ovo Vegetarian (Eat Only Eggs, Cheese and Dairy Animal Products)

CHART 2	1300 veg	1400 veg	1600 veg	1800 veg	2000 veg	2200 veg	2400 veg	2600 veg	2800 veg	3000 veg
Fat grams	≤ 43	≤ 45	≤ 52	≤ 58	≤ 64	≤ 70	≤ 78	≤ 84	≤ 90	≤ 98
Starch*	5	5	6	6	7	8	9	10	11	12
Fruit	2	2	3	3	4	4	4	5	6	6
Vegetable	3+	3+	4+	5+	5+	5+	6+	6+	7+	7+
Dairy	3	3	3	3	3	3	3	3	3	3
M&P**	2	2	2	3	3	3	3	4	4	5

* Include at least half of all starch servings from whole grain products.
** M&P = Meat (beef, poultry, seafood, pork, etc.) and other proteins such as eggs, cheese, nuts.

> **Serving Sizes**
>
> *1 serving of starch* = 1 slice of bread, 1 small roll, 1 small potato, $^1/_2$ cup of cereals, cooked rice, pasta, or starchy vegetables like peas, corn, and beans.
> *1 serving of fruit* = 1 small apple, orange or other similar size whole fruit, $^1/_2$ banana, 15 grapes, $^1/_4$ cup dried fruit, $^1/_2$ cup chopped, cooked, or canned fruit, $^1/_2$ cup juice.
> *1 serving of non-starchy vegetables* = 1 cup raw vegetables, $^1/_2$ cup cooked vegetables, and $^1/_2$ cup vegetable juice.
> *1 serving of dairy* = 1 cup of milk or yogurt.
> *1 serving of meat and other proteins* = 1 ounce of meat such as beef, poultry, pork, fish, oyster, or veal, 2 ounces of other shellfish, 1 ounce of cheese, 1 ounce of nuts, and 1 egg.

SUMMARY

The goal of nutrition therapy for cardiac rehabilitation participants is the adaptation and maintenance of healthy behaviors for a lifetime to improve a participant's cardiovascular risk profile and prevent additional cardiac events. Nutrition therapy begins with an assessment of current dietary practices, followed by identification of targeted areas for change and creation of an implementation plan. Including the services of a registered dietitian in a cardiac rehabilitation program is beneficial in managing the complexities of changing dietary behaviors. Providing support and encouragement for each step a participant makes will foster continued positive changes and cardiac risk reduction.

REFERENCES

1. Balady GJ, Fletcher BJ, Froelicher ES, Hartley LH, Krauss RM, Oberman A, Pollock ML, Taylor B. Cardiac Rehabilitation Programs: A Statement for Healthcare Professionals From the American Heart Association. *Circulation.* 1994;90(3):1602–1610.
2. Ades PA. Cardiac Rehabilitation and Secondary Prevention of Coronary Heart Disease. *NEJM.* 2001;345(12):892–902.
3. American Association of Cardiovascular and Pulmonary Rehabilitation (AACVPR). Certification. Available at http://www.aacvpr.org/certification/, accessed on June 2006.
4. Balady GJ, Ades PA, Comoss P, Limacher M, Pina IL, Southard D, Williams MA, Bazzarre T. Core Components of Cardiac Rehabilitation/Secondary Prevention Programs: A Statement for Healthcare Professionals from the American Heart Association and the American Association of Cardiovascular and Pulmonary Rehabilitation. *Circulation.* 2000;102:1069–1073.
5. Hu FB, Willet WC. Optimal Diets for Prevention of Coronary Heart Disease. *JAMA.* 2002;288(20):2569–2578.
6. Appel LJ, Moore TJ, Obarzanek E, Vollmer WM, Svetkey LP, Sacks FM, Bray GA, Vogt TM, Cutler JA, Windhauser MM, Lin PH, Karanja N. A Clinical Trial of the Effects of Dietary Patterns on Blood Pressure. *NEJM.* 1997;336(16):1117–1124.
7. Zemel MB. The Role of Dairy Foods in Weight Management. *J Am Coll Nutr.* 2005;24(6): 537S–546S.
8. Ornish D, Scherwitz LW, Billings JH, Gould KL, Merritt TA, Sparler S, Armstrong WT, Ports TA, Kirkeeide RL, Hogeboom C, Brand RJ. Intensive Lifestyle Changes for Reversal of Coronary Heart Disease. *JAMA.* 1998;280(23):2001–2007.

9. Howard BV, Van Horn L, Hsia J, Manson JE, Stefanick ML, Wassertheil-Smoller S, Kuller LH, LaCroix AZ, Langer RD, Lasser NL, Lewis CE, Limacher MC, Margolis KL, Mysiw WJ, Ockene JK, Parker LM, Perri MG, Phillips L, Prentice RL, Robbins J, Rossouw JE, Sarto GE, Schatz IJ, Snetselaar LG, Stevens VJ, Tinker LF, Trevisan M, Vitolins MZ, Anderson GL, Assaf AR, Bassford T, Beresford SAA, Black HR, Brunner RL, Brzyski RG, Caan B, Chlebowski RT, Gass M, Granek I, Greenland P, Hays J, Heber D, Heiss G, Hendrix SL, Hubbell FA, Johnson KC, Kotchen JM. Low-Fat Dietary Pattern and Risk of Cardiovascular Disease: The Women's Health Initiative Randomized Controlled Dietary Modification Trial. *JAMA*. 2006;295:655–666.

10. Hu FB, Stampfer MJ, Manson JE, Rimm E, Colditz GA, Rosner BA, Hennekens CH, Willett WC. Dietary Fat Intake and the Risk of Coronary Heart Disease in Women. *NEJM*. 1997;337:1491–1499.

11. Kris-Etherton PM, Harris WS, Appel LJ. Fish Consumption, Fish Oil, Omega-3 Fatty Acids, and Cardiovascular Disease. *Circulation*. 2002;106:2747–2757.

12. American Heart Association. Fish, Levels of Mercury and Omega-3 Fatty Acids. Available at http://www.americanheart.org/presenter.jhtml?identifier=3013797, accessed on June 2006.

13. Jacobs DR Jr, Meyer KA, Kushi LH, Folsom AR. Whole-Grain Intake May Reduce the Risk of Ischemic Heart Disease in Postmenopausal Women: The Iowa Women's Health Study. *Am J Clin Nutr*. 1998;68:248–257.

14. Wolk A, Manson JE, Stampfer MJ, Colditz GA, Hu FB, Speizer FE, Hennekens CH, Willett WC. Long-Term Intake of Dietary Fiber and Decreased Risk of Coronary Heart Disease Among Women. *JAMA*. 1999;281:1998–2004.

15. National Cholesterol Educations Program (NCEP) Expert Panel on Detection, Evaluation, and Treatment of High Blood Cholesterol in Adults (Adult Treatment Panel III). Third Report of the National Cholesterol Education Program (NCEP) Expert Panel on Detection, Evaluation, and Treatment of High Blood Cholesterol in Adults (Adult Treatment Panel III) Final Report. *Circulation*. 2002;106:3143–3421.

16. Krauss RM, Eckel RH, Howard B, Appel LJ, Daniels SR, Deckelbaum RJ, Erdman JW, Kris-Etherton P, Goldberg IJ, Kotchen TA, Lichtenstein AH, Mitch WE, Mullis R, Robinson K, Wylie-Rosett J, St. Jeor S, Suttie J, Tribble DL, Bazzarre TL. AHA Dietary Guidelines: Revision 2000: A Statement for Healthcare Professionals from the Nutrition Committee of the American Heart Association. *Circulation*. 2000;102:2284–2299.

17. Foster GD, Wyatt HR, Hill JO, McGuckin BG, Brill C, Mohammed BS, Szapary PO, Rader DJ, Edman JS, Klein S. A Randomized Trial of a Low-Carbohydrate Diet for Obesity. *NEJM*. 2003;348:2082–2090.

18. Freedman MR, King J, Kennedy E. Popular Diets: A Scientific Review. *Obes Res*. 2001;9 (Suppl 1):1S–40S.

19. Nordmann AJ, Nordmann A, Briel M, Keller U, Yancy WS Jr, Brehm BJ, Bucher HC. Effects of Low-Carbohydrate Vs Low-Fat Diets on Weight Loss and Cardiovascular Risk Factors: A Meta-Analysis of Randomized Controlled Trials. *Arch Intern Med*. 2006;166:285–293.

20. Joshipura KJ, Hu FB, Manson JE, Stampfer MJ, Rimm EB, Speizer FE, Coldita G, Ascherto A, Rosner B, Spiegelman D, Willett WC. The Effect of Fruit and Vegetable Intake on Risk for Coronary Heart Disease.

21. Sacks FM, Sretkey LP, Vollmer WM, Appel LJ, Bray GA, Harsha D, Obarzanek E, Conlin PR, Miller ER III, Simons-Morton DG, Karanja N, Lin PH. Effects on Blood Pressure of Reduced Dietary Sodium and the Dietary Approaches to Stop Hypertension (DASH) Diet. DASH-Sodium Collaborative Research Group. *NEJM* 2001;344:3–100.

4

Weight Management in Patients with Established Cardiovascular Disease

Jonathan K. Ehrman, PhD

CONTENTS

BACKGROUND AND GENERAL INFORMATION

History and Epidemiology

Currently there is no specific treatment strategy for patients who are overweight or obese and participating in cardiac rehabilitation. Although several guidelines mention the need for treatment and provide general recommendations, most programs do not employ targeted weight management strategies *(1,2)*. Studies carried out in the cardiac rehabilitation setting that assessed changes in body weight or variables related to obesity [body fat percentage, lean mass, body mass index (BMI)] have shown mixed results *(2)*. The studies that did demonstrate improvement likely used a multifaceted approach as opposed to exercise alone.

The increase in the prevalence of obesity in the US population almost needs not to be mentioned, as it is highly publicized in both clinical and general populations. However, to establish a baseline from which this chapter will draw upon, we present the following background information.

The definition of BMI is an anthropometric measure of body mass, defined as weight in kilograms divided by height in meter squared. BMI is the primary measure used to categorize individuals according to weight. Table 1 summarizes the accepted cutoff values for BMI when determining whether a person is at an acceptable body weight or whether he/she is overweight or obese *(3)*.

One should note that there are likely individuals who have BMI values that range from a status of overweight to obese I who may not be at increased risk of weight-related diseases as compared with others. But in practice, most of the general public

From: *Contemporary Cardiology: Cardiac Rehabilitation*
Edited by: W. E. Kraus and S. J. Keteyian © Humana Press Inc., Totowa, NJ

Table 1
BMI Categories

BMI (kg/m²)	Status
< 18.5	Underweight
18.5–24.9	Normal or acceptable weight
25.0–29.9	Overweight
30.0–34.9	Obese I
35.0–39.9	Obese II
40.0+	Morbid obesity

would be appropriately classified as at increased risk for weight-related diseases based on their BMI. The relationship between BMI and body fat percentage is positive and significant *(4)*. For the exceptions, Fig. 1 presents a comparison of two individuals with similar BMI values but with likely different weight-related disease risk.

Clinical observation of each person's body type in Fig. 1 suggests that the individual on the left is likely at a lower risk for body weight-related diseases. Given this potential situation, there are additional measures that can be taken to help clarify disease risk. The simplest of these is a waist measurement. Risk is increased when waist circumference exceeds 35 inches (88 cm) for women and 40 inches (102 cm) for men. In the above example, this type of quick measurement would help clarify the risk difference in individuals with the same BMI value. For those with higher BMI categorical values and waist measurements exceeding those mentioned above, the risk of weight-related diseases increases. Waist circumference is likely best at evaluating potential increased risk in those with BMI values ranging from 25.0 to 34.9 kg/m². The question you might ask now is 'why does waist circumference help to identify risk?'

Waist circumference serves two purposes in risk assessment. First, much research indicates that carrying excess weight in the stomach/truncal area indicates an increased risk for coronary artery disease (CAD), diabetes, hypertension, lipid disorders, and metabolic syndrome *(5)*. Additionally, waist circumference is an indirect measure of body fat, and it is the increased body fat that one carries that is related to disease risk. Going back to the example in Fig. 1, it is clear that the individual on the right would have a greater waist circumference and a higher body fat percentage.

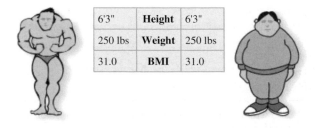

Fig. 1. Comparison of individuals with the same height and weight.

The waist-to-hip ratio may also be used to describe the location of fat accumulation. As with the waist measurement alone, this method identifies those who accumulate fat in the waist area (apple or android body shape) which places a person at increased risk for weight-related disease versus those who accumulate body fat in the hips and thighs (pear or gynoid body shape). The "apple" shape at which one is at increased health risk is a waist-to-hip ratio greater than 0.95 for men and 0.80 for women.

Body composition, and specifically body fat percentage, can be measured more accurately using a number of different methods including water or air displacement, skin-fold thickness, bioelectrical impedance, and dual-energy x-ray absorptiometry (DEXA). Body composition values that refer to an individual as overweight or obese vary slightly depending on the source. Most suggest that a body fat percentage above 20% for men and 30% for women constitutes the beginning standard for overweight or overfat. Morbidly obese individuals with BMIs above 40–50 kg/m^2 can have body fat percentages in the 50–70% range. However, assessment of body fat percentage requires specialized equipment and training, and there can be a large error associated with measurement using any of these methods.

During either a clinic visit or a cardiac rehabilitation program, assessment of BMI and waist circumference is easy and quick to perform, does not require specialized equipment, can be performed by any level of health professional, is not prone to error, and adequately provides both risk assessment and need for weight loss intervention.

Using the BMI definitions, the status of the US population has been described with reference to body weight over the past 45+ years. Data from the National Health and Nutrition Examination Survey (NHANES) provide most of this information. Prior to this, it was the Metropolitan Life Insurance Company that provided much of the weight-related health information with their ideal body weight tables. Table 2 summarizes data from the four NHANES surveys with data that demonstrate a high percentage of individuals classified as overweight since as early as 1960. The trend more recently, as depicted in the NHANES III data, is a rapid rise in the US population that is defined as overweight (6). Fig. 2 presents a similar trend for individuals who can be classified as obese. It is also well-known that minority populations are especially at increased risk for developing obesity.

In 1998, the American Heart Association first listed overweight and obesity as one of seven risk factors for the development of cardiovascular disease. A recent

Table 2
Age-Adjusted Percentage of US Adults Aged 20–74 years with BMI ≥ 25.0 kg/m^2, United States, 1960–1994*

Survey and years	Men	Women	Total
NHES I (1960–1962)	48.2	38.7	43.3
NHANES I (1971–1974)	52.9	39.7	46.1
NHANES II (1976–1980)	51.4	40.8	46.0
NHANES III (1988–1994)	59.3	49.6	54.4

NHES, National Health Examination Survey; NHANES, National Health and Nutrition Examination Survey.
* Results presented in %.

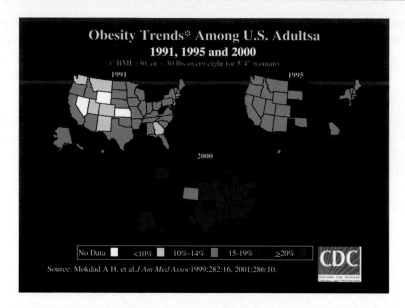

Fig. 2. Obesity trends among US adults. Reproduced with permission *(7,8)*.

report from the American Heart Association titled 'A Nation at Risk: Obesity in the United States' presented data from NHANES III that noted the following relative risk scores for developing heart disease within BMI ranges: BMI < 25, score 1.0; BMI = 25.0–29.9, score 1.39; BMI = 30.0–34.9, score 1.86, and BMI > 35.0, score 1.67. The Seventh Report of the Joint National Committee on Prevention, Detection, Evaluation, and Treatment of High Blood Pressure (JNC-7) reclassified obesity as a major modifiable risk factor for cardiovascular disease *(9)*. And there are many other diseases for which being overweight is strongly associated, including the risk of developing gallstones, some forms of cancer, diabetes, hypertension, osteoarthritis, low back pain, liver disease, sleep apnea, and premature death *(10)*.

Certainly, obesity is prevalent in populations with CAD. Rana et al. *(11)* reported that 58% of a consecutive cohort of post-myocardial infarction patients were classified as either overweight or obese using the BMI classification. They also found a positive and graded relationship of BMI and death in these patients. Cardiac rehabilitation specific populations are also obese. In our experience at Henry Ford Hospital, obesity is observed in 53% and morbid obesity in 13% of patients enrolling in cardiac rehabilitation. Clearly many patients with atherosclerosis are obese, and one can assume that this contributes to complications of CAD and its associated risk factors (e.g., hypertension and diabetes) and comorbidities (e.g., heart attack, angina, and peripheral artery disease). The American Association of Cardiovascular and Pulmonary Rehabilitation (AACVPR) guidelines for weight management in those participating in cardiac rehabilitation include the following *(1)*:

- Interventions should be targeted to those patients whose weight and body composition place them at increased cardiac risk and whose weight may adversely affect other risk factors such as diabetes, abnormal lipids, and hypertension.

- Interventsions should be targeted at men with a BMI $\geq 25 \, \text{kg/m}^2$ and waist > 40 inches (102 cm) and women with a BMI $\geq 25 \, \text{kg/m}^2$ and waist > 35 inches (88 cm) in women.

Pathophysiology

Overweight and obesity, in its simplest terms, is the result of a prolonged imbalance between caloric consumption and expenditure. However, there is much evidence of the multifactorial nature of the disease. Neurologic, physiologic, biochemical, environmental, cultural, and psychosocial factors all interact to drive caloric imbalance. Heredity is also known to play a strong role in the risk of obesity. Because of all these factors, a number of direct and indirect negative effects often occur in these patients.

Obesity is implicated in the metabolic syndrome and various other comorbid conditions that increase the risk of developing CAD, as well as the continued complications associated with established CAD and its comorbidities. Risk factors for CAD that may be affected by obesity include insulin resistance and diabetes, dyslipidemia, hypertension, inflammation, and a prothrombotic state.

1. **Insulin resistance and diabetes**: Both of these related conditions are known to significantly elevate the risk of developing CAD by between 2.5- and 5-fold. However, the mechanisms of obesity leading to these are not well understood. Abdominal obesity specifically elevates risk. Proposed mechanisms include the elevation of free fatty acids in the blood which may affect the skeletal muscles (insulin resistance), the liver (glucose release and insulin clearance), and the pancreas (insulin production) which possibly alone, or in combination, may lead to insulin resistance and/or diabetes. There is evidence that insulin resistance is genetically related *(12)*.
2. **Dyslipidemia**: Often plasma triglycerides, total cholesterol and low-density lipoprotein (LDL) levels are elevated in those who are obese. However, these abnormalities are not always found in the obese. This demonstrates the complicated relationship between obesity and plasma lipoproteins. This also includes lower high-density lipoprotein (HDL) levels. A potential mechanism may be the observed elevated rate of very low-density lipoprotein (VLDL) production in obese individuals which can affect HDL, LDL and triglycerides *(5)*.
3. **Hypertension**: Elevated blood pressure is common in the obese and is related to body weight *(13)*. Again, the relationship is not well understood. Obese individuals are often volume overloaded, possibly due to sodium retention. They may have an impaired vasodilatory capacity, which may be affected also by insulin-related disease. This effect might be related to renal (sodium absorption and renin-angiotensin activity) or sympathetic nervous system function.
4. **Inflammation**: High sensitivity C-reactive protein (hs-CRP) and cytokines are elevated in those who are obese *(14)*. These play a role in inflammation within the arteries, including those with established atherosclerosis. It is not known whether hs-CRP is involved in destabilizing plaque or whether unstable plaque results in increased hs-CRP production.
5. **Prothrombotic status**: Elevated levels of fibrinogen and plasma activator inhibitor (PAI-1) are often elevated in the obese *(15)*. Both factors are related to increased risks of thrombotic events. This alteration in thrombotic state, along with the proinflammatory effects of obesity, may be associated with the increase risk of stroke also seen in obese individuals *(16)*.

These and other potential effects of obesity, including increases in blood volume and cardiac output, increased cardiac work at any level of exertion compared with normal non-obese persons and cardiac hypertrophy/myopathy all can result in the initial genesis of, and ongoing problems associated with atherosclerosis. In addition, there are a number of cardiac electric abnormalities (possibly related to hypertrophy or autonomic nervous dysfunction) that can also occur, many of which are evident on an electrocardiogram (ECG) (e.g., increased heart rate, PR interval, QRS interval, QTc interval, ST segment abnormalities, etc.). Additionally, obesity can result in venous insufficiency (primarily in the massively obese) and endothelial dysfunction as evidenced by increased vasoconstriction. Finally, obesity is the most prevalent modifiable risk factor for sleep apnea *(16)*.

There is evidence that weight loss can modify many of these cardiac risk factors including reducing blood pressure and blood cholesterol levels and improving glucose tolerance *(17)*. Additionally, there are decreases in blood volume, cardiac output, left ventricular mass, resting, and exercise oxygen consumption and improvements in diastolic and systolic left ventricular function, among other positive cardiac changes resulting from weight loss *(16)*. Schotte et al. *(18)* report that for each 1-kg decrease in body weight, there is a dose effect of 1.7 mmHg decrease of diastolic blood pressure. Additionally, a 1.93-mg dL^{-1} total cholesterol, 0.77-mg dL^{-1} LDL, and a 1.33-mg dL^{-1} triglyercide decrease is reported for each 1 kg of weight loss *(19)*. However, there is very little research on the effects of weight loss on these risk factors and the subsequent effect on established CAD morbidity and mortality. And there is especially a lack of data on the effects of weight loss efforts in association with cardiac rehabilitation participation for both the short and the long terms.

TREATMENT STRATEGIES

The Cardiac Rehabilitation Clinical Practice Guidelines from the US Department of Health and Human Services provides an algorithm decision tree for cardiac rehabilitation services which probes whether the patient is overweight and suggests dietary education, counseling, and behavioral intervention as global treatment strategies *(2)*. This strategy is endorsed by the AACVPR in the 4th edition of Guidelines for Cardiac Rehabilitation and Secondary Prevention Programs *(1)*. Most research indicates that the combination of diet, exercise, and behavioral counseling is best for optimal weight loss and the maintenance process. Fig. 3 provides a BMI-based strategy suggesting the intensity of treatment as proposed by the American College of Physicians. Although this strategy is not specific to patients participating in cardiac rehabilitation, it does reflect the current general consensus of the initial treatment approach for obese patients seeking a clinical weight loss approach. The following sections review current state-of-the-art treatment strategies that can be implemented in the cardiac rehabilitation setting.

Medical

Medical treatment can take on several forms. These include diet manipulation, exercise therapy, pharmacologic treatment, and behavioral counseling. Each of these treatments should be implemented and guided by a trained clinician. Prior to developing a treatment program, all patients should be assessed by a physician for underlying

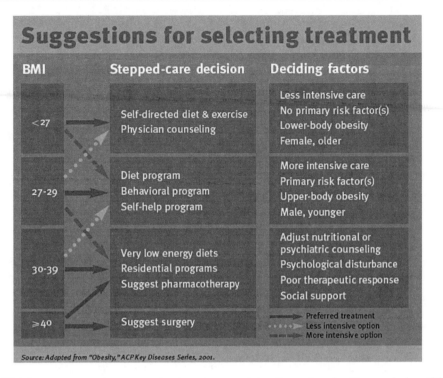

Fig. 3. Weight management program treatment suggestions. Reproduced with permission *(20)*.

metabolic disorders such as hypothyroidism or Cushing's disease. Once these are ruled out or addressed, a comprehensive weight loss treatment strategy can be developed and implemented. Each strategy (diet, exercise, and behavioral) can be delivered by itself, or in conjunction with the other medical treatments, including delivery of all at the same time. The latter strategy is most effective in achieving goals. Prior to providing specific treatment interventions for each weight loss component, weight loss goals should be determined and discussed. Studies show that up to 50% of physicians do not discuss weight control to any degree with their obese and overweight patients *(21)*. Although physicians should be involved in encouraging patients to lose weight, they typically do not emphasize the importance of the cardiac rehabilitation practitioner in the weight loss process.

Goal setting is very important in the initial phases of weight loss. There is strong evidence that losing approximately 5–10% of initial body weight positively impacts the cardiac risk factors associated with obesity *(17)*. This suggests that this range of weight loss would be a reasonable initial goal for most patients. However, research indicates that women, despite targeted education regarding the 5–10% weight loss benefits, indicate that they would be disappointed with a 17% weight loss; and the average desired weight loss is about 25% *(22)*. This may have a negative effect on weight loss success, especially if the treatment program is not tailored to meet the desired outcomes of the patient. On the basis of this type of aggressive goal setting, either more directed education about the positive effects of a lower weight loss total or more aggressive weight loss strategies to achieve desired results should be implemented.

The former might be accomplished using additional focused behavioral strategies such as cognitive behavioral treatment *(23)*.

Developing a weight loss strategy requires knowledge of the individual. At the opening of the 2005 American Heart Association (AHA) Scientific Sessions, President Robert Eckel provided a list of questions that a physician (or cardiac rehabilitation professional) might ask when initially addressing the topics of diet and exercise with their patients (Table 3). Each of these can certainly lead into a discussion using cognitive behavioral strategies.

Cognitive behavorial discussion of weight loss expectations should focus on the establishment of realistic weight loss goals, the discussion of appearance versus health-related benefits of weight loss, the valuing of oneself independent of body weight, and the acceptance of the body weight and appearance that one does achieve during the weight loss phase. In this initial approach, one must be sensitive to the patient's perception of their weight. Using terms such as "obese" and "fatness" have been shown to be less desirable terms when discussing body weight *(25)*. Patients tend to prefer the terms "weight" and "excess weight" and using BMI to discuss their obesity. Table 4 lists discussion points to use with your patients.

Typical weight loss rate goals are suggested to be in the range of 1–2 pounds per week *(10)*. This rate, versus a higher rate, may help to preserve lean body mass, allow for better adherence to lifestyle changes associated with weight loss, and produce less water weight loss *(10)*. However, there is evidence that faster weight loss rates might be best for achieving large weight loss goals and ultimately improve treatment adherence through the reinforcement of significant early weight loss *(26)*. Additionally, there are other strategies such as resistance training that may reduce the rate of lean mass loss during rapid weight loss phases.

Table 3
Suggested 3-Min Lifestyle Interview Questions

Nutrition
How many servings of fruits and vegetables do you eat a day?
How many servings of whole grains do you eat a day?
How many servings of fish do you eat a week?
Do you eat desserts (how often)?
What are your favorite snack foods?
Do you eat because you're hungry or because there is food around?
Do you weigh the most now that you've ever weighed?
Are you interested in losing weight?
Physical Activity
How many steps do you take each day?
Do you have a regular exercise program?
Do you typically take elevators or escalators, or climb the stairs?
Do you park as close as you can to your destination?
What limits your level of physical activity? Have you been evaluated for this?
Would you like to become more active?

Table 4
Talking with Your Patients

Review BMI results
Use open-ended questions or comments and follow-up when appropriate
Ask and define weight loss goals
Respect decisions not to attempt to lose weight at any discussion, but
   suggest that you might discuss again in the future. The patient may not
   be ready to lose weight in the present but may be in the future
Set very specific goals and make them time oriented (e.g., 16 weeks)
Make the treatment program specific to an individual
Suggest professional weight loss help including community based
   programs, and clinical programs staffed by allied health care
   professionals such as registered dietitians, exercise physiologists and
   behavioralists; cardiac rehabilitation programs are excellent locations
   for clinical weight management programs

Adapted from (24).

Although, for most obese individuals, the implementation of dietary, exercise, and behavioral changes will result in significant weight loss, it may be useful to first determine or estimate a patient's daily caloric needs to maintain their weight. Begin by first determining their resting metabolic rate (RMR). Estimating or quantifying the RMR can be used to help develop the initial weight loss plan and to refine the plan during a plateau of weight loss or as a patient nears his/her weight loss goal. There are a number of very specific methods to determine RMR in the units of calories used per day. Indirect calorimetry or gas exchange analysis using a metabolic cart is the simplest of these methods in the clinical setting. However, this requires specialized equipment costing in the range of $20,000–40,000 and must be staffed by skilled health care professionals for accurate and reliable data.

Alternatively, the RMR can be estimated by a number of methods. The Harris-Benedict equation is the most often used of these methods. The equations for men and women are:

$$\text{Men RMR} = 66 + (13.7 \times \text{weight in kg}) + (5 \times \text{height in cm}) - (6.8 \times \text{age in years})$$

$$\text{Women RMR} = 655 + (9.6 \times \text{weight in kg}) + (1.8 \times \text{height in cm}) - (4.7 \times \text{age in years})$$

Once the RMR is determined, the total daily caloric needs can be determined by assessing physical activity level and multiplying the RMR by the appropriate conversion factor. Four physical activity categories and the corresponding conversion factor are listed below.

- If sedentary (little or no exercise, desk job), multiply RMR by 1.2.
- If lightly active (light exercise/sports 1–3 days per week), multiply RMR by 1.375.
- If moderately active (moderate exercise/sports 3–5 days per week), multiply RMR by 1.55.
- If heavy exercise (hard exercise/sports 6–7 days per week), multiply RMR by 1.725.

An even simpler method to determine RMR is to multiply body weight in pounds by 10. The above physical activity conversion factors are again used to determine total daily caloric needs.

For most individuals to achieve a 1–2-pound weight loss per week, a daily caloric deficit of 500–1000 calories per day is required, achieved through a combination of diet manipulation and physical activity/exercise. This is based on the assumption that 1 pound of fat equals approximately 3500 calories. The American College of Sports Medicine (ACSM) suggests a 2000+ calories per week expenditure from exercise *(10)*. This averages nearly 300 calories per day and can be achieved by walking about 3 miles a day. The remainder of the deficit to achieve the 1–2-pound weight loss per week must be accomplished through dietary measures that equate to 350–850 calories per day. This rate of weight loss will often take up to 6 months to achieve a 10% loss.

One should also consider the intensity of weight loss treatment in comparison with patient goals and desired clinical outcomes. For most individuals seeking clinical weight loss, a 5–10% weight loss will keep their BMI above 30kg/m^2 which, although improved and representing a reduction in heart disease risk, still represents an approximately 1.4 times increased risk for heart disease as compared with a BMI under 25kg/m^2. This risk is similar to a diastolic blood pressure of 102 mmHg or a total cholesterol level of 240 mg dL^{-1}. Failure to further treat these risk factors to JNC-7 or Adult Treatment Panel (ATP III) goals might be akin to poor practice or even malpractice. Maybe the treatment of obesity should be considered similarly?

The following is a review of each of the major components of a weight loss program, beginning with diet.

DIET

A number of dietary changes can be simply presented and discussed in the office by a physician. These should ideally take the form of general suggestions for diet modification, unless the physician feels comfortable making more specific recommendations. Some simple tips that are easily understood, easy to implement, and can be discussed by most physicians are summarized in Table 5. If adopted, these changes generally will result in the reduction of caloric intake.

This information can be quickly discussed with a patient and provided in handout form. However, this may result in additional questions from the patient such as "What is a portion size?" or "How do I interpret a food label?" At this point it might be most efficient and effective to refer the patient to a registered dietitian, the professional who specializes in helping patients understand each of these issues and is trained in assisting others with appropriate changes. And certainly more complex diet plans

Table 5
Simple Dietary Suggestions to Result in Weight Loss

Read food labels	Eat smaller portions and limit servings
Choose lower fat foods	Eat less sugar
Eat more fruits and vegetables	Eat more complex carbohydrates
Trim excess fat off of meat	Eat "meatless" several days per week
Replace whole and 2% milk and milk products with skim, 1/2 or 1% milk	

are best developed and presented by registered dietitians. Many cardiac rehabilitation programs either have a dietitian on staff or utilize one periodically for group education. This may be the best place to refer if you do not have access to a dietitian.

Following a specific diet such as the National Cholesterol Education Program (NCEP) Step I or II diets as recommended by the National Institutes of Health (NIH), will likely also achieve some weight loss in obese individuals due to its composition of lower fat and a higher percentage of complex carbohydrate intake than is typically in the diet of an obese individual. Because fat has 9 calories per gram and carbohydrate has 4 calories per gram, it is obvious that these methods will reduce calorie intake. Again, this can be discussed with the patient in an office visit, but it might be best understood and yield the best results if implemented by a registered dietitian.

A more specific plan would be to assign a desired caloric intake that is, as discussed previously, several hundred calories lower than the daily intake required for weight maintenance. The Expert Panel on the Identification, Evaluation, and Treatment of Overweight and Obesity in Adults recommended a 500–1000-calorie per day deficit to achieve the weekly 1–2-pound weight loss (27). In general, a target caloric intake of 1200–1500 per day for women and 1500–2000 per day for men adjusted for age, BMI, and activity level is effective for most individuals (10). These diets are often termed "low-calorie diets" (LCDs).

A common method of achieving these intakes is using the "exchange system", which has been in use for many years by those with diabetes. This process, as developed by a dietitian, allows for a given number of exchanges or servings per day in each of the following six food categories: breads, fruits, vegetables, meats, milk, and fats. The goal is to limit daily food intake to only satisfy the exchanges allowed within each food category. To achieve this, it is best to advise individuals to eat four to six meals, spaced evenly throughout the day. This will help the patient to avoid periods of severe hunger, will allow food to be eaten throughout the day rather than in large amounts, and may help to maintain a consistent metabolic rate throughout the day. Patients should avoid periods of no food intake such as skipping meals (e.g., breakfast). Patients who are very motivated and who understand caloric intake issues such as portion sizes and how to read and use food labels may be counseled to count their own calories throughout the day to achieve the recommended intake. Many free Internet-based tools are available to assist patients with determining the caloric content of various foods (e.g., www.calorielab.com and www.bettermd.net). This method of controlling intake may be more effective in the weight loss process, but it is also more likely to lead to non-adherence in some individuals due to the complexity of determining serving sizes, reading food labels, etc.

Very Low-Calorie Diet (complete meal replacement)

Patients who are extremely obese (BMI $\geq$ 35 or 30 kg/m^2 with comorbid conditions) and who seek a professional weight loss program may be appropriate for the implementation of a very low-calorie diet (VLCD). This diet limits daily calorie intake to 500–800 calories and uses nutritional supplements formulated to be high in protein and low in fat. The principle of the VLCD is the same as of the Atkins diet, in that the VLCD diet depletes liver and skeletal muscle carbohydrate stores, which

Contd.

then requires the body to metabolize fat stores for energy production. However, the composition of the VLCD supplements is very low in fat and thus potential long-term negative effects of a high fat intake, as with the Atkins diet, are avoided. Also, unlike Atkins, the VLCD is only meant to be a short-term, rapid weight loss diet. The rate of weight loss during the initial several months of the VLCD is similar to bariatric surgery.

Medical supervision for patients on the VLCD is required. This includes periodic physician visits to review symptoms, obtain basic lab values (every 4–6 weeks), and adjust medications, especially diuretics, other anti-hypertensives, and anti-diabetes medications. Common medical problems are related to dehydration, low blood glucose levels, and constipation. The risk of gallstones is greatly reduced with the introduction of several grams of fat per day or the use of Ursodiol.

It is important to teach behavior-change techniques during the VLCD as with any comprehensive weight loss program. Patients will be returning to a weight maintenance diet and should use the VLCD phase to learn and apply lifestyle changes as presented elsewhere in this chapter. Typical duration of a VLCD is 12–24 weeks. However, longer durations are common in the morbidly obese as long as medical supervision is maintained. Although VLCDs were associated with a number of arrhythmic cardiac deaths in the late 1970s, increases in protein and micronutrients and careful medical monitoring have essentially eliminated such risk. The VLCD is easily implemented, effective for achieving significant short-term weight loss of up to 20% at 6 months, and very safe if implemented and followed by a trained dietitian and exercise physiologist, as commonly employed in a cardiac rehabilitation program. There is evidence that poorer weight loss maintenance is associated with a VLCD than an LCD, but this rate of recidivism may not be different than any lifestyle intervention (e.g., smoking cessation and exercise).

EXERCISE

It is well accepted that increasing exercise and general physical activity is an important component of the weight management treatment plan. However, exercise alone is generally not effective for weight loss as it requires a great volume of exercise to produce a sufficient energy deficit. For instance, to expend 3500 calories, or the equivalent of 1 pound of fat, one must walk approximately 35 miles. The importance for exercise in the weight loss process is the enhanced rate of weight loss during the weight loss phase (27). Also, exercise is an important predictor of long-term weight loss maintenance as demonstrated by the National Weight Control Registry study (28).

Exercise advice for the obese individual should be encouraged by a physician but is best prescribed by an exercise physiologist experienced in working with these patients. There are many nuances associated with exercise for these patients including issues related to equipment use, orthopedic limitations, appearance and self-consciousness, and adjustment of intensity/frequency/duration levels that need special attention. These patients would be minimally served by a one-on-one session with an exercise physiologist and best served by enrolling in a supervised exercise program, such as that offered in a phase 3 cardiac rehabilitation setting. If a patient is already participating in a phase 2 cardiac rehabilitation program, then they are in a program that is well suited for caring for obese patients with heart disease.

Initially, aerobic-based exercises (e.g., walking, pool use for swimming or water aerobics, cycling, elliptical trainers, etc.) are best for maximizing caloric expenditure. Mode selection is very important for adherence. For some individuals, seated aerobics may be an excellent option to reduce the typical orthopedic limitations these individuals experience including back, hip, knee, and ankle pain. Seated or chair aerobics also can be performed in the comfort of a person's home. Cardiac rehabilitation programs should consider acquiring treadmills that can accommodate 500-pound individuals. Alternatively, larger individuals may use floor space or hallways to perform walking. Larger cycle seats or steps to use to get onto equipment is also useful. When possible, weight-bearing exercise should be performed to maximize caloric expenditure. Once a patient establishes a regular aerobic exercise routine, a resistance-training program may be implemented. These programs, as presented later, provide a stimulus to preserve or increase fat-free mass, improve muscular strength and power, possibly enhance fat mass loss, and may ameliorate declines in RMR *(10)*.

When prescribing exercise, in addition to type of exercise one is concerned with the intensity, duration, and frequency of the program. When working with the extremely obese (BMI $> 40 \, \text{kg/m}^2$), often these individuals have not exercised regularly in years, if ever. Telling these individuals to "go walk a mile a day" would be met with apparent acceptance, but in reality, many are so limited that their effort to ambulate at all may be near their maximal exercise effort. This would result in early frustration and poor adherence. For these individuals, the accumulation of exercise volume in intermittent bouts may be best as an initial exercise strategy. This is defined as the performance of short bouts of exercise (maybe 5–15 min) several times per day to add up to a desired total duration. Current public health recommendations for exercise and physical activity emphasize the benefits of intermittent accumulation. But there are few studies that have assessed the effectiveness of intermittent bouts for weight loss. Early in the exercise process, patients performing intermittent exercise will not likely achieve 2000 calories per week expenditure (and this level is also often difficult for those who can perform continuous exercise).

The duration, frequency, and intensity of exercise combine to determine total exercise volume and thus caloric expenditure. To achieve 2000 calories per week, most individuals will require approximately 60 min daily of moderate-intensity exercise. For those who are able to incorporate a significant amount of daily physical activity, the total intentional exercise volume may be reduced. As stated earlier, as most of these individuals are likely not exercising, the exercise program should be set up in a progressive manner. Typically it is best to begin with a goal of 30 min (continuous or intermittent) of exercise performed on 3 days of the week. Progression should begin with duration and frequency until the ultimate goal of 60 min per day is achieved. An experienced exercise physiologist should be able to work with these patients to determine how they might achieve these goals. Certainly any exercise or physical activity increase is beneficial, and patients should not feel discouraged if they are having a difficult time achieving their ultimate exercise goal.

The intensity of exercise for these patients should follow that typical for a patient participating in a cardiac rehabilitation program. These programs are designed to achieve a moderate intensity that is equivalent to a low of 40–50% of peak VO_2 and as high as 85% of peak VO_2. Most obese individuals who have not recently exercised should begin at the lower end of this range. This is best assessed by the performance of an exercise test, ideally with concomitant gas-exchange analysis using a metabolic cart (i.e., indirect calorimeter). If this is not available, then the intensity level can be set based on a percentage of peak-estimated metabolic equivalents (METs) achieved or by using the heart rate reserve method to determine a training heart rate range. The exercise test is also important in these individuals for common reasons in cardiac rehabilitation including assessment for ischemia, arrhythmias, and hemodynamic decompensation that might be used to limit the exercise intensity.

A recent study of the effect of exercise intensity on weight loss suggests that intensity does not make a difference in the amount of weight lost but that higher intensity exercise is better for improvements in functional capacity and possibly results in an increased daily physical activity level (29). Therefore, from a weight loss perspective, the intensity of exercise should only be increased after patients have achieved a comfortable exercise program on most days of the week for 60 min per session.

Physiologic adaptations to exercise training in cardiac diseased patients who are obese will likely be very similar to the non-obese cardiac rehabilitation population. There is little data assessing the acute and chronic adaptations to exercise in the obese cardiac population. Bader et al. (30) demonstrated an approximately 26% increase in peak-estimated METs in an obese population versus 18% in a normal weight group that performed exercise training in a cardiac rehabilitation program for 10 weeks. Interestingly, others have shown more improvement in non-obese subjects (31). In ischemic patients, one can expect an improved ischemic threshold. Overall, at submaximal work rates, heart rate, blood pressure, and perceived exertion values will be reduced, requiring a progressive increase in absolute exercise work rate to maintain exercise intensity levels. In addition, the National Weight Control Registry shows that exercise is critical for prevention of weight regain (26). These data suggest that a large volume of exercise (80–90 min per day) needs to be performed each day to maintain weight loss.

Resistance exercise training can utilize several different modes. These include calisthenics, elastic bands, machine-type weights, and free weights. The latter may be least desirable due to safety issues. Training programs need not be complex. They should focus primarily on the major muscle groups of the arms, chest, and lower body. Frequency should be 2–3 days per week. Each session duration should allow enough time to perform one to two sets per exercise and between 6 and 12 exercises or lifts per session. If performing more than one set (note that near maximal benefits often occur by performing one set), there should be between 30 s and 1 min of rest. There is little evidence that circuit training, involving calisthenics or other aerobic exercise between exercises, is beneficial in this population. Each set should allow the patient to perform between 10 and 15 repetitions. The resistance utilized in machine or free-weight exercise can be determined using the modified one repetition maximum (RM) assessment. This can be performed by an exercise physiologist. Increases in resistance should be determined by individual perceived exertion once the patient can perform an exercise for 15 repetitions. Resistance exercise not using weights (e.g., elastic bands and calisthenics) should be guided by perceived exertion. These and free- or machine-weight exercises can be performed separately or in conjunction with each other.

Specific resistance exercise for any of these modes is beyond the scope of this chapter. However, almost any exercise physiologist is knowledgeable of these routines and should be able to apply appropriately. Often, resistance training does not occur in phase 2 cardiac rehabilitation but rather in phase 3. However, there is no reason why a motivated individual who has adequately adapted to an aerobic exercise routine cannot perform resistance training during phase 2 cardiac rehabilitation. Resistance training should be limited or not performed in patients with unstable angina, within 6 weeks of bypass surgery, or with uncontrolled hypertension. During the lift, blood pressure will rise substantially. However, total work by the heart does not approach that during aerobic exercise due to the very low heart rate response during resistance training resulting in a lower double product during resistance training than during aerobic exercise.

Pharmacologic Treatment

The use of pharmacologic agents for weight loss should be considered if a patient requires an adjunct to lifestyle modification including diet and exercise or is at a plateau or is having difficulty maintaining weight loss. These uses are supported by the National Heart, Lung, and Blood Institute (NHLBI) in their 1998 report on treating the overweight and obese (NIH). The Food and Drug Administration (FDA) has approved several drugs for short- or long-term use in patients with a BMI $\geq$ 30 (or > 27 if risk factors or comorbid diseases are present). Short-term drugs (< 12 weeks) are those based on phentermine and diethylpropion. Long-term drugs include subutramine and orlistat.

The short-term agents work to suppress appetite, although mechanisms related to neurotransmitter (e.g., norepinephrine, serotonin, and dopamine) actions. Subutramine's mechanism is similar, but its action is to enhance satiety. There is some evidence that these drugs may increase the risk of elevation of blood pressure and heart rate, and therefore, it should be avoided in patients with untreated hypertension, CAD, heart failure, arrhythmias, or stroke (16). Regular monitoring is important and can be easily performed by cardiac rehabilitation staff.

Orlistat inhibits fat absorption in the gastrointestinal tract. It blocks approximately one-third of fat intake. Its important to note that orlistat is not effective in patients eating a low-fat diet. The major side effects are related to gastrointestinal symptoms such as pain, fecal urgency, and loose stools due to evacuation of fatty oils. This latter side effect is unpleasant but may serve as a behavioral mechanism in some individuals to avoid high-fat foods. Orlistat became an over-the-counter product in February 2007 as approved the FDA advisory committee in January 2006. Well-designed studies using these drugs typically produce weight losses in the range of 7–10% (32,33). Sibutramine has also been shown to be beneficial in maintaining weight loss after a VLCD (34).

Behavior Modification

Behavior modification therapy involves the teaching, implementation, and follow-up of techniques designed to increase the likelihood that a lifestyle change will be successful for the long term. Both diet and exercise/physical activity changes are definite lifestyle changes for essentially all overweight individuals attempting to lose weight. Cardiac rehabilitation programs are excellent services for these patients and for the implementation of a weight loss program because the staff (exercise physiologists, dietitians, and others) are trained in behavior modification techniques (cognitive behavioral, motivational interviewing, etc.) designed to help patients reduce the impact of lifestyle-related risk factors on disease progression.

There are a large number of behavioral strategies and tools that can be employed in a weight management setting. Table 6 summarizes some of these with brief explanations. These techniques can be taught in individual or group settings, and frequent contact every 1–2 weeks is desirable (35). Methods of ongoing contact during both the weight loss and the maintenance phases are important to enhance long-term adherence to diet and exercise behaviors and to prevent weight regain (36). Internet options such as email contact or program (see www.bettermd.net) allow for a low-cost method of regular contact that are shown to be effective strategies (37).

Surgical

Bariatric surgery is an option for patients with extreme or clinically severe (versus morbid) obesity. Typically, surgeons request that those seeking surgery have exhausted other weight loss techniques, including clinically based weight management programs.

Table 6
Behavioral Strategies for Weight Management

Goal setting	Both short and long term goals should be realistic and specific
Diet and exercise diary use	Goal is to write down everything that is eaten or performed in exercise with routine self assessment and review by a health professional
Frequent contact	Regular follow-up visits with weight management staff and/or patients physician
Rewards	Often working towards a goal is improved by an incentive
Barrier recognition	A-priori recognition of food and physical activity barriers, with contingency plans in place
Problem solving	Often best used with motivational interviewing during a follow-up visit; it allows the patient to figure out the problem and solution and imparts power to them; may require input from clinicians
Stimulus control	After identifying triggers of lack of diet and exercise adherence, work to limit/eliminate these triggers
Self monitoring	Patients should learn these techniques with respect to 'what, where, when, and how' as it increases awareness and improves ability to change behavior; this monitoring includes food intake, exercise and body weight; recently shown to be very important in long-term maintenance
Social support	Significant others can help to maintain lifestyle changes and provide encouragement which helps with adherence

Criteria for surgery include a BMI ≥ 40 or $35\,\mathrm{kg/m^2}$ with comorbid conditions. Surgery has been shown to provide excellent weight loss success as long as 5 years post-surgery. There are several surgical techniques that can be performed using either open or laparoscopic techniques.

Even though many patients do well after surgery, there is still the risk of subsequent regain of weight or not losing an amount of weight to significantly lower cardiovascular and other health risks. Therefore, selecting well-informed and motivated patients is important. It is also important that all patients receive follow-up with respect to both diet and exercise. Observational studies have demonstrated that patients will lose more weight if they participate in a supervised exercise program, versus on their own, following surgery. Programs such as the phase 3 cardiac rehabilitation model are excellent for these patients as they will learn how to exercise properly and receive counseling by exercise physiologists. Also these programs often have equipment that can support these patients, and the settings of these programs tend to be less threatening than a commercial exercise studio; so patients will likely feel more comfortable during their exercise routine.

SUMMARY

Obesity is very common in patients enrolled in cardiac rehabilitation. These programs are ideally suited to implement a comprehensive weight loss program focusing on diet, exercise, and behavior change. Specific guidelines for weight management in cardiac rehabilitation are lacking. Initial discussion and encouragement from a patient's physician is very important in this process as is subsequent discussions at follow-up. Cardiac rehabilitation programs should work to implement programs delivered by registered dietitians and exercise physiologists who are commonly employed in these programs. Behavior modification should be an integral part of any weight management program, even if aggressive methods such as VLCD or bariatric surgery are indicated.

REFERENCES

1. American Association of Cardiovascular and Pulmonary Rehabilitation. *Guidelines for Cardiac Rehabilitation and Secondary Prevention Programs*, 4th ed. Champaign, IL: Human Kinetics; 2003.
2. Wenger NK, Froelicher ES, Smith LK, et al. *Cardiac Rehabilitation. Clinical Practice Guideline No. 17*. Rockville, MD: U.S. Department of Health and Human Services, Public Health Service, Agency for Health Care Policy and Research and the National Heart, Lung, and Blood Institute. AHCPR Publication No. 96-0672. October 1995.
3. Krauss RM, Eckel RH, Howard B, et al. AHA Dietary Guidelines: Revision 2000: A Statement for Healthcare Professionals from the Nutrition Committee of the American Heart Association. *Circulation*. 2000;102:2284–2299.
4. Gallagher D, Heymsfield SB, Heo M, et al. Health Percentage Body Fat Ranges: An Approach for Developing Guidelines Based on Body Mass Index. *Am J Clin Nutr*. 2000;72:694–701.
5. Grundy SM, Abate N. Obesity. In *Secondary Heart Disease: Systemic Diseases and the Heart*. 2003. http://intl.elsevierhealth.com/e-books/pdf/756.pdf
6. Kuczmarski RJ, Flegal KM. Criteria for Definition of Overweight in Transition: Background And Recommendations for the United States. *Am J Clin Nutr*. 2000;72:1074–1081.
7. Mokdad AH, Serdult MK, Dietz WH, et al. The spread of the obesity epidermic in the united states 1991–1998. *JAMA*, 1999;282(16):1519–1522.

8. Mokdad AH, Bowman BA, Ford ES, et al. The continuing epidemics of obesity and diabetes in the United States. *JAMA*. 2001;286(10):1195–1200.

9. Chobanian A, Bakris GL, Black HR, et al. The Seventh Report of the Joint National Committee on Prevention, Detection, Evaluation, and Treatment of High Blood Pressure: The JNC 7 Report. *JAMA*. 2003;289:2560–2572.

10. Jakicic JM, Clark K, Coleman E, et al. ACSM Position Stand on the Appropriate Intervention Strategies for Weight Loss and Prevention of Weight Regain for Adults. *Med Sci Sports Exerc*. 2001;33:2145–2156.

11. Rana JS, Mukamal KJ, Morgan JP, Muller JE, Mittleman MA. Obesity and the Risk of Death After Acute Myocardial Infarction. *Am Heart J*. 2004;147:841–846.

12. Abate N, Garg A, Peshock RM, et al. Relationship of Generalized and Regional Adiposity to Insulin Sensitivity in Men. *J Clin Invest*. 1995;96:88–98.

13. Brown CD, Higgins M, Donato KA, Rohde FC, Garrison R, Obarzanek E, Ernst ND, Horan M. Body Mass Index and the Prevalence of Hypertension and Dyslipidemia. *Obes Res*. 2000;8:676–677.

14. Klein S, Burke LE, Bray GA, et al. AHA Scientific Statement: Clinical Implications of Obesity with Specific Focus on Cardiovascular Disease. *Circulation*. 2004;110:2952–2967.

15. Juhan-Vague I, Alessi MC. PAI-1, Obesity, Insulin Resistance and Risk of Cardiovascular Events. *Thromb Haemost*. 1997;78:656–660.

16. Poirier P, Giles TD, Bray GA, et al. Obesity and Cardiovascular Disease: Pathophysiology, Evaluation, and Effect of Weight Loss. *Circulation*. 2006;113:898–918.

17. Eckel RH, Krauss RM, for the AHA Nutrition Committee. American Heart Association Call to Action: Obesity as a Major Risk Factor for Coronary Heart Disease. *Circulation*. 1998;97:2099–2100.

18. Schotte D, Stunkard AJ. The Effects of Weight Reduction on Blood Pressure in 301 Obese Patients. *Arch Intern Med*. 1990;150:1701–1704.

19. Dattilo AM, Kris-Etherton PM. Effects of Weight Reduction on Blood Lipids and Lipoproteins: A Meta-Analysis. *Am J Clin Nutr*. 1992;56:320–328.

20. Gumbiner B. Obesity, ACP Key Disease Series, 3rd ed. United States of America: American College of Physicians-American Society of Internal Medicine; 2001.

21. Stafford RS, Farhat JH, Misra B, Schoenfeld DA. National Patterns of Physician Activities Related to Obesity Management. *Arch Fam Med*. 2000;9:631–638.

22. Wadden TA, Womble LG, Sarwer DB, Berkowitz RI, Clark V, Foster GD. Great Expectations: "I'm losing 25% of my weight no matter what you say". *J Consulting Clin Psych*. 2003;71:1084–1089.

23. Ames GE, Perri MG, Fox LD, et al. Changing Weight-Loss Expectations: A Randomized Pilot Study. *Eating Behav*. 2005;6:259–269.

24. Wadden TA, Tsai AG. Weight Management in Primary Care: Can we Talk? *Obes Manag*. 2005;1:9–14.

25. Wadden TA, Didie E. What's in a Name? Patients' Preferred Terms for Describing Obesity. *Obes Res*. 2003;11:1140–1146.

26. Wing RR. Don't Throw Out the Baby with the Bathwater: A Commentary on Very-Low-Calorie Diets. *Diabetes Care*. 1992;15:293–296.

27. National Institutes of Health, National Heart, Lung, and Blood Institute. *Clinical Guidelines on the Identification, Evaluation, and Treatment of Overweight and Obesity in Adults: The Evidence Report*. Bethesda, MD: NIH; 1998.

28. Wing RR, Phelan S. Long-Term Weight Loss Maintenance. *Am J Clin Nutr*. 2005;82(suppl): 222S–225S.

29. Lafortuna CL, Resnik M, Galvani C, Sartorio A. Effects of Non-Specific Vs Individualized Exercise Training Protocols on Aerobic, Anaerobic and Strength Performance in Severely Obese Subjects During a Short-Term Body Mass Reduction Program. *J Endocrinol Invest*. 2003;26:197–205.

30. Bader DS, Maguire TE, Spahn CM, et al. Clinical Profile and Outcomes of Obese Patients in Cardiac Rehabilitation Stratified According to National Heart, Lung and Blood Institute Criteria. *J Cardiipulm Rehabil.* 2001;21:210–217.

31. Lavie CJ, Milani RV. Effects of Cardiac Rehabilitation, Exercise Training, and Weight Reduction on Exercise Capacity, Coronary Risk Factors, Behavioral Characteristics, and Quality of Life in Obese Coronary Patients. *Am J Cardiol.* 1997;79(4):397–401.

32. Jones SP, Smith IG, Kelly F, Gray JA. Long Term Weight Loss with Sibutramine. *Int J Obes.* 1995;19(Suppl 2):60.

33. Sjostrom L, Rissanen A, Andersen T, et al. Randomized Placeto-Controlled Trial of Orlistat for Weight Loss and Prevention of Weight Regain in Obese Patients. *Ter Arkh.* 2000;72(8): 50–54.

34. Apfelbaum M, Vauge P, Zigler O, et al. Long-Term Maintenance of Weight Loss After a Very-Low-Calorie Diet: A Randomized Blinded Trial of the Efficacy and Tolerability of Subutramine. *Am J Med.* 1999;7:189–198.

35. Foreyt JP, Poston WS II. The Role of the Behavioral Counselor in Obesity Treatment. *J Am Diet Assoc.* 1998;98:S27–S30.

36. Perri MG, Nezu AM, Pattie ET, McCann KL. Effect of Length of Treatment on Weight Loss. *J Consult Clin Psychol.* 1989;57:450–452.

37. Tate DF, Wing RR, Winett RA. Using Internet Technology to Deliver a Behavioral Weight Loss Program. *JAMA.* 2001;285;1172–1177.

5

Assessment and Management of Depression in Cardiac Rehabilitation Patients

Krista A. Barbour, PhD

CONTENTS

PREVALENCE OF DEPRESSION IN CARDIAC PATIENTS

The relationship between depression and coronary heart disease (CHD) is well documented *(1)*. Relative to the primary care setting, in which the prevalence is 5–9% *(2)*, depression is highly prevalent in cardiac patients, with estimates ranging from 15 to more than 40% *(3)*. Less is known about the prevalence of depression in patients enrolled in cardiac rehabilitation (CR) programs, but a recent study of patients entering a phase II program found that approximately 26% of patients met diagnostic criteria for a depressive disorder *(4)*.

PROGNOSTIC VALUE OF DEPRESSION IN CHD

Significant evidence exists identifying depression as a powerful and independent risk factor for cardiac outcomes [for a review, see *(3)*], including cardiovascular events [e.g., recurrent myocardial infarction (MI)] *(5)* and mortality *(6)*.

Given the association between depression and cardiac outcomes and the desire to improve the quality of life of depressed patients, assessment of psychological functioning is an essential part of CR programs. Indeed, routine screening for depression has been recommended by the Board of the American Association of Cardiovascular

From: *Contemporary Cardiology: Cardiac Rehabilitation*
Edited by: W. E. Kraus and S. J. Keteyian © Humana Press Inc., Totowa, NJ

and Pulmonary Rehabilitation *(7)*. In the following sections, depression will be defined and commonly utilized methods for assessing depression will be described.

DEFINITIONS OF DEPRESSION

Definitions of "depression" vary from a patient's endorsement of a few key symptoms (e.g., sadness and tearfulness) to that of a clinical diagnosis, such as major depressive disorder (MDD), which is based upon well-defined diagnostic criteria. The diagnostic criteria for MDD, taken from the Diagnostic and Statistical Manual of Mental Disorders-fourth edition *(8)*, are summarized in Table 1.

Although CR patients who meet criteria for MDD merit particular attention by CR staff, it has been shown that even the presence of depressive symptoms that are sub-threshold for MDD also confers increased risk of mortality *(6)*. Thus, it is important to screen all patients entering CR programs.

ASSESSMENT OF DEPRESSION IN THE CARDIAC REHABILITATION SETTING

The gold standard for assessment of mood disorders is a structured diagnostic interview administered by a trained mental health professional. The result of such an interview would be a determination of whether MDD is present. However, such an assessment in most CR settings is impractical and probably not necessary, given the importance of sub-threshold depressive symptoms in relation to patients' quality of life and cardiovascular prognosis. Thus, CR staff need tools designed to quickly screen for degree of depressive symptoms. On the basis of the results of such depression measures, staff can then make decisions about intervention and, if necessary, referral to the appropriate mental health professional.

Table 1
Summary of DSM-IV Diagnostic Criteria for Major Depressive Episode

Five (or more) of the following symptoms are present during the same 2-week period and represent a change from previous functioning [note: at least one of the symptoms has to be either (1) or (2) below]

1 Depressed mood most of the day, nearly every day
2 Diminished interest or pleasure in all or most activities
3 Significant change in weight or appetite
4 Insomnia or hypersomnia
5 Psychomotor agitation or retardation
6 Fatigue or loss of energy
7 Feelings of worthlessness or guilt
8 Diminished ability to think or concentrate
9 Recurrent thoughts of death or suicide

The symptoms cause clinically significant distress or impairment, are not due to the effects of a substance or general medical condition, and are not better accounted for by bereavement or other psychiatric disorder.

Many self-report measures are available to assess the severity of depressive symptoms. These questionnaires generally consist of a series of written questions with multiple-choice responses that patients complete on their own. Widely used examples include the Beck Depression Inventory (BDI) *(9)*, the Center for Epidemiological Studies Depression Scale (CES-D) *(10)*, and the Hospital Depression and Anxiety Scale (HADS) *(11)*. These measures, administered when patients begin participation in CR, provide a picture of the type and severity of depressive symptoms. Staff should pay special attention to responses to items that inquire about suicidal ideation and hopelessness. Patients who endorse such items should be carefully monitored and the appropriate care provider consulted (e.g., the patient's cardiologist or primary care provider).

It is important to remember that self-report questionnaires are not designed to allow for the identification of MDD and are not a substitute for diagnostic clinical interviews. Instead, these screening questionnaires allow CR staff to triage each case and develop a plan at the time of enrollment (i.e., one patient's depressive symptoms may be mild enough to manage within the CR setting, whereas another patient may benefit from referral to a mental health provider for further evaluation of mood). Often, it is not practical for a mental health specialist to assist in the interpretation of these questionnaires; so, specific screening questions have been developed for use by primary care physicians. For example, the Primary Care Evaluation of Mental Disorders (PRIME-MD) is an assessment procedure intended to detect psychiatric disorders in primary care patients *(12)*. Two specific questions from the PRIME-MD may be especially useful in identifying patients who may need to be further evaluated for MDD *(13)* and are included in the Feature Box.

PRIME-MD Depression Screening Questions

During the past month, have you been bothered by

- little interest or pleasure in doing things,
- feeling down, depressed, or hopeless?

Note: A positive screen is indicated if either question is answered with "yes."

MANAGING DEPRESSION IN CR

For depressed patients who are considered appropriate to enter CR (e.g., they are not suicidal, and their depression is not so severe as to prevent active participation), the question arises as to how to manage depressive symptoms that may affect the course of CR participation and adherence. Some common symptoms of depression, such as fatigue and loss of interest in people and activities, may interfere with adherence to CR. In fact, depression is related to lack of adherence to treatment regimens in general *(14)* and CR specifically. For example, results of several studies of depressed patients enrolled in CR programs have demonstrated that depression at program entry is predictive of number of sessions attended as well as drop out *(15,16)*. Thus, identifying and monitoring patients with depression is crucial in the CR setting. These patients may require continued efforts by staff to keep them engaged in the program (see Table 2 for a list of strategies to promote adherence in patients enrolled in exercise programs).

Table 2
Strategies for Enhancing Exercise Adherence in Cardiac Rehabilitation

- Most important, work to establish good rapport with patients. Positive feedback and attention from rehabilitation staff can go a long way toward promoting adherence. (This may be especially true for patients who are depressed.)
- As part of the orientation to cardiac rehabilitation, review with patients their personal barriers to participation (e.g., child care responsibilities and transportation issues). Once barriers have been identified, staff may problem solve with patients about ways to overcome or minimize these obstacles.
- Educate patients about the health and mood benefits of exercise. Elicit from and remind patients of their personal reasons for exercising.
- Many patients benefit from the social support that comes with being involved in cardiac rehabilitation. Interaction with other individuals who are experiencing similar health problems can help to keep patients motivated.
- Patients are more likely to adhere to exercise training if the experience is an enjoyable one. Work with patients to increase their satisfaction with the program (e.g., switching equipment used and increased interaction with other patients).
- Assist patients in the development of realistic exercise goals (e.g., gradual increase in exercise time).
- Encourage patients to reward themselves for participation in exercise. Positive reinforcement for exercise is very important. Even simple rewards (e.g., purchasing a new book or CD) can be powerful motivators.
- Re-establish contact with patients as soon as possible following a cardiac event or hospitalization. Early intervention is crucial in getting patients back on track.
- As much as possible, engage patients' family members. They are often a valuable resource in offering encouragement for patients' participation in exercise.
- Remember that untreated depression is likely to reduce adherence to exercise. Encourage patients to seek treatment for depression if relevant.

TREATMENT OF DEPRESSION IN CARDIAC PATIENTS

In their recent review of psychosocial risk factors in CHD, Rozanski and colleagues *(17)* recommend a stepped care plan of intervention when managing psychologically distressed patients in clinical practice. In this approach, the level of intervention depends on the severity of distress. For example, a patient experiencing a moderate degree of depression may be monitored more closely by staff (e.g., more frequent telephone contact and efforts to enhance motivation and adherence), whereas a patient with more severe depression would be referred to a mental health professional.

Sometimes, a patient's level of depressive symptoms appears to interfere with his/her participation in CR, and it is felt that referral for more intensive intervention is needed. The following section reviews treatments that have been demonstrated to improve depression in cardiac patients.

Pharmacological

One large randomized clinical trial (RCT) *(18)* has been conducted to evaluate the safety and efficacy of the antidepressant medication sertraline in depressed patients with MI or unstable angina. In this trial, 369 patients were randomized to receive either sertraline or placebo for 24 weeks. It was found that sertraline was safe for use in this population, but the medication resulted in only modest improvement in depression. Despite this small effect in the overall study sample, analyses including only those patients with recurrent MDD or severe MDD demonstrated that sertraline was consistently superior to placebo. Thus, it appears that this medication may be a viable treatment option for this subset of depressed cardiac patients.

Evidence-Based Psychological Treatments

Several empirically supported psychological interventions exist for treatment of depression in noncardiac samples. However, only one of these, cognitive behavioral therapy (CBT), has been tested in an RCT of CHD patients diagnosed with MDD *(19)*. In this multi-center trial, 2481 post-MI patients with depression and/or low social support were randomized to the CBT intervention or usual care. CBT was delivered in both individual and group format and was focused on teaching patients about the relationships among thoughts, behavior, and emotion (with the rationale that the modification of thoughts and behaviors can result in an improvement in depression), as well as training in assertive communication. Results indicated that patients in the CBT intervention experienced a significant improvement in depression relative to the usual care group.

Other psychosocial interventions (e.g., stress management) targeting depressive symptoms (not documented MDD) in CHD patients have had mixed results in terms of symptom reduction *(20)*. In sum, evidence suggests that psychological treatment is effective in improving depression in CHD patients.

Several studies have also assessed the degree to which psychological treatments for depression affect health outcomes (e.g., recurrent cardiac events and mortality). The data are mixed in terms of the benefit of these interventions for cardiac outcomes. For example, in the trial of CBT for CHD patients described above, the intervention group did not differ from the usual care group in cardiac outcomes *(19)*. It has been suggested that the failure to affect cardiac prognosis in some studies is due to the modest improvement demonstrated in (or failure to modify) depression scores *(21)*. Additional well-designed RCTs are needed to determine the effect of well-conducted and effective psychological treatment interventions on cardiac outcomes.

Exercise

Exercise training is an integral part of CR programs. In addition to the cardiovascular benefits of aerobic exercise, there has been a growing literature on the psychological benefits of regular exercise. Specifically, evidence exists supporting the value of exercise in reducing depressive symptoms in both healthy and clinical populations *(22)*.

In a community sample of noncardiac patients, exercise was compared to antidepressant medication in the treatment of MDD *(23)*. Patients were randomized to supervised exercise, an antidepressant medication (sertraline), or a combination of exercise and medication. The 16-week exercise treatment consisted of three weekly sessions of aerobic activity. By the end of the treatment period, each of the three treatment groups experienced a significant reduction in depression. The treatments did not differ significantly from one another in efficacy. At 6 months post-treatment *(24)*, it was found that patients assigned to exercise alone endorsed lower rates of depression than did those receiving medication or a combination of exercise and medication. In addition, only 9% of remitted participants in the exercise group relapsed compared with more than 30% of participants in the medication and combination groups. It was also found that 64% of participants who received the exercise treatment continued to exercise following completion of the program. Self-reported exercise among all participants was associated with a 50% reduction in risk of depression 6 months after study completion. These results suggest that aerobic exercise may be a viable alternative to medication in the treatment of MDD.

Several studies have examined the effect of exercise training on depression in cardiac populations. In general, results of these studies indicate significant improvements in depressive symptoms upon completion of exercise training *(22)*. For example, in a sample of over 300 patients enrolled in CR after suffering a cardiac event, 20% of patients reported elevated depressive symptoms. At the end of the 3-month aerobic exercise training period, two-thirds of the initially depressed patients reported resolution of their depressive symptoms. Additionally, the depressed group demonstrated significant improvements in other quality-of-life variables *(25)*. However, it is not clear how much of this improvement can be specifically attributable to the exercise component of the program. Taken together, these results suggest that exercise training ameliorates depressive symptoms in both noncardiac and cardiac populations.

SUMMARY AND FUTURE DIRECTIONS

In sum, depression is quite common in patients with CHD and is a significant risk factor for cardiac outcomes. Patients should be screened for depression at entry to CR programs, using either a few verbal screening questions or a standardized depression questionnaire. Depressed patients enrolled in CR programs will require more attention to insure continued adherence and close monitoring to rapidly intervene should depressive symptoms worsen. Several treatments have shown some success in treating depression in cardiac patients, including antidepressant medication (sertraline), psychological interventions (such as CBT), and exercise training. Patients who endorse significant depressive symptoms should be approached in an empathic manner and encouraged to seek treatment to improve quality of life and cardiac outcomes. (It is often helpful to normalize the experience and treatment of depression when speaking with CHD patients. Patients can be educated regarding the prevalence of depressive symptoms in CHD patients as well as the association between mood and cardiac outcomes.)

Depression in CR

- Important to screen for depression, using an interview or survey tool.
- There are several potential treatment options for individuals who endorse depressed mood.
    CBT under the guidance of a trained professional.
    Antidepressant medications.
    Exercise therapy as a part of CR.
- Extra efforts to monitor and maintain involvement of such patients is optimal.

In future research, more attention should be paid to uncovering the mechanisms of the depression-cardiac outcome relationship. For example, as described earlier, depression also is a predictor of nonadherence, and it is possible that nonadherence accounts for the observed relationship. In addition, many of the studies that have examined treatment of depression in cardiac patients have methodological flaws (e.g., small sample sizes and no control group). Thus, more well-designed depression intervention trials with cardiac patients are needed.

Finally, most of what is known about the relationship between depression and cardiac prognosis has been largely derived from studies in men only (6). It will be important for future clinical trials to focus on women as well as ethnic minorities, who also have been underrepresented in this research. Such studies will inform treatments for depression that are tailored to subgroups of CHD patients.

REFERENCES

1. Wulsin LR, Singal BM. Do Depressive Symptoms Increase the Risk for the Onset of Coronary Disease? A Systematic Quantitative Review. *Psychosom Med.* 2003;65:201–210.
2. Depression Guidelines Panel. Depression in Primary Care: Detection and Diagnosis: Clinical Practice Guideline. Washington, DC: US Department of Health and Human Services, Public Health Service, Agency for Health Care Policy and Research; 1993. AHCPR 93-0550.
3. Lett HS, Blumenthal JA, Babyak MA, Sherwood A, Strauman T, Robins C, Newman MF. Depression as a Risk Factor for Coronary Artery Disease: Evidence, Mechanisms, and Treatment. *Psychosom Med.* 2004;66:305–315.
4. Todaro JF, Shen B, Niaura R, Tilkemeier PL. Prevalence of Depressive Disorders in Men and Women Enrolled in Cardiac Rehabilitation. *J Cardiopulm Rehabil.* 2005;25:71–75.
5. van Melle JP, De Jonge P, Spijkerman TA, Tussen JGP, Ormel J, van Veldhuisen DJ, van den Brink RHS, van den Berg MP. Prognostic Association of Depression Following Myocardial Infarction with Mortality and Cardiovascular Events: A Meta-Analysis. *Psychosom Med.* 2004;66:814–822.
6. Barth J, Schumacher M, Herrmann-Lingen C. Depression as a Risk Factor for Mortality in Patients with Coronary Heart Disease: A Meta-Analysis. *Psychosom Med.* 2004;66:802–813.
7. Herridge ML, Stimler CE, Southard DR, King ML; AACVPR Task Force. Depression Screening in Cardiac Rehabilitation: AACVPR Task Force Report. *J Cardiopulm Rehabil.* 2005;25:11–13.
8. American Psychiatric Association. *Diagnostic and Statistical Manual of Mental Disorders*, 4th ed. Washington, DC: American Psychiatric Association; 1994.
9. Beck AT, Steer RA, Brown GK. *Beck Depression Inventory*, 2nd ed. San Antonio, TX: The Psychological Corporation; 1996.
10. Radloff LS. The CES-D Scale: A Self-Report Depression Scale for Research in the General Population. *J Appl Psychol Meas.* 1977;1:385–401.
11. Zigmond A, Snaith R. The Hospital Anxiety and Depression Scale. *Acta Psychiatr Scand.* 1983;67:361–370.
12. Spitzer RL, Williams JBW, Kroenke K, et al. Utility of a New Procedure for Diagnosing Mental Disorders in Primary Care: The PRIME-MD 1000 Study. *JAMA.* 1994;272:1749–1756.
13. Whooley MA, Avins AL, Miranda J, Browner WS. Case-Finding Instruments for Depression. *J Gen Intern Med.* 1997;12:439–445.
14. DiMatteo MR, Lepper HS, Croghan TW. Depression is a Risk Factor for Noncompliance with Medical Treatment: Meta-Analysis of the Effects of Anxiety and Depression on Patient Adherence. *Arch Intern Med.* 2000;160:2101–2107.
15. Glazer KM, Emery CF, Frid DJ, Banyasz RE. Psychological Predictors of Adherence and Outcomes Among Patients in Cardiac Rehabilitation. *J Cardiopulm Rehabil.* 2002;22:40–46.

16. Turner SC, Bethell HJ, Evans JA, Goddard JR, Mullee MA. Patient Characteristics and Outcomes of Cardiac Rehabilitation. *J Cardiopulm Rehabil*. 2002;22:253–260.

17. Rozanski A, Blumenthal JA, Davidson KW, Saab PG, Kubzansky L. The Epidemiology, Pathophysiology, and Management of Psychosocial Risk Factors in Cardiac Practice: The Emerging Field of Behavioral Cardiology. *J Am Coll Cardiol*. 2005;45:637–651.

18. Glassman AH, O'Connor CM, Califf RM, Swedberg K, Schwartz P, Bigger JT Jr, et al. for the Sertraline Antidepressant Heart Attack Randomized Trial (SADHART) Group. Sertraline Treatment of Major Depression in Patients with Acute MI or Unstable Angina. *JAMA*. 2002;288:701–709.

19. Berkman LF, Blumenthal J, Burg M, Carney RM, Catellier D, Cowan MJ, et al. Enhancing Recovery in Coronary Heart Disease Patients Investigators (ENRICHD). Effects of Treating Depression and Low Perceived Social Support on Clinical Events After Myocardial Infarction: The Enhancing Recovery in Coronary Heart Disease Patients (ENRICHD) Randomized Trial. *JAMA*. 2003;289:3106–3116.

20. Lett HS, Davidson J, Blumenthal JA. Nonpharmacologic Treatments for Depression in Patients with Coronary Heart Disease. *Psychosom Med*. 2005;67:S58–S62.

21. Cossette S, Frasure-Smith N, Lesperance F. Clinical Implications of a Reduction in Psychological Distress on Cardiac Prognosis in Patients Participating in a Psychosocial Intervention Program. *Psychosom Med*. 2001;63:257–266.

22. Brosse AL, Sheets ES, Lett HS, Blumenthal JA. Exercise and the Treatment of Clinical Depression in Adults: Recent Findings and Future Directions. *Sports Med*. 2002;32:741–760.

23. Blumenthal JA, Babyak M, Moore K, Craighead WE, Herman S, Khatri P, Waugh R, Napolitano MA, Forman LM, Appelbaum M, Doraiswamy M, Krishnan KR. Effects of Exercise Training on Older Adults with Major Depression. *Arch Intern Med*. 1999;159:2349–2356.

24. Babyak M, Blumenthal JA, Herman S, Khatri P, Doraiswamy M, Moore K, Craighead WE, Baldewicz TT, Krishnan KR. Exercise Training for Major Depression: Maintenance of Therapeutic Benefit at 10 Months. *Psychosom Med*. 2000;62:633–638.

25. Milani RV, Lavie CJ, Cassidy MM. Effects of Cardiac Rehabilitation and Exercise Training Programs on Depression in Patients After Major Coronary Events. *Am Heart J*. 1996;132:726–732.

6

Managing Stress to Manage Heart Disease

Ruth Q. Wolever, PhD

CONTENTS

BACKGROUND ON THE PSYCHOSOCIAL RISK FACTORS

Five psychosocial risk factors have been consistently linked with the development of heart disease and worse prognosis for those with the disease *(1,2)*: depression, anxiety, social isolation, hostility, and unmanaged stress. Leaders in the field of behavioral cardiology group these psychosocial risk factors into emotional factors (depression, anxiety, anger, or hostility) and chronic stressors (including low social support, low socioeconomic status, work stress, marital stress, and caregiver strain) *(3)*. Others describe the psychosocial factors as stressors themselves *(4)*. However, all agree that they are important in managing cardiovascular disease because they contribute to both the pathogenesis of heart disease and its aggravation by mechanisms independent from those of traditional risk factors *(2)*. The specific roles of depression and anxiety in heart disease are discussed elsewhere in this text, while the significance of hostility and social support are important to mention before delving further into the role of stress.

From: *Contemporary Cardiology: Cardiac Rehabilitation*
Edited by: W. E. Kraus and S. J. Keteyian © Humana Press Inc., Totowa, NJ

The Five Major Psychosocial Risk Factors

Emotional Factors

- Depression
- Anxiety
- Hostility

Chronic Stressors

- Social isolation
- Unmanaged stress

ROLE OF THE TYPE A BEHAVIORAL PROFILE AND HOSTILITY

Since 1959, researchers have studied a series of behaviors that led a 1978 independent panel for the National Institutes of Health to conclude that this cluster of behaviors [termed the "Type A behavioral profile" (TABP)] was an independent risk factor for the development of heart disease (5). The TABP centered around an individual's struggle to achieve or accomplish more and more in less and less time, often in the face of perceived opposition from other people. Prospective studies of incidence showed that otherwise healthy people with this profile were roughly twice as likely to develop some manifestation of heart disease (6,7). However, risk ratios as high as 7.9 were reported for specific groups and circumscribed outcomes: 10-year incidence of myocardial infarction in white collar men (8). Independent researchers also showed that the TABP was strongly associated with the degree of coronary artery blockage in patients (9,10). Researchers began to study the components of the profile separately following the publication of mixed findings on the predictive validity of the TABP in developing heart disease (11,12) as well as in recurrence of such (13–15). Although some of the controversy stemmed from differences in the difficult measurement of the TABP, particularly the interpersonal aspects (16,17), it also became clear that the TABP was not the seminal psychosocial risk factor. Three components have been described: a sense of time urgency (hurry sickness), free-floating hostility, and intense competitiveness.

Researchers at Duke surmised that *hostility and bottled-up anger* may have more damaging effects on the heart, and may increase circulating stress hormones that can have a long-term effect on the cardiovascular system (18). They, as well as other researchers, demonstrated that hostility is an even better predictor of heart disease than is the TABP (19,20). Although there have also been negative findings (21–23), the preponderance of work supports the predictive validity of hostility for heart disease incidence, morbidity and mortality (24,25). Additional work pointed out that hostility is a complex construct with cognitive, affective, and behavioral components. It appears that interactions in these components drive the hostility–heart disease relationship rather than the tendency to experience distressing emotions such as anger, resentment and suspicion (26–28). Moreover, although much of the research on Type A was conducted on White men, the research on hostility has been validated with a wider sociodemographic population and appears to be evident earlier in the disease process. Hostility measures have been linked to findings of subclinical atherosclerosis *(3,27)*.

LOW SOCIAL SUPPORT

The importance of social and emotional connection for both heart disease incidence and prognosis has been well-established for several decades *(1)*. Heart disease patients with lower levels of social connection are three to five times more likely to die prematurely *(29–32)*. In addition, social isolation has been shown to predict mortality in Type A men, whereas high levels of social support are related to lower levels of coronary artery disease *(33)*. Thus, strong social support appears to exert some protective influence over the potential long-term health consequences of the TABP. Many believe that social support is perhaps the most important psychosocial buffer of stress *(30,32)*, and others point to its direct role in heart disease *(1)*.

PSYCHOLOGICAL DISTRESS

One construct that may link the psychosocial risk factors has to do with the presence of *psychological distress*. Indeed research with cardiac patients in the laboratory *(34–36)* and natural environments *(37)* has indicated that mental and emotional stress can result in myocardial ischemia and is associated with a several fold increase in occurrence of subsequent fatal, and nonfatal, cardiac events *(38)*. Specifically, studies of stressful conditions (ranging from earthquakes to emotional stress in daily life) cite relative risks for myocardial infarction and acute cardiac death between 1.8 and 3.0, with an increase in mortality noted between 22 and 34%. Moreover, health researchers have shown that psychological stress can have a deleterious influence on an individual's health status and may also interfere with the performance of health behaviors. High perceived stress has been associated with increased alcohol consumption, smoking, reduced levels of exercise, poor nutritional habits, increased susceptibility to infectious disease processes, and shorter periods of sleep *(30,39,40)*. All of these factors can undermine healing in rehabilitation.

Although they may have separate pathophysiological mechanisms, even the emotional factors are clearly intertwined with the problem of stress. For example, hostility can result from, and lead to, increased interpersonal stress, exacerbating both the frequency and the intensity of the stress response. It is also well established that chronic levels of elevated stress set individuals up for development of depression *(39,41)*.

EFFICACY OF STRESS MANAGEMENT INTERVENTIONS

The robustness of psychosocial findings has led to multiple clinical trials examining the benefits of psychosocial intervention for heart patients. Methodologically, this intervention research is still in its infancy. Treatment of stress as a risk factor in cardiac rehabilitation is quite inconsistent. First, the delivery of stress management or other forms of psychological care is not a standardized part of cardiac rehabilitation *(3,36)*. Where it is standardized, the programs are heterogeneous and make it complex to study the efficacy of such interventions *(42,43)*. Many programs also address multiple psychosocial risk factors through the same modality, and others address one psychosocial risk factor (e.g., stress) through multiple modalities. Either way, it is difficult to discern efficacy for specific approaches for specific risk factors. Nonetheless, several reviews have been conducted to evaluate the efficacy of stress management programs as part of a multi-factorial cardiac rehabilitation program. Each meta-analysis has differed in its selection of studies and thus in its conclusions. Three reviews in the late 1990s demonstrated a positive impact on morbidity and mortality for myocardial infarction patients who participated in a psychological intervention *(43–45)*. The protective effect of the psychological intervention was shown for up to 2 years *(45)*. A Cochrane review was then completed in 2005 using more systematic methodology. Randomized, controlled trials published by December 2001 of adults with coronary heart disease that had at least six months follow-up were included. Of the 36 trials that met such criteria, 18 were identified as having a stress management component (versus other psychological intervention). The authors concluded that there was a reduction in nonfatal re-infarctions in the eight trials reporting this outcome, but no strong evidence was found for an effect on total mortality (based on ten trials), on cardiac mortality (using four trials), or for revascularization (in seven trials) *(46)*. The authors point out that the trials were generally poor in quality and extremely heterogeneous, that the two largest trials had null effects even for nonfatal re-infarction, and that there was statistical evidence of publication bias. Small reductions in anxiety and depression were noted for stress management interventions considered separately *(46)*.

Other reviews demonstrate that the equivocal findings in outcome studies can be explained by the fact that studies which failed to reduce distress also failed to reduce mortality or event recurrence *(42)*. Still others question the potential role of the intensity of relaxation training. For example, in a review of 27 controlled trials, with the exception of reduction in heart rate, outcome effects were small, absent, or not measured when abbreviated relaxation therapy was offered (3 hours or less of instruction). However, when ≥ 9 hours of supervised relaxation training and discussion were provided, improvements were seen in physiological measures (resting heart rate, heart rate variability, exercise tolerance, and high-density lipoprotein cholesterol), psychological outcomes (reduction in state anxiety and depression), cardiac indicators (reduction in angina frequency, arrhythmia occurrence, and exercise-induced ischemia), recurrent cardiac events, and cardiac death *(47)*.

As the greatest impact is seen for those whose distress is reduced, a resource-limited facility should consider stratifying patients based on self-perception of distress. Further support for the use of a patient-centered screening instrument for distress is offered in a study of 26 rehabilitation programs in Germany. Slightly higher predictions for effectiveness in rehabilitation are found when patients' self-assessments of stress are utilized in planning psychosocial interventions and care versus predefined goals, a practice which reportedly is uncommon *(48)*.

KEY COMPONENTS TO STRESS MANAGEMENT

The biggest challenges in providing patients with adequate stress management skills are (i) convincing them of the importance, (ii) providing adequate training and opportunities for guided practice in regulating physiological stress reactivity, and (iii) providing training in shifting perceptions and beliefs to encourage continued stress management and healthy behaviors after the acute crisis passes.

ENGAGING THE PATIENT

Many patients fail to understand the physical impact of stress and its role in heart disease. Patients must be able to link their personal experiences of stress with the physiological mechanisms of heart disease to give stress management credibility and encourage the significant amount of behavioral attention needed to consistently alter stress. Robert Sapolsky's *(39)* theory of stress and heart disease provides an excellent basis to teach patients the rationale for stress management in a tangible and easily understandable way. It may be helpful to explain that we have nearly identical bodies to those of our ancestors 10,000 years ago from the perspective of the autonomic nervous system; yet, our societies are totally different. When faced with a predator, our ancestors needed to physically escape for survival, to either fight or flee (hence the term "fight or flight" response). Patients can easily understand that survival outweighs the body's need for day-to-day functioning when a physical threat is encountered. They gain significant insight when told that despite our physical bodies being quite similar to those of our ancestors, we live in a dramatically different society. When you ask patients what they find stressful, they can begin to understand how grossly different today's stressors are from physical predators; our stressors are more psychological or cognitive in nature rather than physical. When the stressful event is physical in nature, as well as infrequent and time-limited, the sympathetic nervous system response thus provides survival. Once the crisis passes, day-to-day functioning of the body should again become paramount, and the activity of the parasympathetic nervous system governing this increases, generating the "relaxation response" *(49)*. In our current society, however, the stress response is constantly and automatically triggered without adequate engagement of the relaxation response. This process can actually create heart disease or worsen it.

To make this process personally meaningful, it is helpful to have patients imagine that the stressor they face is not an actual predator, but rather being stuck in traffic. The process is, of course, complicated by multiple lifestyle factors and genetics, but the take-home message is the same. It is helpful to teach patients that the impact of repeatedly generating the stress response without allowing the body to recuperate adequately is toxic. When the blood pressure response is chronically triggered *(39,50)*, the smooth inner lining of the arteries becomes damaged throughout the body, particularly at points where one artery branches into two arteries. Whereas the damage is microscopic, the tearing of the lining allows for the accumulation of fatty acids, released into blood for energy, to work their way under the lining and begin to thicken the arterial walls. Elevated levels of blood sugar contribute to the "thickening" process as well by providing starches to the formation of these fatty deposits (called plaques). Add in a high-fat diet and the formation of plaques are amplified. In addition, platelets are released as a function of the stress response *(38)*. In the absence of physical activity (e.g., one is sitting in a car), the clumping together of circulating platelets furthers the disease process by adding to the deposits forming at the tears. It is instructive to explain that even the immune system, which is less functional during times of chronic stress, contributes to the process through the role of inflammation, although the mechanisms for this are just now being studied *(51)*.

The key for patients is to link their personal experiences of the stress response with heart disease. When talking with patients about sources of stress, know that women have significantly different sources from men *(52,53)* and appear to be at even higher risk for psychosocial distress particularly following cardiac hospitalization *(53,54)*. In fact, effective delivery of psychological services necessitates distinct attention to gender differences in perception of stress and outcomes *(42,54)*. All patients, however, must understand that they now have the power to directly impact heart disease by how they choose to cope with stress. For the above example, point out that when sitting in a car, the patient can choose to smoke to relieve tension or to practice deep breathing to lower the stress response. The former choice will further weaken the lining of the vessels and lower "good" cholesterol that will undermine the body's attempt to rid itself of bad cholesterol. The latter will induce the relaxation response. Similarly, the patient can choose to drive through McDonalds and take in a Big Mac and fries or choose to talk to a friend or journal to get a better perspective. The former choice will increase the fatty acids circulating in the blood that can worsen plaque. The latter choice can enhance the immune system. As one more option, point out that after parking the car, the patient can choose to drink a six-pack to take the edge off the worry or frustration or choose to exercise. The former choice can eventually raise blood pressure, whereas the latter will subsequently trigger the relaxation response. Remind them that when our ancestors "fought" or "fled" from stressors, they naturally performed exercise that our industrial, ever-efficient society makes easy to avoid (e.g., we drive rather than walk, use electronic devices to perform manual labor, etc.). Explain that *choices* in how to cope with stress tend to relate to lifestyle. Nutrition and exercise are thoroughly covered in other chapters of this text.

To reiterate the bottom line, we can count on our bodies and minds to trigger the stress response in reaction to multiple stimuli. On the contrary, because our environments are so demanding in terms of sensory stimuli, the parasympathetic system's "relaxation and recuperation response" will not be automatically triggered; it must be consciously generated.

STRESS MANAGEMENT

Although there are multiple models of stress management *(42,55)* beyond the scope of this chapter, there are two aspects that are central for cardiac rehabilitation patients: (i) the regular elicitation of the relaxation response and (ii) learning to shift perceptions and beliefs that tend to increase the frequency of the stress response and undermine healthy behavior patterns. It is helpful for patients to understand that they must create the relaxation response on a daily basis. The metaphor of a cup is useful, with the liquid in the cup representing one's stress level. If the cup is full, any small drop causes overflow. That small drop may be another driver behaving erratically, a child asserting autonomy, or a spouse who has not picked up the laundry. If the level of stress in the cup is lower, the "drops" can be handled with greater flexibility and thoughtful choice. As "overflowing" undermines health, it is imperative to have multiple ways to lower the cup on a daily basis. First, it is important for patients to understand that ample and safe exercise, healthy nutrition, and adequate sleep are important ways to "lower the cup." Next, it is important to teach them multiple ways to generate the relaxation response.

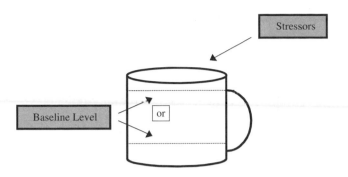

TECHNIQUES FOR ELICITING THE RELAXATION RESPONSE

There are various techniques that evoke the relaxation response. Although several are more evidence-based than others, the most effective technique for a given patient is the one that he/she will use repeatedly. As all active relaxation techniques alter sympathetic activity, decrease oxygen consumption, reduce respiration rate, and lower heart rate and blood pressure, many believe that no single technique is superior to another (56). As more sophisticated methodology emerges to clearly specify the micro-mechanisms behind the relaxation response, we may find that certain approaches are better for certain conditions. Transcendental meditation, for example, has been claimed to be superior to relaxation techniques for the reduction of trait anxiety, and an excellent case is made for its use with heart disease patients (57). At this point in the science, however, it appears that the selection of a specific relaxation technique to practice is less important than the fact that it gets practiced routinely. In fact, one review of cardiac rehabilitation programs that taught stress management noted that those programs that included a minimum number of 9 hours of relaxation training provided the strongest impact on well-being as well as health indices (47). Provision of training for only 3 hours was only minimally effective.

Skills to train patients on the generation of the relaxation response include breathwork, progressive muscle relaxation (PMR), various forms of meditation, and self-hypnosis. Breathwork is perhaps the easiest and shortest way to help patients experience the relaxation response. First, patients can easily understand the behavioral rationale-once they understand that the breath, unlike most body systems, is under both voluntary and involuntary control. As respiration is closely connected to heart rate, they can actually drop their heart rates by slowing the breathing rate. This, in turn, will lower blood pressure and subsequently alter the body's automatic cascade of stress hormones. Second, learning breathing techniques can help give patients back a sense of control. Loss of control of one's own body is a salient part of cardiac events and continues to be a significant driver of stress after the event. By utilizing proper breathing techniques, one can learn to down-regulate the sympathetic nervous system and regain a sense of control. Third, simple techniques such as diaphragmatic breathing and the 4-7-8 breath are straightforward and easy to teach (58). They are best offered as an immediate tool and as an introduction to learning more intensive techniques. Such simple breathing techniques alone, however, are necessary, but not sufficient, because they are rarely practiced consistently for sufficient time periods on a daily basis. Clinical experience suggests that 20 minutes of practice one to two times per day is needed, although no empirical work is available to support this common recommendation.

Most patients experience deep breathing as a pleasant state, although the more tightly wound Type A patient may find it uncomfortable to slow down and focus on breathing until the skill is mastered. Such patients tend to initially downplay the importance of breathwork and may feel awkward learning breathing skills when they believe that breathing should be automatic. It is important to underline that in the hectic pace of life, slow and deep breathing is not automatic, and learning to breathe in a way that triggers the relaxation response is essential.

A somewhat longer, and highly useful approach to achieve the relaxation response is PMR. Originated by Edmund Jacobson and later abbreviated by Wolpe and others, PMR is the most common relaxation technique used in the peer-reviewed stress management literature. PMR is a systematic tensing and releasing of 16 large muscle groups. While attending to a specific muscle group, muscles are tensed for a brief period (5–7 seconds) and then released/relaxed for 30 seconds. With practice, one initially learns to combine the active tensing and releasing of the 16 muscle groups down to four, thus allowing the experience of total body relaxation in a relatively short time. Later training allows one to passively reach the same state of relaxation through the use of the mind rather than active use of the muscles (59). This skill is easily learned and utilized to reduce the general level of sympathetic arousal but does take consistent practice and training time. Forty minutes of practice per day is originally recommended, and this gradually reduces to about 20 minutes at least once per day after 4–6 weeks of training. Stress management research to date indicates that PMR demonstrates the strongest impact on physiologic outcome variables. PMR has been shown to reduce hypertension, reduce chronic pain in various medical conditions, and help manage mood states of anxiety and depression (60).

A third practice that induces rest and recuperation response is meditation. Although there are many forms of meditation, there are several forms that have received the greatest degree of attention from medical researchers: transcendental meditation, Benson's respiratory one meditation, and mindfulness meditation. Although the psychophysiological mechanisms of meditation are currently under intense study and there are some equivocal findings, most agree that meditation reduces oxygen consumption, decreases heart and respiration rates, diminishes blood lactate levels, elevates mood states, improves immune functioning, changes brain wave activity, and improves hormone levels (60). Furthermore, unlike other relaxation practices, regular meditation practice has been found to lead to positive behavior change outside of the meditative state (60,61) that is extremely useful for cardiac rehabilitation participants.

Methods of Inducing the Relaxation Response

- Breathwork.
- PMR.
- Meditation.
- Hypnosis and self-hypnosis.
- Guided imagery.

Breathwork, PMR, some types of meditation (not mindfulness), and hypnosis are easily and commonly augmented by the use of guided imagery, a technique whereby individuals use their "mind's eye" to visualize a place of comfort, relaxation, safety, and serenity that they remember. By accessing all of the senses associated with that memory, individuals re-experience relaxation, thus reducing sympathetic nervous system arousal. Although it has not been specifically studied with cardiac patients, the benefits of imagery have been shown in treatment of various disorders including headaches, breast cancer, diabetes, skin ailments, arthritis and severe burns *(60)*.

One other approach that has been unequivocally shown to deepen the relaxation state is hypnosis/self-hypnosis *(62)*. Although not well studied in cardiac patients, the effectiveness of hypnosis has been demonstrated in the treatment of multiple medical conditions presumably through its ability to engage the relaxation response. Such conditions include angina, hypertension, migraine, insomnia, chronic pain, duodenal ulcers, irritable bowel syndrome, and nausea associated with chemotherapy and pregnancy *(55)*.

Thus, breathwork, PMR, meditation, guided imagery, and self-hypnosis are all valuable tools for eliciting the relaxation response. The key for patients is daily practice of such techniques. Understanding the interests and abilities of patients is central to help them choose the best way to engage the relaxation response.

SHIFTING PERCEPTIONS AND BELIEFS

The stress response is triggered when one perceives a threat or challenge to goals or well-being. Thus, individuals may avoid or lessen a stress response by learning to interpret stimuli and events differently. Even more importantly, individuals can learn to decrease stress from internal sources (e.g., thoughts and beliefs) that are often outside of awareness and perpetuated unknowingly. The human mind constantly provides a "running commentary" on life, full of judgments and reviews of our environment, behaviors, feelings, sensations and thoughts. For example, "I have to remember to call my sister. I cannot believe that guy is driving so crazily. I wonder what Bill learned in his review. Oh, cute shoes." Interestingly, the running commentary can perpetuate unhealthy perceptual patterns unless they are brought into conscious awareness. Meditation, mentioned above as a way to engage the relaxation response, is an excellent tool to use to bring this running commentary into awareness. Once in awareness, the automatic thoughts can be reworked, shifting habitual ways of thought.

One significant driving force behind the running commentary is belief systems, most of which are also out of awareness. People assign meaning to perceived stimuli based on their beliefs. In other words, patients' beliefs set the stage for perception and inter-pretation of events in the world; thoughts then determine how stressful a situation is perceived to be. Is the driver "out to get you" or "distracted by his/her own worries?" Is the slow-moving line due to "some incompetent clerk who doesn't appreciate your time" or "a new learner with a first job trying to better him/herself?" (D. Ulmer, personal communication, December 1995) who was seminal in the Recurrent Coronary Prevention Project *(63)* described the impact of a common belief for people with a TABP: "My worth is dependent on how much and how well I accomplish." Such a belief can set up a negatively reinforcing cycle that leads individuals to set unrealisti-cally high goals, feel pressured, move at a highly rapid pace, experience and express frustration at common setbacks, and ultimately emotionally isolate themselves in the pursuit of achievements. When emotional connection is lacking, individuals with this belief do not gain a sense of self-worth from interpersonal relationships, from a feeling of being loved, or even a recognition of character traits. So, they default to the compensatory belief that their worth stems from achievements, thus further ingraining both the belief system and the behavior patterns *(64)*.

Beliefs that can significantly increase stress or undermine healthy behavior patterns for cardiac patients

- Failure is a sign of weakness.
- If I make a mistake, something bad will happen.
- I must be better than everyone else to be good enough.
- I must take care of everyone else before I take care of myself.
- I must be liked by everyone.
- I must do everything perfectly.
- I must be rational and in control at all times.
- I can only depend on myself.

The good news is that training in cognitive reframing techniques helps individuals recognize how their perceptions, thoughts, and beliefs influence their appraisal of situations and ultimately their behavior. Through cognitive reframing or restructuring, individuals learn to reinterpret situations in a manner that reduces stress. Over time, they can reframe the ways they habitually perceive things as well as reformulate general belief systems. The steps to changing automatic thoughts are actually simple, but sticking to them is much more difficult than it sounds. There is a large body of research on this process, and these steps are clearly effective if practiced over time. Furthermore, the impact of beliefs on health and happiness has been well documented *(65–68)*. The more environmental and social support one has in this process, the easier it will be. The steps are to

- Recognize automatic thoughts and appraisals.
- Challenge them from a truly curious, rather than judgmental, perspective, noticing the impact of the interpretation on stress levels and subsequent behavior.
- Consider possible alternative appraisals, whether they are believed. Discuss them with an objective, trusted person who is willing to point out other perspectives (e.g., a mentor, coach, or therapist).
- Weigh the evidence for each alternative and imagine the impact of that alternative interpretation.
- Choose a realistic alternative that would lead to lower stress.
- Repeat it over and over. The more the environment and others support the new alternative perception or belief, the easier it will be to ingrain the new idea.
- Apply the new appraisal in multiple situations, looking for evidence that it may be true.
- Over time, notice that the mind offers the new appraisal automatically.

CONCLUSIONS

Psychosocial risk factors have been consistently linked to the pathogenesis of heart disease and prognosis. Unmanaged stress is one of these factors and plays a significant role in the others. Although the efficacy research on stress management in cardiac rehabilitation is fraught with methodological issues, it appears that psychological interventions that are successful in reducing distress are also successful in reducing morbidity and mortality. Key components for providing adequate stress management interventions include engaging patients through linking the process of heart disease to their own experiences, helping them to understand the power they have in slowing or reversing the process through the choices they make in coping responses, providing adequate training and opportunities for guided practice in generating the relaxation response, and teaching patients to shift perceptions and beliefs that tend to increase stress and undermine healthy coping.

REFERENCES

1. Hemingway H, Marmot M. Evidence Based Cardiology: Psychosocial Factors in the Aetiology and Prognosis of Coronary Heart Disease. Systematic Review of Prospective Cohort Studies. *BMJ*. 1999;318:1460–1467.
2. Shen BJ, Wachowiak PS, Brooks LG. Psychosocial Factors and Assessment in Cardiac Rehabilitation. *Eura Medicophys*. 2005;41:75–91.
3. Rozanski A, Blumenthal JA, Davidson KW, Saab PG, Kubzansky L. The Epidemiology, Pathophysiology, and Management of Psychosocial Risk Factors in Cardiac Practice: The Emerging Field of Behavioral Cardiology. *J Am Coll Cardiol*. 2005;45:637–651.
4. Pickering T, Clemow L, Davidson K, Gerin W. Behavioral Cardiology Has Its Time Finally Arrived? *Mt Sinai J Med*. 2003;70:101–112.
5. Coronary-Prone Behavior and Coronary Heart Disease: A Critical Review. The Review Panel on Coronary-Prone Behavior and Coronary Heart Disease. *Circulation*. 1981;63:1199–1215.
6. Rosenman RH, Brand RJ, Jenkins D, Friedman M, Straus R, Wurm M. Coronary Heart Disease in Western Collaborative Group Study. Final Follow-Up Experience of 8 1/2 Years. *JAMA*. 1975;233:872–877.
7. Haynes SG, Feinleib M, Kannel WB. The Relationship of Psychosocial Factors to Coronary Heart Disease in the Framingham Study. III. Eight-Year Incidence of Coronary Heart Disease. *Am J Epidemiol*. 1980;111:37–58.
8. Haynes SG, Feinleib M. Type A Behavior and the Incidence of Coronary Heart Disease in the Framingham Heart Study. *Adv Cardiol*. 1982;29:85–94.
9. Blumenthal JA, Williams RB Jr, Kong Y, Schanberg SM, Thompson LW. Type A Behavior Pattern and Coronary Atherosclerosis. *Circulation*. 1978;58:634–639.
10. Frank KA, Heller SS, Kornfeld DS, Sporn AA, Weiss MB. Type A Behavior Pattern and Coronary Angiographic Findings. *JAMA*. 1978;240:761–763.
11. Shekelle RB, Hulley SB, Neaton JD, Billings JH, Borhani NO, Gerace TA, Jacobs DR, Lasser NL, Mittlemark MB, Stamler J. The MRFIT Behavior Pattern Study. II. Type A Behavior and Incidence of Coronary Heart Disease. *Am J Epidemiol*. 1985;122:559–570.
12. Ragland DR, Brand RJ. Type A Behavior and Mortality from Coronary Heart Disease. *N Engl J Med*. 1988;318:65–69.
13. Jenkins CD, Zyzanski SJ, Rosenman RH. Risk of New Myocardial Infarction in Middle-Aged Men with Manifest Coronary Heart Disease. *Circulation*. 1976;53:342–347.
14. Dimsdale JE, Gilbert J, Hutter AM Jr, Hackett TP, Block PC. Predicting Cardiac Morbidity Based on Risk Factors and Coronary Angiographic Findings. *Am J Cardiol*. 1981;47:73–76.
15. Haynes S, Matthews K. Review and Methodologic Critique of Recent Studies on Type A Behavior and Cardiovascular Disease. *Ann Behav Med*. 1988;10:47–59.

16. Booth-Kewley S, Friedman HS. Psychological Predictors of Heart Disease: A Quantitative Review. *Psychol Bull.* 1987;101:343–362.
17. Miller TQ, Turner CW, Tindale RS, Posavac EJ, Dugoni BL. Reasons for the Trend Toward Null Findings in Research on Type A Behavior. *Psychol Bull.* 1991;110:469–485.
18. Williams RB Jr, Haney TL, Lee KL, Kong YH, Blumenthal JA, Whalen RE. Type A Behavior, Hostility, and Coronary Atherosclerosis. *Psychosom Med.* 1980;42:539–549.
19. Barefoot JC, Dahlstrom WG, Williams RB Jr. Hostility CHD Incidence, and Total Mortality: A 25-Year Follow-Up Study of 255 Physicians. *Psychosom Med.* 1983;45:59–63.
20. Shekelle RB, Gale M, Ostfeld AM, Paul O. Hostility, Risk of Coronary Heart Disease, and Mortality. *Psychosom Med.* 1983;45:109–114.
21. Helmer DC, Ragland DR, Syme SL. Hostility and Coronary Artery Disease. *Am J Epidemiol.* 1991;133:112–122.
22. McCranie EW, Watkins LO, Brandsma JM, Sisson BD. Hostility, Coronary Heart Disease (CHD) Incidence, and Total Mortality: Lack of Association in a 25-Year Follow-Up Study of 478 Physicians. *J Behav Med.* 1986;9:119–125.
23. Hearn MD, Murray DM, Luepker RV. Hostility, Coronary Heart Disease, and Total Mortality: a 33-Year Follow-Up Study of University Students. *J Behav Med.* 1989;12:105–121.
24. Matthews KA. Coronary Heart Disease and Type A Behaviors: Update on and Alternative to the Booth-Kewley and Friedman (1987) Quantitative Review. *Psychol Bull.* 1988;104:373–380.
25. Miller TQ, Smith TW, Turner CW, Guijarro ML, Hallet AJ. A Meta-Analytic Review of Research on Hostility and Physical Health. *Psychol Bull.* 1996;119:322–348.
26. Dembroski TM, MacDougall JM, Williams RB, Haney TL, Blumenthal JA. Components of Type A, Hostility, and Anger-In: Relationship to Angiographic Findings. *Psychosom Med.* 1985;47:219–233.
27. Julkunen J, Salonen R, Kaplan GA, Chesney MA, Salonen JT. Hostility and the Progression of Carotid Atherosclerosis. *Psychosom Med.* 1994;56:519–525.
28. Suarez EC, Williams RB Jr. Situational Determinants of Cardiovascular and Emotional Reactivity in High and Low Hostile Men. *Psychosom Med.* 1989;51:404–418.
29. Berkman LF, Syme SL. Social Networks, Host Resistance, and Mortality: A Nine-Year Follow-Up Study of Alameda County Residents. *Am J Epidemiol.* 1979;109:186–204.
30. Cohen S, Wills TA. Stress, Social Support, and the Buffering Hypothesis. *Psychol Bull.* 1985;98:310–357.
31. Orth-Gomer K, Unden AL. Type A Behavior, Social Support, and Coronary Risk: Interaction and Significance for Mortality in Cardiac Patients. *Psychosom Med.* 1990;52:59–72.
32. Ornish D. *Love & Survival: The Scientific Basis for the Healing Power of Intimacy*, 1st ed. New York: HarperCollins; 1998.
33. Blumenthal JA, Burg MM, Barefoot J, Williams RB, Haney T, Zimet G. Social Support, Type A Behavior, and Coronary Artery Disease. *Psychosom Med.* 1987;49:331–340.
34. Jiang W, Babyak M, Krantz DS, Waugh RA, Coleman RE, Hanson MM, Frid DJ, McNulty S, Morris JJ, O'Connor CM, Blumenthal JA. Mental Stress-Induced Myocardial Ischemia and Cardiac Events. *JAMA.* 1996;275:1651–1656.
35. Krantz DS, Quigley JF, O'Callahan M. Mental Stress as a Trigger of Acute Cardiac Events: The Role of Laboratory Studies. *Ital Heart J.* 2001;2:895–899.
36. Pashkow FJ. Is Stress Linked to Heart Disease? The Evidence Grows Stronger. *Cleve Clin J Med.* 1999;66:75–77.
37. Gullette EC, Blumenthal JA, Babyak M, Jiang W, Waugh RA, Frid DJ, O'Connor CM, Morris JJ, Krantz DS. Effects of Mental Stress on Myocardial Ischemia During Daily Life. *JAMA.* 1997;277:1521–1526.
38. Stalnikowicz R, Tsafrir A. Acute Psychosocial Stress and Cardiovascular Events. *Am J Emerg Med.* 2002;20:488–491.

39. Sapolsky RM. *Why Zebras Don't Get Ulcers : An Updated Guide to Stress, Stress-Related Diseases, and Coping*. New York: W.H. Freeman and Co.; 1998.

40. Hafen BQ. *Mind/Body Health : The Effects of Attitudes, Emotions, and Relationships*. Boston: Allyn and Bacon; 1996.

41. Gold PW, Goodwin FK, Chrousos GP. Clinical and Biochemical Manifestations of Depression. Relation to the Neurobiology of Stress (2). *N Engl J Med*. 1988;319:413–420

42. Linden W. Psychological Treatments in Cardiac Rehabilitation: Review of Rationales and Outcomes. *J Psychosom Res*. 2000;48:443–454.

43. Dusseldorp E, van Elderen T, Maes S, Meulman J, Kraaij V. A Meta-Analysis of Psychoeducational Programs for Coronary Heart Disease Patients. *Health Psychol*. 1999;18:506–519.

44. Jones DA, West RR. Psychological Rehabilitation After Myocardial Infarction: Multicentre Randomised Controlled Trial. *BMJ*. 1996;313:1517–1521.

45. Linden W, Stossel C, Maurice J. Psychosocial Interventions for Patients with Coronary Artery Disease: A Meta-Analysis. *Arch Intern Med*. 1996;156:745–752.

46. Rees K, Bennett P, West R, Davey SG, Ebrahim S. Psychological Interventions for Coronary Heart Disease. *Cochrane Database Syst Rev*. 2004;CD002902.

47. van Dixhoorn J, White A. Relaxation Therapy for Rehabilitation and Prevention in Ischaemic Heart Disease: A Systematic Review and Meta-Analysis. *Eur J Cardiovasc Prev Rehabil*. 2005;12:193–202.

48. Farin E, Follert P, Jackel WH. [Therapy Goal Setting in Patients with Psychological Stress in Orthopaedic and Cardiac Rehabilitation]. *Rehabilitation (Stuttg)*. 2002;41:389–400.

49. Benson H. *The Relaxation Response*. New York: Morrow; 1975.

50. Carels RA, Sherwood A, Blumenthal JA. Psychosocial Influences on Blood Pressure During Daily Life. *Int J Psychophysiol*. 1998;28:117–129.

51. Wilson EM, Diwan A, Spinale FG, Mann DL. Duality of Innate Stress Responses in Cardiac Injury, Repair, and Remodeling. *J Mol Cell Cardiol*. 2004;37:801–811.

52. Buchner B, Kleiber C, Stanske B, Herrmann-Lingen C. [Stress and Heart Disease in Women]. *Herz*. 2005;30:416–428; quiz 429–430.

53. Davidson PM, Daly J, Hancock K, Moser D, Chang E, Cockburn J. Perceptions and Experiences of Heart Disease: A Literature Review and Identification of a Research Agenda in Older Women. *Eur J Cardiovasc Nurs*. 2003;2:255–264.

54. Abbey SE, Stewart DE. Gender and Psychosomatic Aspects of Ischemic Heart Disease. *J Psychosom Res*. 2000;48:417–423.

55. Quillian-Wolever RE, Wolever ME. Stress Management at Work. In *Handbook of Occupational Health Psychology*, JC Quick and LE Tetrick (eds.). Washington, DC: Americal Psychological Association; 2003;355–375.

56. Benson H, Klipper M. *The Relaxation Response*. New York: Avon Books; 1975.

57. King MS, Carr T, D'Cruz C. Transcendental Meditation, Hypertension and Heart Disease. *Aust Fam Physician*. 2002;31:164–168.

58. Weil A. Week Four; Week Five. In *8 Weeks to Optimum Health*. New York: Random House; 1997, 108, 122.

59. Bernstein DA, Borkovec TD, Hazlett-Stevens H. *New Directions in Progressive Relaxation Training: A Guidebook for Helping Professionals*. Westport, CT: Praeger; 2000.

60. Freeman L. Relaxation Therapy. In *Mosby's Complementary & Alternative Medicine: A Research-Based Approach*, L. Freeman and G. Lawlis (eds.). St. Louis, MO: Mosby; 2001: xxiv, 532.

61. Kabat-Zinn J. University of Massachusetts Medical Center/Worcester. Stress Reduction Clinic. *Full Catastrophe Living : Using the Wisdom of Your Body and Mind to Face Stress, Pain, and Illness*. New York: Delacorte Press; 1990.

62. Lichstein KL. *Clinical Relaxation Strategies* (Wiley Series on Personality Processes). New York: Wiley; 1988.

63. Mendes de Leon CF, Powell LH, Kaplan BH. Change in Coronary-Prone Behaviors in the Recurrent Coronary Prevention Project. *Psychosom Med.* 1991;53:407–419.
64. Ulmer D. *Personal Communication from the Clinical Institute of Behavioral Medicine*, R. Wolever (ed.). Berkeley, CA; 1996.
65. Beck A, Rush J, Shaw B, Emory G. *Cognitive Therapy of Depression.* New York: Guilford Press; 1979.
66. Ellis A, Harper RA. *A New Guide to Rational Living.* Englewood Cliffs, NJ: Prentice-Hall; 1975.
67. Burns D. *The Feeling Good Handbook.* New York, NY: Plume Book; 1989.
68. Seligman MEP. *Learned Optimism.* New York: A.A. Knopf; 1991.

7 Use of Readiness for Change in Cardiac Rehabilitation Programs

Charlotte A. Collins, Meghan L. Butryn, and Ernestine G. Jennings

Contents

Cardiovascular disease constitutes the major cause of morbidity and mortality in industrialized nations. Because multiple health behaviors influence the cardiovascular system and making changes to long-term lifestyle patterns are difficult, effective behavior change interventions are an essential part of the cardiac rehabilitation (CR) program, which employs a comprehensive approach to cardiovascular disease risk factor modification *(1)*. CR programs actively use behavioral approaches to increase patient participation and adherence in sustainable behavior change efforts. Most patients come to CR after a major cardiovascular health crisis with the need to address multiple modifiable behavioral risk factors, such as physical inactivity, active smoking history, poor dietary habits, excessive weight, and stress. In addition, patients may need to control other medical conditions that affect cardiovascular health, such as hypertension and diabetes, that are in turn a consequence of poor behavioral choices. However, helping patients adhere to treatment and make all the necessary lifestyle changes remains a continuing challenge for healthcare professionals in the clinical setting in general and the CR setting in particular. Most health care providers recognize that it is not enough to simply mention the need for change in the clinic environment. Approaches

From: *Contemporary Cardiology: Cardiac Rehabilitation*
Edited by: W. E. Kraus and S. J. Keteyian © Humana Press Inc., Totowa, NJ

to initiate, achieve, and sustain effective behavior change based on the Transtheoretical Model of Intentional Behavior Change (TTM) *(2)* and Motivational Interviewing (MI) *(3)* techniques are emerging as promising alternatives to more traditional behavior change approaches.

TRANSTHEORETICAL MODEL OF BEHAVIOR CHANGE

At the heart of the TTM is the assertion that behavior change is an incremental process that involves specific and varied tasks *(2)*. The model was first developed to address smoking cessation and maintenance using psychotherapeutic approaches. It has subsequently and effectively been applied to a broad array of behavioral issues *(4)*. The TTM defines the change process as a progression through five stages of change: precontemplation, contemplation, preparation, action, and maintenance *(2,4–6)*. In the first stage, precontemplation, individuals are highly ambivalent about changing their behavior and do not intend to take action toward behavior change in the next 6 months. In the contemplative stage, individuals recognize that a problem exists and seriously about their behavior; however, they are not yet committed. Individuals in the preparation stage are convinced that the advantages of change outweigh the disadvantages and are ready to act within the next 30 days. In the action stage, individuals are successfully altering a behavior for a period of time anywhere between 1 day and 6 months *(7)*. After 6 months of sustained change, individuals progress to the maintenance stage. The TTM also recognizes that relapse is possible, even likely, when moving through these five stages (relapse).

Stages of Change (TTM)
• Precontemplation.
• Contemplation.
• Preparation.
• Action.
• Maintenance.
• Relapse.

The TTM offers an integrative framework for understanding the change process, whether in the initiation, modification, or cessation phase. The change stages provide a paradigm in which to view the change process, allowing clinicians to understand the progression, use motivational strategies to facilitate movement through the stages toward sustainable change, and plan interventions with their patients addressing the myriad of interactions of behavior changes which are a necessary part of a successful CR program. The stages of change are a component of the TTM model that has played an integral role in the development of interventions for behavior change using a motivational approach *(8–10)*.

MOTIVATIONAL INTERVIEWING

MI is a client-centered, directive method for enhancing intrinsic motivation to change by exploring and resolving ambivalence *(3)*. MI provides important tools to promote health behavior change. Recognizing how motivated a patient is to change a behavior allows the clinician to address patient goals and barriers to change. Health care providers can use the principles of MI to increase motivation, moving the patient through the change process without reinforcing resistance or disagreement. The technique has been shown to have positive effects on treatment retention and adherence in several areas of health behavior change *(11)*.

MI is a counseling style that was developed as an alternative to more traditional treatment methods which tend to use more direct persuasion *(12)*. It involves a partnership between client and provider that honors the client's perspective and own areas of expertise. The practitioner provides an atmosphere that is conducive rather than coercive to change, as can be the case with prescriptive advice *(3)*. This perspective differs from traditional treatment paradigms that view provider–patient disagreement as a "state of denial" on the part of the patient. MI views provider–patient disagreement as an opportunity to address ambivalence through eliciting and selectively reinforcing "change talk," thereby moving the person toward change. In this approach, the resources and motivation for change are presumed to reside within the client. In contrast to advice giving and traditional behavior change counseling, the MI practitioner strategically uses the client's own responses to elicit and reinforce talk directed toward change. The "spirit" of the interaction can be likened to a dance, wherein the practitioner leads a delicately balanced collaborative effort *(3)*.

This client-centered approach focuses on an individual's present interests and concerns. Specifically, MI interactions focus on increasing motivation by using an empathic style to reduce resistance, develop discrepancy, and support the patient *(13)*. The counselor actively explores patient barriers and provides a structure for change. The principles underlying MI help to translate the spirit of the approach into behavioral strategies that guide the practitioner. The first principle in MI is *expressing empathy*, which is demonstrated through active listening techniques. Empathic exchanges can often prevent resistance from developing. The second principle, *developing discrepancy*, involves understanding and amplifying differences between the patient's current behavior and his/her goals, values, and self-image *(3)*. The practitioner's objective is to tip the balance in the direction of change. The third principle is *responding to resistance*. Resistance is seen as the signal to change strategies rather than to push the patient harder as in more confrontational approaches. The final principle, *supporting self-efficacy*, refers to the belief that the patient is the ultimate decision maker. The practitioner acknowledges that the client has the ability to make the change using his own resources.

Principles in MI

- Expressing empathy.
- Developing discrepancy.
- Responding to resistance.
- Supporting self-efficacy.

Health care settings, such as CR, represent an important channel for delivering MI, as health care providers can capitalize on the "teachable moment" during which patients may be more receptive to modifying behaviors *(14)*. Assessing motivation for change allows the provider to choose stage-appropriate interventions and develop a collaborative relationship with the patient. Discussing a patient's ambivalence allows the clinician to explore barriers to treatment and work with the patient to develop an effective treatment plan for behavior change. Additionally, reinforcing "change talk" during intervention facilitates development of strategies that can help maintain change.

MI has been tested with several health behaviors in the context of health promotion *(15)*. Although MI appears to perform best when used as a prelude to more intensive substance abuse treatment, it has been shown to be effective in the area of treatment adherence, diet and exercise change, HIV-risk reduction, and other health-promoting behaviors *(11,16,17)*. Treatment retention and adherence significantly improve when MI is added to interventions, and these improvements may be responsible for other positive outcomes. If MI is offered as a stand-alone intervention, long-term effects may need to be enhanced by booster sessions or stepped care. When it is used as a prelude to treatment, however, its effects appear to endure across time, suggesting a synergistic result of MI and other treatment procedures *(17)*. Even very brief (5–10 min) intervention models have been used successfully to address specific health behaviors such as smoking cessation and dietary changes *(18,19)*. These newer approaches, such as behavior change counseling, incorporate the TTM and principles of MI in an effort to increase motivation for change in 5–30-min interventions and are designed for use by various health care providers *(10)*.

EFFECTIVENESS OF MOTIVATION-BASED APPROACHES FOR CR

Few studies have examined the effectiveness of MI or stages-of-change approaches with CR patients, but those that have been conducted demonstrate promising results. For instance, patients enrolled in a standard, 12-week outpatient CR program, who also participated in three brief sessions of MI, significantly increased their physical activity scores from pre- to post-treatment, and the proportion of participants who were very inactive decreased from 43 to 11% *(20)*. Although these results indicate that participants made substantial improvement, without a control group it is difficult to determine what value was added specifically by the MI component of treatment.

Several studies that used randomized designs with CR patients provide additional evidence that motivation-based approaches promote behavior change superior to that produced by standard treatment. In one study, which demonstrates the effectiveness of MI for initial behavior change, CR patients who were randomly assigned to participate in MI in combination with standard treatment had greater improvements at post-treatment in self-reported stress, physical activity, and dietary fat intake than those who received standard treatment alone *(21)*. A second study indicates the success of MI in the maintenance of behavior change. Patients who had successfully completed 11 weeks of CR were then randomly assigned to participate in a 30-min session based on the TTM. After 4 weeks, those who participated in the MI session showed significantly greater increases in their self-reported leisure physical activity than those who did not participate *(22)*. A third study, conducted with cardiac patients who had chronic heart failure, randomly assigned participants to three groups: traditional exercise, MI, or a combination of the two interventions. At post-treatment, those who received MI alone or in combination with the exercise program reported greater increases than exercise-only participants in the level and type of activities in which they were engaged, and patients in all three conditions increased the distance covered in a 6-min walk test *(23)*. These preliminary studies demonstrate that MI and approaches based on the TTM have the potential to result in outcomes that are superior to those achieved with standard CR, particularly with regard to physical activity.

EFFECTIVENESS OF MOTIVATION-BASED APPROACHES WITH OTHER POPULATIONS

Additional research needs to be conducted with CR patients to more clearly define the capabilities of MI or stages-of-change interventions. Until more data are collected, the field can be guided by preliminary research that has been conducted on the effectiveness of these approaches in promoting behavior change with groups similar to those targeted in CR. Such studies include those that use these approaches to target multiple cardiac risk factors, physical activity, or dietary change in populations other than CR, such as in primary or secondary prevention programs addressing cardiovascular disease risk. The findings from these studies have implications for reducing disease risk in the CR population.

USE OF MI IN REDUCING CARDIAC RISK FACTORS

Motivation-based approaches have been examined as a tool for promoting lifestyle change in patients at elevated cardiovascular risk. In a randomized controlled trial conducted with patients at increased risk of coronary heart disease, stages-of-change intervention participants received between three and five individual sessions and telephone calls aimed at reducing smoking, decreasing fat intake, and increasing physical activity *(24)*. At 4- and 12-month follow-up, greater reductions in number of cigarettes smoked per day and dietary fat intake and greater increases in physical activity were reported by intervention participants than control participants. Systolic blood pressure for intervention participants declined more at post-treatment than for control participants. However, there were no differences between groups at follow-up in diastolic blood pressure, total serum cholesterol, or body mass index (BMI).

In another study aimed at lifestyle change, hypertensive patients were randomly assigned to treatment as usual (usual care) or MI provided in either (i) six sessions or (ii) one session and five phone calls. At post-intervention, the six-session MI participants had greater decreases in blood pressure and weight than those who received usual care, and the one-session MI participants had greater decreases in salt and alcohol intake relative to those who received usual care *(25)*. However, a study that used a similar design, conducted with patients who had hypertension, type 2 diabetes, or coronary artery disease, found that at post-intervention and at follow-up 6 months later, change in blood pressure, fat intake, serum cholesterol, and BMI did not significantly differ between groups *(26,27)*. Taken together, these studies suggest that, although MI and stages-of-change approaches can promote behavior change in patients at elevated cardiovascular risk, it is difficult to produce change in biological markers.

USE OF MI IN PHYSICAL ACTIVITY PROMOTION

Other interventions have specifically targeted physical activity with MI or stages-of-change approaches and have shown promising results. In one intervention conducted at an urban general medical practice, intervention participants who received either one session or six sessions of MI reported greater increases in physical activity at post-treatment than controls, but differences were not maintained at 1-year follow up *(28)*. Studies also have targeted physical activity in diabetic patients. In one study, diabetic participants who received a 3-month stage-matched intervention reported greater improvement in physical activity level at post-treatment than participants who received standard education about physical activity *(29)*. In another study, diabetic participants who received one session of exercise consultation based on the TTM had greater increases in physical activity at 5 weeks, as measured by accelerometers, than those who received standard education about physical activity *(30)*.

Additional stages-of-change interventions for physical activity promotion conducted with print-based media have consistently found that MI or stages-of-change approaches can promote initial increases in physical activity, but evidence regarding maintenance of these changes is mixed *(31,32)*.

USE OF MI IN PROMOTING DIETARY CHANGE

Changes in dietary intake, another common target of change for CR patients, might also be promoted with motivation-based approaches. Some research has examined dietary change in patients at elevated cardiovascular risk. In one study, patients with hyperlipidemia who were randomly assigned to a three-session, bimonthly MI dietary intervention had significant reductions at post-treatment in consumption of total fat and saturated fat, energy intake, and BMI. However, these changes were not significantly different from those observed in participants who received standard dietary care. Serum cholesterol did not significantly change in either group *(33)*, although this may be due more to the lack of the effectiveness of the intervention to change cholesterol in the study population than to the failure of adopting the promoted behavior itself. In another study, patients with elevated cholesterol, a high-fat diet, and a diagnosis of diabetes or hypertension who received stage-matched counseling from a physician and dietician over a period of 6 months were twice as likely as participants who received usual care to be in a post-preparation stage for dietary change at post-treatment *(34)*. Fat intake was significantly lower in the intervention group than in the usual care group at 6 months but not at 12 months.

Other research has examined dietary change in participants with particular demographic characteristics. A study found that providing adolescent participants who had elevated low-density lipoprotein levels with two MI sessions resulted in a significant reduction in calories from fat and dietary cholesterol and advanced their stage of change at post-treatment; however, no control group was available for comparison *(35)*. A study conducted with African-American adults found that participants randomly assigned to receive self-help materials and three telephone sessions of MI for dietary change over the course of 1 year increased their self-reported fruit and vegetable intake at post-treatment more than those who received only self-help or standard education materials *(36)*. Finally, a study conducted with post-menopausal females found that those who received three sessions of MI in addition to a standard dietary intervention reduced fat consumption more than those who received standard treatment alone *(37)*. The literature on motivation-based approaches for dietary intake suggests that such interventions could be useful for changing eating behaviors in CR patients.

CONCLUSIONS AND FUTURE DIRECTIONS

Interventions involving MI and stages of change models have potential to provide substantial benefits to individuals with cardiovascular disease. MI offers providers a tool to enhance motivation toward behavior change, particularly with patients who are identified as lacking commitment or ability to change. The evidence that MI is most effective with those individuals less ready to change *(15)* only increases the potential benefits. And, although MI may require training and more time than traditional approaches, it allows for targeted interventions that may prove time and energy efficient.

The use of MI in CR settings presents unique challenges. First and foremost, intervention with MI may need to involve multiple members of a patient's health care team. In fact, MI may be most advantageous when used to get patients to CR following an acute coronary syndrome event. Therefore, determining which health care providers can effectively deliver these interventions and how much training is necessary will be important. Furthermore, patients in CR may not be interested in behavior changes that are targeted by the staff or may prioritize the changes differently. This situation may lead to frustration by staff members who are interested in measurements of improvement over the course of treatment. Additionally, some behavior changes such as increasing exercise is actually a complex of different behaviors with significant external influences, only some of which can be addressed in a CR setting. Finally, given the natural time restraints and multiple responsibilities of the members of CR staff, MI may not be seen as the most efficient approach to eliciting behavior changes by members of the CR team. However, newer interventions that are targeted and brief have the potential to overcome prioritization discrepancies and time restraints *(10)*.

One open question is which of the many potential possible behavior targets of any given patient should be addressed first. Clearly, it might be overwhelming to a CR patient to address smoking cessation, dietary modification, a physically inactive lifestyle, and excessive psychological stress all at the same time, while the patient is struggling to recover from a life changing event. Thus, should the provider address the behavior for which the patient is further along the continuum of the stages of change or the one with the greatest perceived health risk to the patient (e.g., smoking)? This issue would be a fruitful line for further investigation.

MI and stages-of-change approaches clearly have the potential to improve outcomes for CR patients *(38)*. The available research indicates that when added to standard CR, these interventions can promote changes in physical activity, diet, and stress levels *(21)*, although it is not yet apparent how well these changes can be maintained. Research on health behavior change with other populations provides additional support for the use of MI and stages-of-change approaches in CR. When these approaches are used to target multiple lifestyle factors in populations at increased cardiovascular risk, they can prompt changes in physical activity and dietary intake, but they are less effective at modifying biological markers of risk, such as cholesterol, blood pressure, and BMI.

Physical activity and dietary intake have each been successfully targeted with these approaches in other special populations (e.g., those with diabetes), but evidence is again mixed about the effectiveness of these approaches over longer periods of time.

Future research is necessary in several essential areas. More studies need to examine the effectiveness of MI and stages-of-change approaches in producing both initial behavior change and maintenance of behavior change for CR patients. Initial issues include the fact that few measurements of stages of change have been validated and specific stage-based interventions have not been extensively evaluated *(39)*. Furthermore, randomized controlled trials with large samples and longer follow-up periods will be particularly valuable, as will studies that use objective measures of outcome such as attendance rates, medication adherence, accelerometer data, and 6-min walk test performance. Dose–response research should be conducted to determine how intensive these interventions must be to evoke behavior and biological marker change. In this literature, there is great variability in the number and length of intervention sessions, as well as whether time is spent in session on other intervention components, but no clear dose–response effect has emerged. Order of addressing specific behaviors, as noted above, is a potentially important issue for further work. Future researchers in this area should take care to clearly describe such details about the interventions they deliver. It also will be useful to determine whether there are characteristics that identify patients who most benefit from these interventions.

Increasing attention to the value of CR in recovery from acute coronary events and the need to demonstrate improved health outcomes of CR patients create an opportunity for new approaches to promote behavior change. Studies offer preliminary evidence that MI and the TTM may prove useful in attracting patients to CR, improving attendance while enrolled in CR, and increasing health behavior changes during and after CR. Additionally, MI interventions may result in improved provider–patient relationships and consumer satisfaction, which is an underdeveloped and potentially powerful selling point to providers and health care agencies *(40)*. As in other areas of behavioral health, the use of MI and the TTM in CR settings continues to increase, although the development of specific interventions is still in the early phases. Despite many proponents of these approaches, until further research delineates the effectiveness for specific behaviors and in specific settings, it is not clear whether MI and TTM interventions will become the standard of care in CR.

REFERENCES

1. American Association of Cardiovascular and Pulmonary Rehabilitation. *Guidelines for Cardiac Rehabilitation and Secondary Prevention Programs*, 4th ed. Champaigne, IL: Human Kinetics; 2004.
2. Prochaska J, DiClemente C. Stages and Processes of Self-Change for Smoking: Toward an Integrative Model of Change. *J Consult Clin Psychol.* 1983;51:390–395.
3. Miller W, Rollnick S. *Motivational Interviewing: Preparing People for Change*, 2nd ed. New York: Guilford Press; 2002.
4. Prochaska J, Velicer W, Rossi J, et al. Stages of Change and Decisional Balance for 12 Problem Behaviors. *Health Psychol.* 1994;13:39–46.
5. DiClimente C, Prochaska J. Processes and Stages of Change: Coping and Competence in Smoking Behavior Change. In *Coping and Substance Abuse*, S. Shiffman and T. Wills (eds.). New York: Academic Press; 1985:319–342.

6. DiClimente C, Prochaska J. Toward a Comprehensive, Transtheoretical Model of Change: Stages of Change and Addictive Behaviors. In *Treating Addictive Behaviors*, 2nd ed., W. Miller and N. Heather (eds.). New York: Plenum Press; 1998:3–24.

7. Weinstein N, Rothman A, Sutton S. Stage Theories of Health Behavior: Conceptual and Methodological Issues. *Health Psychol.* 1998;17:290–299.

8. DiClemente C. Motivation for Change: Implications for Substance Abuse. *Psychol Sci.* 1999;10:209–213.

9. Miller W, Rollnick S. *Motivational Interviewing: Preparing People for Change.* New York: Guilford Press; 1991.

10. Rollnick S, Mason P, Butler C. *Health Behavior Change: A Guide for Practitioners.* London: Churchill Livingstone; 1999.

11. Burke B, Arkowitz H, Menchola M. The efficacy of Motivational Interviewing: A Meta-Analysis of Controlled Clinical Trials. *J Consul Clin Psychol.* 2003;71:841–861.

12. Rollnick S, Butler C, Stott, N. Helping Smokers Make Decisions: The Enhancement of Brief Intervention for General Medical Practice. *Patient Educ Couns.* 1997;31:191–203.

13. Rollnick S, Miller W. What is Motivational Interviewing? *Behav Cogn Psychother.* 1995;23:325–334.

14. Rigotti N. Efficacy of Smoking Cessation Program for Hospital Patients. *Arch Intern Med.* 1997;157:2653–2660.

15. Miller W. Enhancing Patient Motivation for Health Behavior Change. *J Cardiopulm Rehabil.* 2005;25:207–209.

16. Dunn C, Deroo L, Rivara F. The Use of Brief Interventions Adapted from Motivational Interviewing Across Behavioral Domains: A Systematic Review. *Addiction.* 2001:96:1725–1742.

17. Hattema J, Steele J, Miller W. Motivational Interviewing. *Annu Rev Clin Psychol.* 2005;1:91–111.

18. Ockene J, Quirk M, Goldberg R, et al. A Residents Training Program for the Development of Smoking Intervention Skills. *Arch Intern Med.* 1988;148:1039–1045.

19. Rosal M, Ebbeling C, Lopgren I, Ockene J, Ockene I, Hebert J. Facilitating Dietary Change: The Patient-Centered Counseling Model. *J Am Diet Assoc.* 2001;101:332–341.

20. Scales R, Akalan C, Miller JH, Lueker RD. Can a Health Educator Improve Physical Activity with Motivational Counseling in a Clinical Setting? *Med Sci Sports Exerc.* 2003;35:S144.

21. Scales R, Atterbom HA, Lueker RD. Impact of Motivational Interviewing and Skills-Based Counseling on Physical Activity and Exercise. *Med Sci Sports Exerc.* 1998;30:S92.

22. Hughes AR, Gillies F, Kirk AF, Mutrie N, Hillis WS, MacIntyre PD. Exercise Consultation Improves Short-Term Adherence to Exercise During Phase IV Cardiac Rehabilition. *J Cardiopulm Rehabil.* 2002;22:421–425.

23. Brodie DA, Inoue A. Motivational Interviewing to Promote Physical Activity for People with Chronic Heart Failure. *J Adv Nurs.* 2005;50;518–527.

24. Steptoe A, Kerry S, Rink E, Hilton S. The Impact of Behavioral Counseling on Stage of Change in Fat Intake, Physical Activity, and Cigarette Smoking in Adults at Increased Risk of Coronary Heart Disease. *Am J Public Health.* 2001;91:265–269.

25. Woollard J, Beilin L, Lord T, Puddey I, MacAdam D, Rouse I. A Controlled Trial of Nurse Counseling on Lifestyle Change for Hypertensives Treated in General Practice: Preliminary Results. *Clin Exp Pharmacol Physiol.* 1995;22:466–468.

26. Woollard J, Burke V, Beilin LJ, Verheijden M, Bulsara MK. Effects of a General Practice-Based Intervention on Diet, Body Mass Index and Blood Lipids in Patients at Cardiovascular Risk. *J Cardiovasc Risk.* 2003;10:31–40.

27. Woollard J, Burke V, Beilin LJ. Effects of General Practice-Based Nurse-Counselling on Ambulatory Blood Pressure and Antihypertensive Drug Prescription in Patients at Increased Risk of Cardiovascular Disease. *J Hum Hypertens.* 2003;17:689–695.

28. Harland J, White M, Drinkwater C, Chinn D, Farr L, Howel D. The Newcastle Exercise Project: A Randomized Controlled Trial of Methods to Promote Physical Activity in Primary Care. *BMJ*. 1999;319:828–832.

29. Kim CJ, Hwang AR, Yoo JS. The Impact of Stage-Matched Intervention to Promote Exercise Behavior in Participants with Type 2 Diabetes. *Int J Nurs Stud*. 2004;41:833–841.

30. Kirk AF, Higgins LA, Hughes AR, Fisher BM, Mutrie N, Hillis S, MacIntyre PD. A Randomized Controlled Trial to Study the Effect of Exercise Consultation on the Promotion of Physical Activity in People with Type 2 Diabetes: A Pilot Study. *Diabet Med*. 2001;18:877–882.

31. Bock BC, Marcus, BH, Pinto BM, Forsyth LH. Maintenance of Physical Activity Following an Individualized Motivationally Tailored Intervention. *Ann Behav Med*. 2001;23:79–87.

32. Marshall AL, Bauman AE, Owen N, Booth ML, Crawford D, Marcus BH. Population-Based Randomized Controlled Trial of a State-Targeted Physical Activity Intervention. *Ann Behav Med*. 2003;25:194–202.

33. Ni Mhurchu C, Margetts BM, Speller V. Randomized Clinical Trial Comparing the Effectiveness of Two Dietary Interventions for Patients with Hyperlipidaemia. *Clin Sci*. 1998;95:478–487.

34. Verheijden MW, Van der Veen JE, Bakx JC, Akkermans RP, Van der Hoogen HJM, Van Staveren WA, Van Weel C. Stage-Matched Nutrition Guidance: Stages of Change and Fat Consumption in Dutch Patients at Elevated Cardiovascular Risk. *J Nutr Educ Behav*. 2004;36:228–237.

35. Berg-Smith SM, Stevens VJ, Brown KM, Van Horn L, Gernhofer N, Peters E, Greenberg R, Snetselaar L, Ahrens L, Smith K. A Brief Motivational Intervention to Improve Dietary Adherence in Adolescents. *Health Educ Res*. 1999;14:399–410.

36. Reniscow K, Jackson A, Wang T, De AK, McCarty F, Dudley WN, Baranowski TA. A Motivational Interviewing Intervention to Increase Fruit and Vegetable Intake Through Black Churches: Results of the Eat for Life Trial. *Am J Public Health*. 2001;91:1686–1693.

37. Bowen D, Ehret C, Pedersen M, Snetselaar L, Johnson M, Tinker L, Hollinger D, Lichty I, Bland K, Sivertsen D, Ocken D, Staats L, Beedoe JW. Results of an Adjunct Dietary Intervention Program in the Women's Health Intervention. *J Am Diet Assoc*. 2002;102:1631–1637.

38. Hancock K, Davidson P, Daly J, Webber D, Chang E. An Exploration of the Usefulness of Motivational Interviewing in Facilitating Secondary Prevention Gains in Cardiac Rehabilitation. *J Cardiopulm Rehabil*. 2005;25:200–206.

39. Adams J, White M. Why Don't Stage-Based Activity Promotion Interventions Work? *Health Educ Res*. 2005;20:237–243.

40. Prochaska J. Staging: A Revolution in Helping People Change. *Manag Care*. 2003;12(Suppl 9):6–9.

8 Smoking Cessation: The Prescription that Every Smoker Should be Given

Jennifer Davis, MS

CONTENTS

The burden that smoking places on health is easy to recognize. Cigarette smoking is the primary preventable cause of illness and death in the United States. Statistics are alarming, including the more than 400,000 deaths attributed to cigarette smoking per year *(1)*. Also a leading cause of cardiovascular morbidity and mortality, cigarette smoking accounts for approximately 115,000 heart disease-related deaths and 27,000 deaths in the United States from strokes each year *(2)*.

According to the US Surgeon General, smoking is the "most important of the known modifiable risk factors for CHD" *(3)*. Observational studies approximate that stopping smoking decreases the risk of "subsequent mortality and further cardiac events among patients with CHD by as much as 50%" *(4)*. Smoking cessation may have a more significant effect than any other intervention or treatment on reducing the risk of mortality in patients with coronary heart disease (CHD) who are smokers *(4)*. However, even though the benefits of smoking cessation are clear, physicians and other health care providers are not effectively addressing this problem. This is evident when considering that even though smoking cessation may be more effective at reducing cardiovascular morbidity and mortality, in recent years, it has not received as much attention as secondary preventive therapies, including lipid-lowering therapies. This may be due in part to the higher-time burden required by providers to address this problem, when compared to a pharmacological therapy. On the basis of the potential risk reduction, it is not only appropriate but essential

From: *Contemporary Cardiology: Cardiac Rehabilitation*
Edited by: W. E. Kraus and S. J. Keteyian © Humana Press Inc., Totowa, NJ

for physicians and health care providers to consider smoking cessation an important treatment to provide to patients who smoke.

This chapter will outline the epidemiology of cigarette smoking, the pathophysiology of smoking and heart disease, and treatment interventions and guidelines to assist health care providers in with smoking cessation in the cardiac rehabilitation setting.

EPIDEMIOLOGY OF SMOKING AND HEART DISEASE

Prevalence

An estimated 45 million Americans and at least 1.2 billion people worldwide use tobacco regularly *(5)*. This number remains astoundingly high despite the awareness of the dangers of cigarette smoking and the efforts made toward smoking cessation education and treatments. Table 1 *(6)* summarizes the prevalence of smoking within adults 18 years and older living in the United States.

PREVALENCE OF HEART DISEASE IN SMOKERS

Cigarette smoking increases the risk that an individual will develop several atherosclerotic syndromes. These include stable angina, acute coronary syndromes, sudden death, stroke, and aortic and peripheral atherosclerosis *(7)*. Cigarette smokers have a two to four times increased risk of developing heart disease *(8)*, double the risk of stroke *(9,10)*, and up to ten times the risk of developing peripheral vascular disease compared with nonsmokers *(11)*. Not only do smokers have an increased morbidity, they are also more likely to die years before nonsmokers *(12)*. Male smokers die an average of 13.2 years earlier than nonsmokers, and female smokers die an average of 14.5 years earlier than nonsmokers *(12)*.

Did You Know?

- Heavy smokers are not the only people at increased risk of CHD. Even light smokers are found to have increased risk of CHD. Research shows that women who smoked one to four cigarettes per day had a relative risk of 2.5 of fatal CHD *(13)*.
- Studies have also shown that passive smokers, or those exposed to second hand smoke, are at increased risk of cardiovascular morbidity and mortality *(14)*.

PATHOPHYSIOLOGY OF SMOKING AND HEART DISEASE

Owing to the complexity of over 4000 combined chemicals in a cigarette, it is impossible to suggest that the entire picture of how cigarette smoking leads to, or worsens, cardiovascular disease is understood. However, it is clear that inhaling tobacco smoke from cigarettes leads to several immediate and long-term physiologic changes in the body, specifically within the heart and blood vessels. These changes indirectly promote the atherosclerotic process throughout the arteries of the entire body including the heart, brain, and peripheral circulation. Therefore, heart disease, stroke, and peripheral artery disease are significantly increased by smoking.

Table 1

Prevalence of Smoking. Percentage of persons aged ≥ 18 years who were current smokers*, by sex and selected characteristics — National Health Interview Survey, United States, 2003

Characteristic	Men (n = 13,427) %	(95% CI[†])	Women (n = 17,425) %	(95% CI)	Total (N = 30,852) %	(95% CI)
Race/Ethnicity[§]						
White, non-Hispanic	24.3	(±1.0)	21.2	(±0.9)	22.7	(±0.7)
Black, non-Hispanic	25.5	(±2.5)	18.3	(±1.8)	21.5	(±1.6)
Hispanic	22.1	(±2.0)	10.3	(±1.1)	16.4	(±1.2)
American Indian/Alaska Native[¶]	42.0	(±15.9)	37.3	(±14.7)	39.7	(±11.9)
Asian**	17.5	(±4.5)	6.5	(±2.2)	11.7	(±2.5)
Education[††]						
0–12 (no diploma)	32.4	(±2.1)	21.2	(±1.9)	26.6	(±1.4)
< 8 years	23.4	(±2.9)	11.8	(±2.0)	17.6	(±1.8)
9–11 years	40.6	(±3.4)	28.5	(±3.0)	34.0	(±2.3)
12 years (no diploma)	35.2	(±7.7)	23.7	(±5.8)	29.3	(±4.6)
GED (diploma)[§§]	43.4	(±5.9)	45.6	(±5.8)	44.4	(±4.1)
12 years (diploma)	29.2	(±2.0)	22.1	(±1.5)	25.4	(±1.2)
Associate degree	21.9	(±2.9)	18.2	(±2.1)	19.8	(±1.7)
Some college (no degree)	23.7	(±1.8)	20.4	(±1.3)	21.9	(±1.1)
Undergraduate degree	13.6	(±1.8)	11.0	(±1.5)	12.3	(±1.1)
Graduate degree	8.1	(±1.6)	6.7	(±1.5)	7.5	(±1.1)
Age group (years)						
18–24	26.3	(±2.6)	21.5	(±2.3)	23.9	(±1.8)
25–44	28.4	(±1.4)	22.8	(±1.2)	25.6	(±1.0)
45–64	23.9	(±1.5)	20.2	(±1.4)	22.0	(±1.0)
≥ 65	10.1	(±1.4)	8.3	(±1.1)	9.1	(±0.9)
Poverty level[¶¶]						
At or above	24.2	(±1.0)	19.1	(±0.9)	21.7	(±0.7)
Below	33.0	(±3.1)	28.8	(±2.5)	30.5	(±2.1)
Unknown	21.2	(±1.6)	16.0	(±1.3)	18.4	(±1.0)
Total	24.1	(±0.8)	19.2	(±0.7)	21.6	(±0.6)

* Persons who reported smoking at least 100 cigarettes during their lifetimes and who reported at the time of interview smoking every day or some days. Excludes 402 respondents whose smoking status was unknown.

[†] Confidence interval.

[§] Excludes 310 respondents of unknown or multiple racial/ethnic categories or whose race/ethnicity was unknown.

[¶] Wide variances among estimates reflect small sample sizes.

** Does not include Native Hawaiians or other Pacific Islanders.

[††] Among persons aged ≥ 25 years; excludes 409 persons with unknown years of education.

[§§] General Educational Development.

[¶¶] Calculated on the basis of U.S. Census Bureau 2002 poverty thresholds.

Two chemicals in cigarettes, nicotine and carbon monoxide, are thought to be responsible for many of these pro-atherogenic changes, and the increased risk of heart disease associated with smoking. Nicotine is a stimulant that directly and immediately increases the myocardial workload. Nicotine is also a vasoconstrictor, therefore leading to elevations in blood pressure. Additional vasoconstriction occurs when nitric oxide biosynthesis is inhibited by smoking. The combined effect of increase in heart rate (HR) and systolic blood pressure (SBP) leads to an obvious increase in the HR × SBP double-product, a known predictor of myocardial oxygen demand.

In parallel to the unfavorable effects of nicotine, carbon monoxide present in cigarette smoke binds to hemoglobin with greater affinity than oxygen and reduces the oxygen-carrying capacity of hemoglobin, inducing a state of actual tissue hypoxia. This results in a lower oxygen supply to a myocardium working at a higher load. Hypoxia also appears to stimulate the atherosclerotic process. Over time, the arterial lumens progressively narrow. Additionally, nicotine induces the release of cholesterol from adipocytes into the blood stream, increasing the likelihood of cholesterol deposition in arterial walls. This shows that cigarette smoking indirectly promotes atherosclerosis though various mechanisms. Another mechanism is likely its effects on lipid profile. "Smokers have significantly higher serum cholesterol, triglyceride, and low-density lipoprotein levels, but high-density lipoprotein is lower in smokers than in nonsmokers" (15).

Smoking also raises the plasma level of fibrinogen and increases platelet activity, which increases thrombogenicity. As the atherosclerotic process progresses, decreased blood flows through stenosed arteries and the effects of smoking increase the likelihood of plaque rupture and thrombus formation, resulting in myocardial infarction (MI), stroke, or extremity gangrene (16). Therefore, although cigarette smoking may not directly cause atherosclerosis, it is a strong predictor of MI. This may be because smoking increases the risk of thrombotic events in people who already have atherosclerosis (17). In fact, autopsy studies do not show a higher vascular surface area affected by atherosclerosis than nonsmokers (17). This finding is supported by the Pathobiological Determinants of Atherosclerosis in Youth (PDAY) study, in which "the extent of coronary atherosclerosis did not correlate significantly with serum thiocyanate (a marker of exposure to smoke, measured postmortem) but, evaluated microscopically, established plaques appeared to be more rapidly progressing and thus reaching an advanced stage of the disease earlier" (17).

In summary, as is shown above, "smoking contributes to CHD risk independently of other risk factors" through the multiple changes that smoking initiates throughout the body. However, "this does not mean that smoking is an independent cause of CHD. Cigarette smoking is pathogenetically a cholesterol-dependent risk factor and acts synergistically with other risk factors, substantially increasing the risk of CHD" (17).

Smoking Cessation and Heart Disease Risk Reduction

The evidence that health suffers significantly under the influence of smoking is overwhelming. However, the evidence that health risks significantly improve with smoking cessation is equally impressive. It is estimated that stopping smoking decreases the risk of "subsequent mortality and further cardiac events among patients with CHD by as much as 50%" (4) and is associated with a decreased risk of total mortality of

Table 2
Benefits of Smoking Cessation

Short-term benefits	Long-term benefits
Blood pressure returns to presmoking levels within 20 min	Lung function improves up to 30% within 2–3 months
Carbon monoxide levels drop within hours	Risk of coronary heart disease is reduced by 50% after 1 year
Money is saved each day by not buying cigarettes	Risk of stroke is similar to that of a nonsmoker within 5–15 years
Sense of smell and taste improve within days	Patient enjoys increased self-esteem due to quitting smoking
Patient earns greater self-respect because of a real sense of accomplishment in quitting	

36% (4). The evidence that smoking cessation quickly and significantly reduces cardiac risk and mortality indicates that the smoking-related causes are rapidly reversible (17). The risk reduction from smoking cessation has been shown to be at least as great as other secondary preventive therapies, such as use of statins for cholesterol lowering (a 29% reduction), aspirin (15%), B-blockers (23%), or angiotensin-converting enzyme inhibitors (23%) (4).

The Benefits of Quitting

The benefits of quitting smoking are both immediate and ongoing. The World Health Organization indicates that within 1 year of smoking cessation, CHD risk decreases by 50%. "Within 15 years, the relative risk of dying from CHD for an ex-smoker approaches that of a long-time (lifetime) nonsmoker" (18). Stopping smoking also significantly decreases the risk of stroke over time. Smokers who have quit have the same risk of stroke as nonsmokers after 5–15 years of quitting (12). Table 2 (19) summarizes additional short-term and long-term benefits of smoking cessation.

Owing to the undeniable short-term and long-term benefits of quitting smoking on health, it is essential to motivate patients toward quitting as soon as possible and to also educate older patients that it is never too late to quit smoking.

> Health risks are improved even if a smoker does not quit completely. When the amount of cigarettes smoked is decreased, the risk of heart disease is reduced. Research shows that if all smokers decreased their amount of cigarettes smoked to 10 cigarettes per day, this could lead to a CHD reduction of 5.2% for men and 4.5% for women (20).

PROVIDING SUCCESSFUL SMOKING CESSATION TREATMENT INTERVENTIONS

To most effectively motivate and assist patients to quit smoking, it is important to understand the numerous factors that maintain their personal smoking habit and to provide various intervention modalities to deal with these factors. Tobacco dependence encompasses physical addiction, psychological addiction, and habit, as well as sensory stimulation and association with pleasure. Therefore, successful smoking cessation interventions must address physical, psychological, and sensory stimulation issues for each individual. The components of a successful cessation intervention include, but are not limited to, accurate assessment of smoking and of tobacco dependence, assessment of willingness and readiness to quit smoking, motivation of patients toward quitting if they are not willing or ready, creation of an appropriate and evidence-based cessation plan that incorporates necessary supportive components (including, but to limited to, behavioral counseling, social support, and pharmacotherapies), and relapse prevention. The following sections will provide more in-depth information about the above components.

Components of a Successful Smoking Cessation Plan

- Assessment of dependence components
- Assessment of stage of change (willing and readiness to stop smoking – see Chapter 7)
- Creation of a smoking cessation plan
    Provision of supportive social constructs (family, friends, and work colleagues)
    Possible counseling
    Possible pharmacotherapies
- Relapse prevention strategies

Assessment of Smoking and Tobacco Dependence

The first step in effectively treating smoking is to consistently identify, document, and treat tobacco users. By effectively identifying tobacco users and their willingness to quit, clinicians can identify intervention methods that are both appropriate and available (depending on the patient's financial and community resources). Simply asking patients about their smoking status at each patient visit allows for clinicians to understand their patient's interest in quitting, readiness to quit, and the support necessary for them to quit successfully. Strategies for consistently gathering, documenting, and updating this information are to either expand the number of vital signs collected to include smoking status or place an appropriate tobacco use sticker on patient charts.

Assessing Willingness to Quit and Readiness to Quit Smoking

Once a patient has been identified as a smoker, their willingness to quit should be assessed. Willingness to quit directs the treatment intervention appropriate for each person. According to the Treating Tobacco Use and Dependence: Clinical Practice Guideline *(21)*, every patient who uses tobacco should be offered at least one of the appropriate and available treatments for smoking cessation. This is true for both patients who are currently willing to quit and those who are unwilling to quit at this time. Fig. 1 *(21)* demonstrates what treatment should be offered depending on a person's willingness to quit.

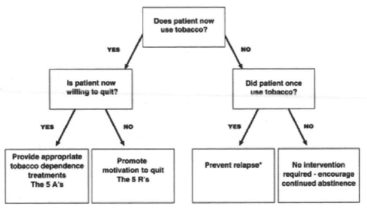

Fig. 1. Algorithm to guide clinical tobacco intervention.

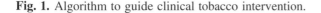

- Many smokers report an understanding of the dangers of smoking and a desire to quit.
- About 35% of smokers report having made at least one serious attempt to quit within the last year *(22)*, and 80% have tried to quit at some point in their smoking history *(23)*.
- Having a cardiac event increases the chances a person will attempt to quit.
- In comparison with the general population, 8% *(3)*, the percentage of smokers who quit after a cardiac event is significantly greater, 35–75%, *(24)*.
- There remains a significant amount of people with heart disease who either continue to smoke or relapse after a period of being smoke free *(25)*.

Smoking Cessation When the Patient is Willing to Quit

All patients willing to try to quit tobacco use should be provided with treatments that are identified as effective *(21)*. For those willing to quit, using the "5As," Ask, Advise, Assess, Assist, and Arrange, can deliver brief and effective intervention. These five steps, summarized in Table 3 *(21)*, promote asking about and systematically identifying all tobacco users at every visit; advising all tobacco users to quit in a clear, strong, and personalized manner; assessing the patient's willingness to make a quit attempt; and assisting in providing aid to the patient in quitting.

For patients with a recent heart disease episode, significant symptoms or severe disease, this can be an especially effective time to offer smoking cessation interventions. Severity of heart disease or of a cardiac event appears to increase motivation to quit smoking as well as is an important predictor in stopping *(26)*. Studies have shown that 20–60% of smokers quit after the diagnosis of acute MI *(25)*. There is also an influence of severity of disease on smoking cessation. This was demonstrated by Frid et al. *(24)* by showing a relationship between the number of diseased vessels [0-vessel (21%), 1-vessel (47%), 2-vessel (56%), and 3-vessel disease (76%)] and the likelihood of remaining smoke-free long term. Additionally, the proximity of the smoking cessation intervention to the cardiac event positively influenced smoking cessation probability. One study showed that when a smoking patient's coronary arteriography was done after

Table 3
Brief Strategies: Helping the Patient Willing to Quit*

Action	Strategies for Implementation

Ask – systematically identify all tobacco users at every visit

Implement an office-wide system that ensures that, for every patient at every clinic visit, tobacco-use status is queried and documented[†].	Expand the vital signs to include tobacco use or use an alternative universal identification system[‡].

Advise – strongly urge all tobacco users to quit

In a clear, strong, and personalized manner, urge every tobacco user to quit.	Advice should be:
	Clear – "I think it is important for you to quit smoking now and I can help you. Cutting down while you are ill is not enough."
	Strong – "As your clinician, I need you to know that quitting smoking is the most important thing you can do to protect your health now and in the future. The clinic staff and I will help you."
	Personalized – Tie tobacco use to current health/illness and/or its social and economic costs, motivation level/readiness to quit, and/or the impact of tobacco use on children and others in the household.
	Encourage all clinical staff to reinforce the cessation message and support the patient's quit attempt.

Assess – determine willingness to make a quit attempt

Ask every tobacco user if he/she is willing to make a quit attempt at this time (e.g., within the next 30 days).	Assess patient's willingness to quit:
	If the patient is willing to make an attempt to quit at this time, provide assistance.
	If the patient will participate in an intensive treatment, deliver such a treatment or refer to an intensive intervention.
	If the patient clearly states he/she is unwilling to make an attempt to quit at this time, provide a motivational intervention.
	If the patient is a member of a special population (e.g., adolescent, pregnant smoker, and racial/ethnic minority), consider providing additional information.

Assist – aid the patient in quitting

Help the patient with a plan to quit.	A patient's preparations for quitting (STAR): Set a quit date, ideally, the quit date should be within 2 weeks.

Provide practical counseling (problem solving/skills training).	Tell family, friends, and coworkers about quitting and request understanding and support. Anticipate challenges to planned quit attempt, particularly during the critical first few weeks; these include nicotine withdrawal symptoms. Remove tobacco products from your environment; prior to quitting, avoid smoking in places where you spend a lot of time (e.g., work, home, and car). Abstinence – total abstinence is essential; "not even a single puff after the quit date." Past quit experience – review past quit attempts including identification of what helped during the quit attempt and what factors contributed to relapse. Anticipate triggers or challenges in upcoming attempt – discuss challenges/triggers and how patient will successfully overcome them. Alcohol – drinking alcohol is highly associated with relapse; the patient should consider limiting/abstaining from alcohol during the quit process. Other smokers in the household – the presence of other smokers in the household, particularly a spouse or partner, is associated with lower abstinence rates. Patients should encourage significant others to quit with them. If others continue to smoke, they should be asked to smoke outdoors and not in the quitter's presence.
Provide intratreatment social support.	Provide a supportive clinical environment while encouraging the patient in his/her quit attempt; "my office staff and I are available to assist you."
Help patient obtain extratreatment social support.	Help patient develop social support for his/her attempt to quit in his/her environments outside of treatment: "ask your spouse/partner, friends and coworkers to support you in your quit attempt."
Recommend the use of approved pharmacotherapy except in special circumstances.	Recommend the use of pharmacotherapies found to be effective in the guideline; explain how these medications increase smoking cessation success and reduce withdrawal symptoms; the first-line pharmacotherapy medications include the following: bupropion SR, nicotine gum, nicotine inhaler, nicotine nasal spray, and nicotine patch.
Provide supplementary materials.	Sources – federal agencies, nonprofit agencies, or local/state health departments. Type – culturally/racially/educationally/age appropriate for the patient. Location – readily available at every clinician's workstation.

their MI and on the same hospitalization, their rate of remaining abstinent 6 months later was significantly higher (74%) compared with patients with angina without a history of MI (49% abstinence) or those who had an MI in the recent past and were admitted for additional diagnostic evaluation (52% abstinence) after intervention. *(26)*. Whereas other studies have confirmed that severity of disease predicts success in quitting smoking, this study shows that those with the most severe disease were more likely to respond to smoking cessation intervention, as well as the importance of offering treatment as close to the event time as possible. It may be that those with more severe symptoms or requiring more procedures are unable to maintain denial about the risks associated with smoking and/or their own disease state. It is necessary to reach patients and offer smoking cessation intervention during the teachable moments to increase the likelihood of smoking cessation success.

Smoking Cessation When the Patient Is Unwilling to Quit

Patients may not be willing to quit for various reasons including misinformation about the risks of smoking, denial or lack of understanding of the personal relevance of smoking on their health, fears or concerns about quitting, demoralization after previous failed attempts, or other reasons. Inquiring about their lack of willingness to quit allows the health care provider to better understand why the patient is unmotivated and then provide a brief intervention designed to increase their motivation to quit. Using the "5Rs," Relevance, Risks, Rewards, Roadblocks, and Reception, can help to increase the patient's willingness and readiness to quit. Table 4 *(21)* further describes the "5Rs". Motivating patients toward quitting and using the "5Rs" are most likely to be successful if the clinician is understanding and empathetic with the patient, allows for patient autonomy, does not engage in arguing, and supports the patient in believing that they are capable of quitting smoking *(27)*.

Recognizing Tobacco Dependence as a Chronic Disease

When motivating or assisting a patient in smoking cessation, it is important to understand that smoking is known to be a chronic addiction similar to other addictive substances (e.g., alcohol and drugs) with a vulnerability to relapse, requiring repeated intervention. It often takes several quit attempts before previous smokers remain abstinent. This places a responsibility on the "clinician to provide ongoing counseling, support, and appropriate pharmacotherapy, just as for other chronic diseases such as hypertension or hypercholesterolemia" *(27)*. It is essential to use appropriate smoking cessation interventions with every patient visit to increase the patient's opportunity to successfully quit smoking. If a patient relapses or is unwilling to quit, they should not be labeled noncompliant or unmotivated and the issue of smoking no longer addressed. Instead, this should be noted as part of their addiction, and the treatment team should provide interventions geared toward increasing their motivation to quit smoking in the future.

Creating a Smoking Cessation Plan

As previously noted, smoking addiction is complex and includes physical addiction, psychological addiction and, as more recently recognized, sensory stimulation that reinforces both the physical and the psychological addiction. Therefore, it is essential

Table 4
Enhancing Motivation to Quit Tobacco: The 5Rs

Motivation	*Description*
Relevance	Encourage the patient to indicate why quitting is personally relevant, being as specific as possible. Motivational information has the greatest impact if it is relevant to a patient's disease status or risk, family or social situation (e.g., having children in the home), health concerns, age, gender, and other important patient characteristics (e.g., prior quitting experience, personal barriers to cessation).
Risks	The clinician should ask the patient to identify potential negative consequences of tobacco use; the clinician may suggest and highlight those that seem to be the most relevant to the patient; the clinician should emphasize that smoking low-tar/low-nicotine cigarettes or use of other forms of tobacco (e.g., smokeless tobacco, cigars, and pipes) will not eliminate these risks. Examples of risks are: • Acute risks: shortness of breath, exacerbation of asthma, harm to pregnancy, impotence, infertility, increased serum carbon monoxide. • Long-term risks: heart attacks and strokes, lung and other cancers (larynx, oral cavity, pharynx, esophagus, pancreas, bladder, and cervix), chronic obstructive pulmonary diseases (chronic bronchitis and emphysema), long-term disability, and need for extended care. • Environmental risks: increased risk of lung cancer and heart disease in spouses; higher rates of smoking by children of tobacco users; increased risk for low birth weight, Sudden Infant Death Syndrome (SIDS), asthma, middle ear disease, and respiratory infections in children of smokers.
Rewards	The clinician should ask the patient to identify potential benefits of stopping tobacco use, the clinician may suggest and highlight those that seem to be the most relevant to the patient. Examples of rewards follow: • Improved health. • Food will taste better. • Improved sense of smell. • Save money. • Feel better about yourself. • Home, car, clothing, and breath will smell better. • Can stop worrying about quitting. • Set a good example for kids. • Have healthier babies and children. • Not worry about exposing others to smoke. • Feel better physically. • Perform better in physical activities. • Reduced wrinkling/aging of skin.

(Continued)

Table 4 (Continued)

Motivation	Description
Roadblocks	The clinician should ask the patient to identify barriers or impediments to quitting and note elements of treatment (i.e., problem-solving and pharmacotherapy) that could address barriers. Typical barriers might include: • Withdrawal symptoms. • Fear of failure. • Weight gain. • Lack of support. • Depression. • Enjoyment of tobacco.
Repetition	The motivational intervention should be repeated every time an unmotivated patient visits the clinic setting; tobacco users who have failed in previous quit attempts should be told that most people make repeated quit attempts before they are successful.

for successful smoking cessation interventions to target each of these components of a smoking habit. The following section will look at approaches useful in treating the physical dependence, the psychological dependence, and habit, as well as sensory stimulation.

Dealing with the Physical Addiction of the Smoking Act

There are a number of things to consider when treating the physical addiction to tobacco. First, it is necessary to determine how much nicotine the person is experiencing daily. A rule of thumb is that if a person smokes less than ten cigarettes per day and/or if they do not smoke within the first few hours of the day, they do not have a strong physical addiction to nicotine. However, there is individual variation. Physical addiction level is essential in planning an appropriate quit approach. If a patient is physically dependent on cigarettes, they will benefit from pharmacotherapy and may be more successful using a nicotine reduction approach to quit smoking.

Pharmacotherapy

Historically, clinicians have been hesitant to prescribe pharmacotherapy to their patients who smoke and often wait for failed cessation attempts before suggesting pharmacotherapies. This may be because physicians underestimate the addictive qualities of cigarettes, the degree to which their patients have developed dependence, and the relative likelihood of overcoming tobacco dependence when pharmacotherapy is used. Pharmacotherapies may also be withheld due to the misconception that they are only necessary for heavy smokers.

Except when contraindicated, one or a combination of the recommended pharmacotherapies should be used with all patients who are tobacco dependent and attempting to quit smoking. There are seven pharmacotherapies that have been approved by the US Food and Drug Administration (FDA) for smoking cessation and these are considered to be first-line treatments. These are buproprion SR, varenicline nicotine gum, nicotine inhaler, nicotine nasal spray, nicotine patch, and the nicotine lozenge, which are further described in Table 6 *(21)*. There are also two second-line pharmacotherapies, clonidine and nortriptyline, that are shown to be effective, however have not been approved by the FDA for smoking cessation. Clonidine has primarily been prescribed as an antihypertensive medication, and nortriptyline is used primarily as an antidepressant.

Each of the recommended medications has been shown to significantly increase the success of short-term and long-term smoking abstinence. Although each of the pharmacotherapies is found to increase rate of smoking abstinence, using a combination of the nicotine patch with other forms of nicotine replacement therapy (NRT) (e.g., transdermal patch, nicotine gum, nicotine inhaler, nicotine nasal spray, and nicotine lozenge) is more effective than using only one form of nicotine replacement. For patients who are unable to quit using NRT, they should be encouraged to use a combination of approved pharmacotherapics NRT. For example, combining bupropion SR with NRT. Guidelines for prescribing pharmacotherapies are included in Table 5 *(21)* and Table 6 *(21)*. Special consideration is necessary for special populations (e.g., smoking less than ten cigarettes per day, pregnant and breastfeeding women, adolescents).

Behavioral Approaches to Smoking Cessation

There are three behavioral approaches to smoking cessation: quitting "cold turkey," brandswitching to lower nicotine level cigarettes, and cutting back on the number of cigarettes smoked per day.

When choosing the approach to quitting, consider the following:

- How addicted to nicotine is the patient?
- How many cigarettes per day are they smoking?
- How many previous attempts have there been to quitting?
- How severe is the tobacco dependence?
- What are the daily smoking habits?
- What is the current access to cigarettes?
- What is the recent health history?
- Is the patient currently hospitalized?

All of these considerations can help in determining which quit style will be most effective.

Cold turkey, or quitting without gradually reducing nicotine level, may be most successful for patients who have received negative news about their cardiac health or have just experienced a cardiac event or procedure. Furthermore, patients who are hospitalized or have a significant cardiac event may find quitting cold turkey to be easier than at other times. This can be due to not being able to have cigarettes for several days while hospitalized and therefore overcoming the physical withdrawal process as part of the hospitalization. Other reported reasons are the decreased desire to smoke while experiencing uncomfortable or painful cardiac symptoms as well as not being able to deny the negative health consequences smoking is having on their health.

Table 5
Clinical Guidelines for Prescribing Pharmacotherapy for Smoking Cessation*

Question	Answer
Who should receive pharmacotherapy for smoking cessation?	All smokers trying to quit except in the presence of special circumstances; special consideration should be given before using pharmacotherapy with selected populations: those with medical contraindications; those smoking < 10 cigarettes per day, pregnant and adolescent smokers.
What first-line pharmacotherapies are recommended?	All seven of the FDA-approved pharmacotherapies for smoking cessation are recommended including bupropion SR, varenicline, nicotine gum, nicotine inhaler, nicotine nasal spray, nicotine lozenge, and the nicotine patch.
What factors should a clinician consider when choosing among the five first-line pharmacotherapies?	Because of the lack of sufficient data to rank-order these seven medications, choice of a specific first-line pharmacotherapy must be guided by factors such as clinician familiarity with the medications, contraindications for selected patients, patient preference, previous patient experience with a specific pharmacotherapy (positive or negative), and patient characteristics (e.g., history of depression and concerns about weight gain).
Are pharmacotherapeutic treatments appropriate for lighter smokers (e.g., 10–15 cigarettes per day)?	If pharmacotherapy is used with lighter smokers, clinicians should consider reducing the dose of first-line pharmacotherapies.
What second-line pharmacotherapies are recommended?	Clonidine and nortriptyline.
When should second-line agents be used for treating tobacco dependence?	Consider prescribing second-line agents for patients unable to use first-line medications because of contraindications or for patients for whom first-line medications are not helpful; monitor patients for the known side effects of second-line agents.
Which pharmacotherapies should be considered with patients particularly concerned about weight gain?	Buproprion SR and nicotine replacement therapies, in particular nicotine gum, have been shown to delay, but not prevent, weight gain.
Which pharmacotherapies should be considered with patients with a history of depression?	Buproprion SR and nortriptyline appear to be effective with this population.

Should nicotine replacement therapies be avoided in patients with a history of cardiovascular disease?	No. Nicotine replacement therapies are safe and have not been shown to cause adverse cardiovascular effects; however, the safety of these products has not been established for the immediate (2 weeks) post-MI period, with serious arrhythmias, or in patients with severe or unstable angina.
May tobacco dependence pharmacotherapies be used long-term (e.g., 6 months or more)?	Yes. This approach may be helpful with smokers who report persistent withdrawal symptoms during the course of pharmacotherapy or who desire long-term therapy; a minority of individuals who successfully quit smoking use ad libitum NRT medications (i.e., gum, nasal spray, and inhaler) long-term; the use of these medications long-term does not present a known health risk; additionally, the FDA has approved the use of bupropion SR for a long-term maintenance indication.
May nicotine replacement pharmacotherapies ever be combined?	Yes. There is evidence that combining the nicotine patch with either nicotine gum or nicotine nasal spray increases long-term abstinence rates over those produced by a single form of NRT.

FDA, Food and Drug Administration; MI, myocardial infarction; NRT, nicotine replacement therapy.
* Fiore MC, Bailey WC, Cohen SJ, et al. Treating Tobacco Use and Dependence: clinical practice guideline. Rockville, MD: US Department of Health and Human Services, Public Health Services, 2000.

These are considered teachable moments and can be opportunities where patients will be more open and receptive to smoking cessation interventions.

Brandswitching, also known as the "warm chicken" *(28)* approach to quitting smoking, is a method of gradually reducing the amount of nicotine delivered to the body. This enables the body to adjust to lower levels of nicotine over time and reduces the negative experience of intense withdrawal symptoms, thus making the quitting process easier. This can be a good strategy for people with strong nicotine dependence or those smoking higher nicotine level cigarettes. Brandswitching is operationalized by determining the amount of nicotine delivered by the type of cigarettes the participant is currently smoking and then switching to a lower level of nicotine cigarette. If a patient is smoking a 1.7-mg nicotine cigarette, it would be recommended to switch to a 0.9-mg nicotine cigarette and then a 0.5-mg nicotine cigarette, then a 0.2-mg nicotine cigarette before quitting completely. The patient would plan to spend about 1 week at each level and to set their quit date approximately 1 week after switching to the lowest nicotine level cigarette. As the patient switches levels, they are beginning to lose the association of cigarettes bringing the same nicotine response and pleasure that they previously did. It is important for the patient not to smoke more cigarettes per day or to smoke cigarettes longer, or cover up the filter ventilation holes, which would increase the nicotine delivered.

Table 6
Clinical Use of Pharmaceutical Agents for Smoking Cessation (21)

Pharmacotherapy/dosage	Duration	Availability	Cost for 30-day supply[†]	Precautions/ contra- indications	Adverse effects
First-line agents					
Nicotine gum, 2-mg gum (up to 24 pieces per day) for smokers of 1–24 cigarettes per day	Up to 12 weeks	OTC only	$38.00 for 108 2-mg pieces, $45.00 for 108 4-mg pieces		Mouth soreness and dyspepsia
Nicotine transdermal patch, 21 mg/24 h, 14 mg/24 h, 7 mg/24 h, 15 mg/16 h	4 weeks, then 2 weeks, then 2 weeks, 8 weeks	Rx and OTC	$84.00 for 28 21-mg patches, $90.00 for 28 7-mg patches[‡]		Local skin reaction and insomnia
Nicotine nasal spray, 8–40 doses per day	3–6 months	Rx only	$44.00 for bottle		Nasal irritation
Nicotine inhaler, 6–16 cartridges per day	Up to 6 months	Rx only	$43.00 for box of 10 cartridges		Local irritation of mouth and throat
Nicotine lozenge* 2 mg or 4 mg up to 20 dose per day	12 weeks	OTC only			Mouth soreness, local irritation of throat, hiccups, and heartburn/ indigestion
Sustained-release Bupropion hydrochloride, 150 mg every morning for 3 days then 150 mg twice daily (begin treatment 1–2 weeks before quitting)	7–12 weeks; maintenance up to 6 months	Rx only	$98.51 for 60 tablets	History of seizure or eating disorders	Insomnia and dry mouth

Drug, dosage	Duration	Availability	Cost	Precautions	Side effects
Varenicline, .5mg once daily for days 1–3, then .5mg twice daily for days 4-7, then 1mg twice daily for days 8-end of treatment.	12-weeks; maintenance for an additional 12 weeks.	Rx only		Safety and effective of varenicline in pediatric patients has not been established; therefore, it is not recommended for use in patients under 18 years of age.	Nausea, sleep disturbance, constipation, flatulence, and vomiting
Second-line agents					
Clonidine, 0.15–0.75 mg/day	3–10 weeks	Rx only (oral formulation or transdermal patch)	$9.00–12.00 for 60 tablets, $40.00–111.00 for 4 patches	Rebound hypertension	Dry mouth, drowsiness, dizziness, and sedation
Nortriptyline hydrochloride, 75–100 mg/d	12 weeks	Rx only	$9.50–13.50 for 30 capsules	Risk of arrhythmias	Sedation and dry mouth

Rx, prescription; OTC, over the counter.

The information contained here is not comprehensive. Readers should see package inserts for additional information. Prices given are based on May 24, 2002, prices at drugstore.com (see http://www.drugstore.com) and a national chain pharmacy in Chicago, IL. First-line pharmacotherapy agents have been approved for smoking cessation by the Food and Drug Administration (FDA); second-line pharmacotherapy agents have not been approved for smoking cessation.

 * The nicotine lozenge was approved by the FDA October 2002.
 † Prescription medication is often significantly less expensive when purchased through online pharmacies than from their "brick-and-mortar" counterparts.
 ‡ Generic brands of the nicotine transdermal patch may be less expensive.

Cutting back is performed by reducing the total amount of cigarettes smoked per day. This approach yields conflicting results. Many people find that they are able to give up smoking certain cigarettes in their typical daily routine. For example, they might give up the first cigarette of the day or stop smoking while in the car or inside their home. Gradually they are able to reduce the amount to a few per day or quit completely. However, decreasing the amount of cigarettes per day can actually increase the positive association and reward effect of each cigarette *(29)* and make it more difficult for the person to quit completely. With this approach, it is important to not smoke cigarettes longer or to cover up the filter ventilation holes, which would increase the nicotine delivered.

Regardless of the quit approach taken, it is important to choose an approach and to set a quit date that the patient believes will allow for success. If the person previously had a negative experience with one approach, it may be helpful to choose an alternative approach the next time. When choosing the quit date, try to choose a lower stress day. However, there is no magic day when quitting will be perfectly easy. So, if a patient says they want to wait until things are less stressful, push them to think through when that will be and to set the quit date, even if it is several weeks or months in the future. Also encourage them to set goals to support their ability to quit between now and their quit date.

Cleaning house. Prior to the quit date, the patient should take time to eradicate cigarettes and smoking from the environment. Removal and disposal of ashtrays, lighters, and cigarettes is key. Also, carpets and car upholstery should be steam cleaned, clothes washed, and coats dry cleaned if they smell like cigarette smoke. Everything the patient can do to remove smoking from their life prior to their quit date will make quitting easier. Once the quit date has arrived, remind the patient of their commitment and that they can never have one puff. Explain that smoking is a chronic addiction and that even having one puff can lead to relapse.

SPECIAL ISSUES DURING THE ACTION STAGES

Effects of Smoking Rate

Heavy smokers typically have more difficulty stopping smoking and are likely to experience more severe withdrawal symptoms *(29)*. This trend generalizes to smokers who have heart disease as well. Heavy smoking is a predictor for those who continue smoking or relapse after having a cardiac event *(29)*. The increased difficulty is likely influenced by an increased nicotine addiction as the amount of cigarettes smoked per day increases. Not only are an increased number of nicotine receptors activated, and activated more frequently, these nicotine receptors may in turn stimulate the dopaminergic reward system. "Activating the dopaminergic reward systems has the potential to alter mood and cognition, and reinforce the smoking habit" *(29)*. This suggests that the level of nicotine dependence/amount of cigarettes smoked should influence the strategy a smoker uses in quitting smoking. For example, if a person has high nicotine dependence, using NRT, decreasing the amount of cigarettes smoked per day over time, or brandswitching to lower nicotine level cigarettes may increase their success at quitting *(29)*, in comparison with quitting "cold turkey."

Planning for Withdrawal Symptoms

As the body adjusts to decreased nicotine and other chemicals from cigarettes, the body experiences withdrawal. Symptoms include coughing, sweating, lightheadedness or dizziness, changes in sleep and energy level, increased anxiety and restlessness, difficulty concentrating, depression, frustration, irritability, constipation or diarrhea, and cravings for tobacco *(28)*. Withdrawal symptoms are usually most intense after the first few days of quitting and typically subside within 2–4 weeks *(28)*. Recognizing withdrawal symptoms as signs of the body healing and recovering from smoking can help the person to remain positive and to better tolerate these symptoms. Withdrawal cravings for tobacco can be intense, however only last an average of 3–5 min. Learning coping strategies to get through a few minutes of a craving is essential to make the withdrawal process easier and to remain smoke free during this time period.

Dealing with Psychological Addiction

Counseling and behavioral therapies have been found to be effective and are thought to be the most central aspect of smoking cessation intervention *(30)* and should be used with all patients who are attempting tobacco cessation. Because smoking is a learned behavior, an important component of smoking cessation is to increase awareness of factors that trigger and are associated with smoking and then to make changes *(30)* or to learn how to better cope with these. Strategies that can be helpful in this change process include identifying environmental cues that lead to the urge to smoke and substitution of smoking with healthier activities; cognitive restructuring to challenge negative or destructive thoughts that support and maintain smoking behaviors; realizing the effect of personal habits (such as smoking) on health and the personal ability to improve health; learn stress management and relaxation skills to help cope with stress, anxiety, depression, and withdrawal symptoms and cravings; as well as setting up rewards for abstinence *(29)*. Another important goal of counseling is to treat depression, anxiety, and anger or hostility, if the patient is symptomatic of these, because these psychological factors negatively influence the probability of successfully stopping smoking.

Increasing Awareness of Triggers to Recidivism

Dealing with the smoking habit requires that persons increase their awareness of the routines, people, places, and situations that trigger them to smoke and to change or modify these. This may mean that if a person typically smokes while drinking a glass of wine in the evening, then they stop drinking wine in the evening for a while, or permanently. If they use smoking as a reason to take breaks from work during the day, they need to find other ways to take breaks, such as going for a brief walk down the hall. If they smoke in the car on the way to or from work as a way to relax, they could listen to calming music or to a book on tape instead. It is important when taking smoking out of certain routines that the person replace it with another behavior, so that the needs smoking was meeting are still getting met – and met in a healthier way.

Challenging Destructive Thinking

Without realizing it, people often engage in destructive thinking that maintains smoking and prevents a person from successfully quitting smoking. Ways of thinking that are negative and limit the person's ability to make positive changes need to be challenged and more accurately and positively reframed. For example, a person may think that because they have not been able to quit in the past, they will not quit this time. This belief should be challenged to help the person realize that past failure does not necessarily predict future failure. You might ask, "What if in the past you did not have all of the information, tools and support that were necessary to be successful? What if I told you that we could create a plan to make sure you had all of the information, tools and support this time? What would you need in order to be successful this time? Would that make you more likely to be successful?" Often people are not aware of the limitations their thinking imposes on them. Helping patients recognize when they are engaging in ways of thinking that limit their ability to use their full potential, and to challenge destructive thinking, can help to remove this roadblock and can increase their success.

Stress management and relaxation training and skill building are also important goals of counseling. Stress is commonly reported as a reason people return to smoking. It is necessary to learn coping strategies to deal with life stress before, during, and after stress happens. This may entail learning to prevent stress by not taking on additional responsibilities. If an unresolved task is causing stress, it may be important to plan how you can tackle this, so that it no longer drains your energy. You may also need to learn assertive communication skills to get your needs met or to set boundaries with others. Additionally, learning and regularly practicing relaxation skills, such as deep breathing and meditation can also help manage stress, anxiety, withdrawal symptoms, and cravings.

Using health locus of control is another important factor influencing both motivation to quit smoking and long-term smoking abstinence. External locus of control (belief that what happens is outside of his/her own control or behavior) versus internal locus of control (belief that what happens is inside of his/her own control or behavior) is an important factor in whether a person believes that smoking, or any negative health behavior, has a negative effect on their health and is therefore important to quit smoking. Ockene et al. *(25,26)* found that patients hospitalized with coronary artery disease (CAD) who had high external locus of control were less likely to accept responsibility for the effect their lifestyle had on their current health status. Being able to help a smoking patient shift from perceiving their current health as simply happening as a result of fate, or factors completely outside of their control, and helping them to realize the impact of lifestyle, and specifically smoking, on their health is important. If they believe that their behaviors influence their health, they may be more likely to improve them *(29)*.

Psychological factors such as depression, anxiety, and anger or hostility are more prevalent in smokers compared with nonsmokers *(29)*. It is unclear if this symptomology initiates the smoking habit, or if smoking increases the symptomology over time. These emotional states may be triggers for smoking as well as make it more difficult for people to feel motivated to quit or believe in the possibility of quitting successfully. Therefore, treating depression, anxiety, and anger and hostility is important to increase smoking cessation success. It is also likely that people with depression, anxiety, and hostility have "ineffective personal relationships" *(29)*. Therefore, improving social relationships and the necessary social skills may improve smoking cessation success in these people. Treatment for these psychological states may need to include both counseling and psychopharmacology. This group may respond well to buproprion SR.

Depression, Coronary Disease, and Smoking

An estimated 20% of smokers are depressed *(31)*. Depression decreases the success rate of smoking cessation and increases relapse *(31)*. One possible reason is that nicotine's stimulant effects decrease depressive symptomology, and therefore, smokers with depression are medicating with nicotine *(32)*. Smoking may then become a learned response to alleviate depressive symptoms *(31)*. In addition, withdrawal symptoms of depression have been shown to be more extreme in smokers with a pre-existing depression. This makes smoking cessation even more difficult with this group. Also, markers of depression are lack of motivation, low self-esteem and feelings of hopelessness, and helplessness *(29)*. These characteristics of depression are likely to decrease a depressed smoker's initiation of stopping smoking. For these reasons, it is essential for treatment of depression, or depressive symptoms, to be addressed when helping people, especially smokers with a history of depression, in their attempt to quit. Treatment may include antidepressants and counseling.

Establishing and Maintaining Support

Social support can be a powerful predictor of almost any change a person wishes to make. It has been a known predictor in increasing smoking cessation success as well *(29)*. Not only is it important to have social support, it seems that whether a person's support system includes smokers influences their success as well. Shiffman found that people who were successful at quitting smoking were less likely to list smokers among their 20 closest friends. On the contrary, people whose spouse remained a smoker always relapsed *(33)*. Successfully quitting may require that other people in the household who smoke also quit. The person quitting may also need to decrease time with smokers or find smoke-free activities to do with supports who smoke. In addition to support from those close to the person, support of physicians treatment providers is also essential for both quitting smoking and remaining smoke-free. It is important for treatment providers to reach out to smokers and those who have recently quit and to offer ongoing support.

Creating a Reward System

Many people do not set up rewards for quitting smoking, instead believe that quitting is something they should do and not something they should be rewarded for doing. However, the reward system can be a powerful motivator, and it can continue to provide enthusiasm and positive reinforcement for reaching quit smoking goals. There are several ways to set up rewards for quitting smoking. Using the money saved by not smoking to purchase rewards or to take a vacation is a common one. However, rewards do not have to cost much. They could consist of pats on the back, going to a movie, earning a bit of free time to use as they please, etc. Other examples of how to set up rewards include setting up rewards for reaching lower-level nicotine cigarettes, smoking fewer cigarettes, replacing smoking with healthier behaviors, or for anniversaries of being smoke-free. Make sure to set clear goals and establish the reward in advance for reaching these goals.

Delivery Method

Using multiple interventions that address the physical and psychological addiction and focusing on the multiple reasons that maintain smoking behavior can strengthen an intervention's success *(26)*. Written materials, both audio and video media, self-help materials, face-to-face counseling with a health professional, and individual and group sessions have been used in stop-smoking programs *(29)*. A positive approach in patient education and counseling, as compared with fear based, tends to be more motivational *(27,29)*. There is also a dose–response relationship between intensity of tobacco dependence counseling and success of quitting smoking, with their effectiveness increasing as the intensity of the treatment increases (e.g., minutes of contact) *(21)*. However, even brief tobacco dependence treatment is effective *(21)*. Therefore, even if clinicians and treatment providers do not have a substantial amount of time to provide smoking cessation interventions, brief intervention by the clinician can increase the chance the patient will attempt to quit and increase the probability of their success. Clinical interventions as brief as a few minutes can increase the likelihood of successful smoking cessation. Additionally, because of the limitations on the amount of time clinicians may have to provide smoking cessation counseling, it is recommended to incorporate various health care professionals to deliver the smoking cessation message. Physicians, physician assistants, nurses, medical assistants, counselors, and smoking cessation specialists can help to reinforce the smoking cessation message and to provide the necessary follow-up support.

Managing Withdrawal Symptoms

Once the person stops smoking, they should be prepared to manage withdrawal symptoms. Educating the patient that withdrawal symptoms are actually signs that their body is healing can help to change this from a negative experience to a more positive and tolerable experience. To help manage and reduce withdrawal symptoms recommend the following: regular exercise, eating a well-balanced diet (to avoid blood sugar crashes and irritability and fatigue), decrease caffeine (nicotine speeds up the metabolism of caffeine; therefore, once nicotine is decreased, the effects of caffeine will be more pronounced), drink plenty of water, and making sure to keep busy to decrease the focus on not smoking and withdrawal symptoms.

Relapse Prevention

For patients who have recently quit smoking, it is essential to keep in mind the chronic addictions model and to provide relapse prevention with these patients. This includes reminding the patients of their decision to quit, the immediate and ongoing benefits of quitting, and assisting in problem solving any obstacles they are experiencing or concerned about. Table 7 *(21)* further describes components of relapse prevention. It may be that this is most necessary during the 3-month period immediately after quitting, because this is the most common time of relapse. Arranging for follow-up visits or phone calls to provide relapse prevention during the first 2 weeks of quitting and also within the 3-month period of quitting can promote successfully

Table 7
Components of Relapse Prevention

Intervention	*Responses*

Interventions that should be part of every encounter with a patient who has quit recently. Every former tobacco user undergoing relapse prevention should receive congratulations on any success and strong encouragement to remain abstinent.

When encountering a recent quitter, use open-ended questions designed to initiate patient problem-solving (e.g., "How has stopping tobacco use helped you?").

The clinician should encourage the active discussion of the benefits the patient may derive from cessation, success the patient has had in quitting, problems encountered or anticipated threats to maintaining abstinence.

Problems	*Solutions*
Lack of support for cessation	Schedule follow-up visits or phone calls with the patient
	Help the patient identify sources of support within his/her environment
	Refer the patient to an appropriate organization that offers cessation counseling or support
Negative mood or depression	If significant, provide counseling, prescribe appropriate medications, or refer the patient to a specialist
Strong or prolonged withdrawal symptoms	If the patient reports prolonged craving or other withdrawal symptoms, consider extending the use of an approved pharmacotherapy or adding/combining pharmacologic medications to reduce strong withdrawal symptoms
Weight gain	Recommend starting or increasing physical activity; discourage strict dieting
	Reassure the patient that some weight gain after quitting is common and appears to be self-limiting
	Emphasize the importance of a healthy diet with plenty of fruits and vegetables
	Maintain the patient on pharmacotherapy known to delay weight gain (e.g., bupropion SR, nicotine replacement therapies, particularly nicotine gum)
	Refer the patient to a specialist or program
Flagging motivation/feeling deprived	Reassure the patient that these feelings are common
	Recommend rewarding activities
	Probe to insure that the patient is not engaged in periodic tobacco use
	Emphasize that beginning to smoke (even a puff) will increase urges and make quitting more difficult

quitting smoking. While relapse is most common within the first 3 months of quitting, it is important to acknowledge that relapse can occur at any time. Thus, ongoing questioning of the patient's quit smoking status as well as encouragement and support is beneficial.

SMOKING CESSATION IN THE FUTURE

Although continual progress is being made in understanding the burden of smoking on health, in the research of various smoking cessation interventions, and in reaching out to smokers, smoking remains a problem without definitive solutions. The number of smokers, and more specifically smokers with heart disease, remains disturbingly high and even those who do attempt to quit are likely to relapse. More research needs to be done to find more effective ways of reaching smokers, motivating smokers, creating effective treatment interventions, and using pharmacotherapies in order to more appropriately treat tobacco dependence and increase the probability of successfully quitting smoking.

There are numerous smoking cessation interventions and medications already created that have not been studied enough to prove effectiveness and/or safety by the FDA and therefore are not considered evidence-based or first-line standard of care. However, these appear to be promising. These include new medications, more appealing delivery methods of NRT, research regarding sensory receptor stimulation and that smoking appears to have, and unconventional therapies, such as hypnosis.

One controversy in the field is how appealing to make NRT. Current methods may not be easy enough or appealing enough for smokers to use them as prescribed or intended and are therefore not as effective. Making NRT more appealing (better tasting or easier to ingest like in a beverage) could increase compliance with taking the medication as intended and increase treatment effect. On the contrary, some researchers worry that this could lead to people quitting smoking and becoming addicted to the NRT instead. Although this would not be ideal, it is still likely to decrease health risks.

CONCLUSIONS

Tobacco dependence is a chronic addiction, similar to drugs and alcohol, with a high probability for relapse. Long-term motivation and treatment of the physical and psychological addiction is necessary. Providing smoking cessation interventions that address both parts of this addiction are likely to yield increased success as they help the smoker deal with many of the factors of their smoking habit.

There are a number of treatments known to be effective and evidence-based for smoking cessation. These should become a standard of care by clinicians and treatment providers. Health care providers have a vital role and a responsibility to help their patients quit smoking. They also have a unique opportunity to help patients understand the unnecessary risks they are placing on their health, as well as the ability to provide treatment interventions that can significantly increase their health and quality of life. Making smoking cessation a primary focus of preventive care as well as rehabilitation after a cardiac event can take advantage of teachable moments where the patient is more likely to be invested in making healthy lifestyle changes. Treatment providers can also provide education and necessary support to help move patients toward quitting as well as provide ongoing support and reinforcement for patients who have recently quit.

REFERENCES

1. Centers for Disease Control and Prevention. Cigarette Smoking Among Adults – United States, 2000. *MMWR Morb Mortal Wkly Rep.* 2002;51(29):642–645.
2. U.S. Department of Health, and Human Services. *The Health Benefits of Smoking Cessation: A Report of the Surgeon General.* Atlanta, GA: US Department of Health and Human Services. Public Health Service, Centers for Disease Control, Center for Chronic Disease Prevention and health Promotion, Office of Smoking and health; 1990, DHHS Publication No. (CDC) 90–8416.
3. U.S. Department of Health and Human Services. *The Health Consequences of Smoking: Cardiovascular Disease. A Report of the Surgeon General.* Rockville, MD: U.S. Department of Health and Human Services. Public Health Service, Office of the Assistant Secretary for Health, Office on Smoking and Health; 1983, DHHS Publication No. (PHS) 84–50204.
4. Critchley JA, Capewell S. Mortality Risk Reduction Associated with Smoking Cessation in Patients with Coronary Heart Disease – A Systemic Review. *JAMA.* 2003;290(1):86–97.
5. US Department of Health and Human Services. *Healthy People 2010: Understanding and Improving Health,* 2nd ed. Washington, DC: US Department of Health and Human Services; 2001. Available at http://www.healthypeople.gov
6. CDC. Cigarette smoking among adults – United States, 2003. *MMWR.* 2005;54:509–513.
7. Black HR. Smoking and Cardiovascular Disease. In *Hypertension: Pathophysiology, Diagnosis and Management,* 2nd ed., JH Laragh and BM Brenner (eds.). New York: Raven Press Ltd; 1995: 2621–2647.
8. U.S. Department of Health and Human Services. *Reducing the Health Consequences of Smoking – 25 Years of Progress: A Report of the Surgeon General.* Atlanta, GA: U.S. Department of Health and Human Services, CDC; 1989. DHHS Pub. No. (CDC) 89–8411. Accessed: February 2004.
9. Novotny TE, Giovino GA. Tobacco Use. In *Chronic Disease Epidemiology and Control,* RC Brownson, PL Remington, and JR Davis (eds.). Washington, DC: American Public Health Associa- tion; 1998:117–148.
10. Ockene IS, Miller NH. Cigarette Smoking, Cardiovascular Disease, and Stroke: A Statement for Healthcare Professionals from the American Heart Association. *J Am Heart Assoc.* 1997;96(9): 3243–3247.
11. Fielding JE, Huston CG, Eriksen MP. Tobacco: Health Effects and Control. In *Public Health and Preventive Medicine,* KF Maxcy, MJ Rosenau, JM Last, RB Wallace, and BN Doebbling (eds.). New York: McGraw-Hill; 1998:817–845.
12. U.S. Department of Health and Human Services. *The Health Consequences of Smoking: A Report of the Surgeon General.* U.S. Department of Health and Human Services. Centers for Disease Control and Prevention, National Center for Chronic Disease Prevention and Health Promotion, Office on Smoking and Health; 2004
13. Bartecchi CE, et al. The Human Costs of Tobacco Use. *N Engl J Med.* 1994;330;907–912.
14. He J, Vupputuri S, Allen K, et al. Passive Smoking and the Risk of Coronary Heart Disease: A Meta-Analysis of Epidemiologic Studies. *N Engl J Med.* 1999;340:920–926.
15. Ambrose JA, Barua RS. The Pathophysiology of Cigarette Smoking and Cardiovascular Disease: An Update. *J Am Coll Cardiol.* 2004;43:1731–1737.
16. *Cigarettes: What the Warning Label Doesn't Tell You.*American Council on Science and Health, 1996. Action on smoking and Health contributors. In: Smoking, The Heart and Circulation Fact Sheet no.6 – ASH, [online]. Available: URL://www.ash.org.uk/html/factsheet/html/fact06.html
17. Falk E, Fuster V. Atherogenesis and its Determinants. In *Hurst's The Heart,* 10th ed., V Fuster, RW Alexander, and RA O'Rourke (eds.). New York: McGraw-Hill; 2001:1065–1093.
18. World No – Tobacco Day 1998. American Heart Association contributors. Learn and Live: Statistical Fact Sheet – populations: 2007 Update: Tobacco use, [online]. Available: http://www. americanheart.org/downloadable/heart/11686/2193463JNTL07.pdf

19. Jorenby DG. Smoking Cessation Strategies for the 21st Century. *Circulation*. 2001;104:e51–e52.
20. McPherson K, Britton A, Causer L. Coronary Heart Disease. Estimating the Impact of Changes in Risk Factors. London: Nation Heart Forum, The Stationery Office, 2002.
21. Fiore MC, Bailey WC, Cohen SJ, et al. *Treating Tobacco Use and Dependence. Clinical Practice Guideline.* Rockville, MD: U.S. Department of Health and Human Services; 2000. Public Health Service.
22. Hatziandreu EJ, Pierce JP, Lefkooulou M, et al. Quitting Smoking in the United States in 1986. *J Natl Cancer Inst*. 1990;82:1402–1406.
23. U.S. Department of Health and Human Services. *Reducing the Health Consequences of Smoking: 25 Years of Progress; A Report of the Surgeon General.* Rockville, MD: US Department of Health and Human Services, Public Health Service, Centers for Disease Control, Center for Chronic Disease Prevention and Health Promotion, Office on Smoking and Health, 1989; DHHS Publication No. (CDC) 89–8411.
24. Frid D, Ockene IS, Ockene JK, Merriam P, Goldberg R, Kristeller J, et al. Severity of Angiographically Proven Coronary Artery Disease Predicts Smoking Cessation. *Am J Prev Med*. 1991;7(3): 131–135.
25. Ockene JK, Hosmer D, Rippe J, Williams J, Goldberg RJ, DeCosimo D, et al. Factors Affecting Cigarette Smoking Status in Patients with Ischemic Heart Disease. *J Chronic Dis*. 1985;48(12): 985–994.
26. Ockene J, Kristeller JL, Robert G, Ockene I, Merriam P, Barrett S. Smoking Cessation and Severity of Disease: The Coronary Artery Smoking Intervention Study. *Health Psychol*. 1992:11(2),119–126.
27. Anderson JE, Jorneby DE, Scoot WJ, Fiore MC. Treating Tobacco Use and Dependence: An Evidence-Based Clinical Practice Guideline for Tobacco Cessation. *Chest*. 2002;121;932–941.
28. Shipley RH. *QuitSmart Stop Smoking Guide: With the QuitSmart System It's Easier Than You Think!* Durham, NC: QuitSmart Stop Smoking Resources, Inc.; 2006.
29. McKenna K, Higgins H. Factors Influencing Smoking Cessation in Patients with Coronary Artery Disease. *Patient Educ Couns*. 1997:32:197–205.
30. Jensen MA. Understanding Addictive Behaviors: Implications for Health Promotion Programming. *Am J Health Promot*. 1987;3:48–57.
31. Anda RF, Williamson DF, Escobedo LG, Mast EE, Giovino A, Remington PL. Depression and the Dynamics of Smoking: A National Perspective. *J Am Med Assoc*. 1990;264(12):1541–1545.
32. Huges JR, Hatsukami DK, Mitchell JE, Dahlgren LA. Prevalence of Smoking Among Psychiatric Outpatients. *Am J Psychiatry*. 1986;143:993–997.
33. Shiffman S. Relapse Following Smoking Cessation: A Situational Analysis. *J Consult Psychol*. 1982;50:71–86.

9 Utility of Graded Exercise Testing in the Cardiac Rehabilitation Setting

William E. Kraus, MD

CONTENTS

In the cardiac rehabilitation setting, a graded exercise test (GXT) might be obtained for risk stratification and prognostication, for diagnostic reasons (e.g., to test for residual ischemia in the setting of recurrent symptoms following an invasive therapeutic cardiovascular procedure), for therapeutic reasons (development of an exercise prescription), or to quantify functional capacity – at baseline or in response to exercise training.

Reasons for Obtaining a GXT in Cardiac Rehabilitation

- *Diagnosis* – evaluation of ischemia following event or procedure.
- *Prognosis* – following event.
- *Exercise prescription* – when entering a cardiac rehabilitation (CR) program.
- *Evaluation of functional capacity* – following exercise training.

THE GXT FOR DIAGNOSTIC PURPOSES

In most cardiovascular settings, the primary reason for obtaining a GXT, sometimes referred to an exercise tolerance test (ETT), is to confirm or refute the diagnosis of functionally significant occlusive coronary artery disease in the setting of symptoms suspicious of stable angina pectoris. The consensus guidelines and literature supporting this indication are thoroughly addressed in the official guidelines of the American Heart Association and American College of Cardiology *(1)*, which are periodically updated, and the methods for performing this test are addressed in the subsequent chapter (see Chap. 10). However, in the cardiac rehabilitation setting, extremely rarely is GXT performed for a *de novo* diagnosis of occlusive coronary artery disease. Rather,

From: *Contemporary Cardiology: Cardiac Rehabilitation*
Edited by: W. E. Kraus and S. J. Keteyian © Humana Press Inc., Totowa, NJ

following an invasive corrective procedure (percutaneous coronary intervention or coronary artery bypass grafting) for the correction of occlusive disease, the cardiac patient might experience recurrent symptoms that are reminiscent or suggestive of cardiac angina. In such settings, it is reasonable to consider performing a GXT with electrocardiogram (ECG) monitoring to screen for exercise-induced ischemia. This may occur early in the setting of a cardiac rehabilitation program (e.g., indicative of incomplete revascularization) or later in the course (e.g., restenosis following angioplasty or stenting). If ischemia is documented, often the patient will be referred to for more extensive studies and perhaps a repeat revascularization procedure.

The Positive Exercise ECG Tracing

The diagnosis of functionally occlusive coronary artery disease is made on the basis of the exercise ECG. At our institution, we use the following criteria to read the test as "positive" for such a condition. The criteria are designed to optimize the balance between sensitivity and specificity in a population with a relatively high rate of cardiovascular risk factors. The ST segments have to be depressed 0.1 mV compared with the PR interval for the same beat, with a configuration that is down-sloping or flat at a point in the complex that is 0.08 ms from the conclusion of the QRS complex in a lead tracing with no baseline ST depression. Additionally, this configuration has to be consistent and evident in at least three successive complexes to avoid findings due to motion artifacts. The finding has to be in at least one of the 12 standard ECG leads, other than III and aVR. A lone finding in lead III is not considered to be valid, but rather it has to be accompanied by a similar finding in leads II or aVF. In lead tracings with baseline ST depression, the tracing has to meet "double criteria" to be considered positive, where the ST tracing has to be depressed beyond baseline by an additional 0.2 mV. That is, if the ST segment tracing is already 0.05 mV below the resting PR interval at baseline, then to meet double criteria, the tracing has to be 0.25 mV below the PR interval during the exercise test.

There are several additional caveats. To reduce the prevalence of false-positive tests, we consider the exercise ECG as being uninterpretable if there is baseline ST changes due to left ventricular hypertrophy or left bundle branch block, or if the subject is taking digitalis and related medications. A test is considered interpretable in the lateral precordial leads (V4–V6) and in the limb leads in the presence of right bundle branch block. We have observed a high prevalence of false-positive tests if the subject is using exogenous estrogens. This is likely due to the fact that the chemical structure of estrogenic hormones resembles that of digitalis. Higher levels of endogenous estrogens are also likely the cause of the higher rate of false-positive testing in middle-aged women, although this has never been conclusively proven. One might suggest that it is prudent to proceeding directly to a functional imaging study instead of obtaining a simple GXT in women on exogenous estrogen therapy if one is obtaining the test for diagnostic reasons. Many of these considerations are summarized in an excellent text by Ellestad on the subject dealing with the interpretation of the exercise ECG (2). Included are examples of resting and exercise ECG reports, should they be of potential use to the reader (Fig. 1A,B).

IV. Pre Study ECG

ECG *(check one)* ○ Normal ○ Abnormal ○ Not Available
If Abnormal

Rhythm *(check all that apply)*	P Wave *(check all that apply)*	Axis *(check one. if applicable)*	Conduction *(check all that apply)*
❏ AIVR ❏ Atrial fibrillation ❏ Atrial flutter ❏ AV sequential pacing ❏ Ectopic atrial tachycardia ❏ Nodal rhythm ❏ NSR ❏ Paced rhythm ❏ Sinus bradycardia ❏ Sinus tachycardia ❏ SVT ❏ Ventricular pacing	❏ LAE ❏ RAE	○ Normal ○ LAD ○ RAD	❏ 1° AV Block ❏ 2° AV Block - Type I ❏ 2° AV Block - Type II ❏ 3° AV Block ❏ Incomplete LBBB ❏ LBBB ❏ Left Ant Hemiblock (LAD > -30°) ❏ Left Post. Hemiblock (RAD > +120°) ❏ Nonspecific IVCD ❏ RBBB ❏ Incomplete RBBB ❏ WPW

Arrhythmias *(check all that apply)*	QRS Complex *(check all that apply)*	ST-T Waves *(check all that apply)*	
❏ Couplets ❏ PAC's ❏ PJC's ❏ PVC's ❏ Ventricular tachycardia	❏ Anterior MI ❏ Inferior MI ❏ LVH ❏ Lateral MI ❏ Posterior MI ❏ RVH	❏ Early repolarization ❏ Low voltage ❏ LV ischemia ❏ Nonspecific ST-T changes ❏ Poor R wave progression ❏ Prolonged QTc ❏ Secondary repolarization changes (LVH, RBBB) ❏ Secondary repolarization changes (RVH) ❏ ST elevation (persistent) c/w LV aneurysm ❏ ST elevation c/w acute infarction ❏ ST elevation c/w acute pericarditis ❏ Subendocardial injury ❏ Transient ST elevation c/w variant angina	

IV. Interpretation (to be filled out by M.D./P.A.)

ECG Interpretation: *(check one)*			
○ Positive	❏ When interpretation was Initially positive	❏ Maximum net exercise ST Depression	❏ Maximum net exercise ST Elevation
	In stress or recovery? *(check one)* ○ Stress ○ Recovery	Max ST depression - _____ mV	Max ST elevation + _____ mV
	Heart rate was _____ bpm	In Leads: *(check all that apply)*	In Leads: *(check all that apply)*
	ST depression - _____ mV	❏ I ❏ II ❏ III ❏ aVR ❏ aVL ❏ aVF ❏ V1 ❏ V2 ❏ V3 ❏ V4 ❏ V5 ❏ V6	❏ I ❏ II ❏ III ❏ aVR ❏ aVL ❏ aVF ❏ V1 ❏ V2 ❏ V3 ❏ V4 ❏ V5 ❏ V6
	ST change type initially? *(check one)* ○ Depression ○ Elevation	Resting ST depression ≥ .05mV in above leads? ○ Yes ○ No	Resting ST elevation ≥ 0.05 mV in above lead(s)?
	In Leads: *(check all that apply)* ❏ I ❏ II ❏ III ❏ aVR ❏ aVL ❏ aVF ❏ V1 ❏ V2 ❏ V3 ❏ V4 ❏ V5 ❏ V6	ST depression is downsloping? ○ Yes ○ No	○ Yes ○ No
○ Negative	Adequate or Inadequate *(check one)* ○ Adequate (peak HR is within 5 beats of THR) ○ Inadequate (THR not reached, no exercise ECG changes)	Variable horizontal ST depression, nondiagnostic? ○ Yes ○ No	
○ Uninterpretable	Uninterpretable due to: *(check all that apply)* ❏ Resting and further exercise ST elevation only in leads with pathologic Q waves and/or residual ST segment coving from prior MI ❏ Exercise induced conduction disturbance ❏ Exercise induced conduction disturbance (not Right Bundle Branch Block) ❏ Rest and Exercise IVCD ❏ Rest and Exercise IVCD (not Right Bundle Branch Block) ❏ Rest and Exercise paced ventricular rhythm ❏ Resting IVCD/paced rhythm disappears with exercise but significant ST segment changes are present on the exercise ECG. ❏ Baseline ST changes ❏ Paroxysmal atrial tachycardia ❏ Increased ventricular arrhythmia ❏ Lead fell off ❏ Patient fell ❏ Artifact ❏ LVH repolarization ❏ Digoxin effect		

V. Additional Comments   Interpreted by: _____

Interpreting MD *(check one)*

Fig. 1. Example of a ECG report form for graded exercise testing.

Interpretations of the Exercise ECG

- Criteria for positive test
    ST segments depressed 0.1 mV in the absence of baseline changes
    * Three successive beats
    * Flat or down-sloping 0.08 ms
    * Any one or more of 10 leads excluding III and aVR
    Meets "double criteria" in presence of baseline ST depression
- Uninterpretable in the presence of
    LBBB, LVH with strain, digitalis
- High prevalence of false positives (i.e., use caution) in the presence of
    exogenous estrogen use, LVH without strain, middle-aged women

THE GXT FOR PROGNOSTIC PURPOSES

Cardiorespiratory Fitness

Cardiorespiratory fitness, as measured by a graded ETT, provides strong and independent prognostic information about overall – and especially cardiovascular – morbidity and mortality. Cardiorespiratory fitness is a valid prognostic indicator in apparently healthy individuals, in at-risk individuals with diabetes mellitus, metabolic syndrome, and hypertension, and in patients with cardiovascular disease, such as those that present to a cardiac rehabilitation program *(3–9)*. However, despite the profoundly important prognostic information provided by simple clinical assessments of fitness, they are rarely used in the clinical setting and often ignored in the exercise-testing laboratory. There is an undue emphasis on the exercise ECG, whose diagnostic interpretation was just discussed. Table 1 indicates, for women and men, the expected fitness level in metabolic equivalents (METs). Owing to its increasingly recognized value, we have begun to report the fitness classification on our clinical GXT reports. This can be used as a valuable marker to follow longitudinally the changes in risk stratification in individuals in cardiac rehabilitation programs.

The Exercise ECG for Prognostic Purposes

There is a rich literature from the 1980s regarding the use of the exercise ECG – specifically, the timing during the GXT at which it turns positive – and the prognostic implications of such for making clinical decisions. In one set of investigations, it has been well documented that after myocardial infarction, a submaximal test can be used to determine medium- and long-term risk of recurrent ischemic events and cardiovascular death. Additionally, GXT information can be used to determine the likelihood of left main and three-vessel coronary artery disease (sometimes referred to as "surgical disease").

Table 1
Cardiorespiratory Fitness Classifications for Women and Men
[Metabolic Equivalents (METs)] *(10)*

AGE (years)	Low	Below average	Average	Above average	High
Women					
20–29	≤ 8.0	8.1–9.9	10.0–12.4	12.5–13.9	≥ 14.0
30–39	≤ 7.7	7.8–9.6	9.7–11.9	12.0–13.6	≥ 13.7
40–49	≤ 7.1	7.2–9.0	9.1–11.6	11.7–13.0	≥ 13.1
50–65	≤ 6.0	6.2–8.2	8.3–10.5	10.6–11.9	≥ 12.0
Men					
20–29	≤ 10.9	11.0–12.5	12.6–14.8	14.9–16.2	≥ 16.3
30–39	≤ 9.7	9.8–11.3	11.4–13.6	13.7–14.8	≥ 14.9
40–49	≤ 8.6	8.7–10.2	10.3–12.5	12.6–13.6	≥ 13.7
50–59	≤ 7.1	7.2–9.0	9.1–11.3	11.4–12.5	≥ 12.6
60–69	≤ 6.0	6.1–7.6	7.7–10.2	10.3–11.3	≥ 11.4

In a publication from our institution during this period, the Duke Treadmill Score was developed and subsequently reached broad popularity for prognostic purposes *(7)*. In work from our institution and others, it was observed that a limited GXT performed within the first several weeks following a myocardial infarction could determine whether follow-up testing was indicated to identify surgical disease. If the exercise ECG of a GXT was positive or symptoms developed before a heart rate (HR) of 120 bpm, this implied a 22% likelihood of the patient having three-vessel occlusive coronary disease or left main coronary artery disease *(11)*. This would often prompt further studies in the coronary catheterization laboratory with anticipation of coronary artery surgery. Soon, these criteria were shown to be relevant for all individuals suspected of having occlusive coronary artery disease *(12)*. We have been employing these standards for test interpretation for over 20 years. Unfortunately, with the ready availability of invasive diagnostic and therapeutic catheterization laboratories at many institutions, this practice has fallen out of favor, and the GXT is rarely used today as prognostic test in the development of a therapeutic plan.

The Use of the GXT for Therapeutic Purposes – Modifying the Exercise Prescription

The GXT also has utility to follow progress and modification of the exercise prescription with exercise training. It is for this purpose that the Center for Medicare and Medicaid Services (CMS) recognizes the need to reimburse for a GXT both prior to and following an approved period (36 sessions) of cardiac rehabilitation. The principles underlying this practice in the coronary patient is summarized in Fig. 2.

It is a principle of exercise physiology that there is a linear relationship between HR and workload from rest to the ventilatory threshold – when the oxygen demands of the exercise workload exceeds oxygen supply to the working muscles. After a period of exercise training, there occur three observable physiologic responses that characterize the "training effect." These three responses are illustrated in Fig. 2: (i) resting bradycardia – where the resting HR is lower following exercise training; (ii) a training bradycardia – a relative bradycardia at each successive workload to HR maximum; and (iii) an increase in maximum workload (measured as peak VO_2 with a metabolic cart). This physiology is particularly pertinent to individuals with occlusive coronary artery disease and angina pectoris. With a fixed lesion, the angina threshold (HR at which angina occurs) is reproducible and corresponds to a given workload. In Fig. 2, before and following exercise training, the angina threshold is approximately 115 bpm. The maximum workload at the angina threshold is 6 METs prior to training and 10 METs following, representing a 66% increase in exercise tolerance following exercise training.

It should be noted that these responses are specific to the muscles being exercise trained, and therefore, careful attention should be given to the exercise prescription and the muscle groups that will be commonly used in the activities of daily living when the angina threshold is likely to be exceeded. For example, if the individual of interest works in a job that requires primarily upper body work, then consideration should be given to exercise training primarily the upper body during the cardiac rehabilitation period to provide the greatest increase in exercise tolerance in the work setting *(12)*.

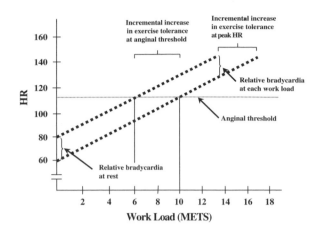

Fig. 2. Utility of Exercise Training in Individuals with Angina. The upper line represents the relationship between work load (in metabolic equivalents – METs) and HR prior to a period of exercise training. For an individual with a fixed obstructive lesion the angina threshold tends to occur at a given hear rate (in this case 115 beats per minute). This corresponds to a limiting work load of 6 METs. However, after a period of training within cardiac rehabilitation, the curve (lower) demonstrates several characteristics relative to the pre-training curve (e.g., relative bradycardia at rest, a relative bradycardia at each work load and a potential for increase in maximal work capacity). In addition, there is a significant increase at the work load achieved at the angina threshold. In this case example, angina is not experienced post training until the patient achieves 10 METs, representing a significant increase in angina free work capacity following exercise training.

CONCLUSIONS

In conclusion, GXT is a useful clinical tool with prognostic, diagnostic, and thera-peutic uses. Careful attention to the use of this tool in the cardiac rehabilitation program can increase the utility of program components to modify risk for subsequent events. More attention should be given to the use of the fitness assessment in the clinical environment.

REFERENCES

1. AHA/ACC. ACC/AHA 2002 Guideline Update for Exercise Testing: Summary Article. A Report of the American College of Cardiology/American Heart Association Task Force on Practice Guidelines (Committee to Update the 1997 Exercise Testing Guidelines). *Circulation*. 2002;106:1883–1892.
2. Ellestad MH, Selvester RH, Mishkin FS, James FW, Muzami K. *Exercise Electrocardiography*, 4th ed. Philadelphia, PA: F.A. Davis Company; 1996.
3. Blair SN, Kampert JB, Kohl HWI, et al. Influences of Cardiorespiratory Fitness and Other Precursors on Cardiovascular Disease and All-Cause Mortality in Men and Women. *JAMA*. 1996;276:205–210.
4. Blair SN, Kohl HWI, Paffenbarger RS Jr, Clark DG, Cooper KH, Gibbons LW. Physical Fitness and All-Cause Mortality: A Prospective Study of Healthy Men and Women. *JAMA*. 1989;262:2395–2401.
5. Kraus WE, Douglas PS. Where Does Fitness Fit In? *N Engl J Med*. 2005;353:517–519.
6. Lee S, Kuk JL, Katzmarzyk PT, Blair SN, Church TS, Ross R. Cardiorespiratory Fitness Attenuates Metabolic Risk Independent of Abdominal Subcutaneous and Visceral Fat in Men. *Diabetes Care*. 2005;28:895–901.

7. Mark DB, Hlatky MA, Harrell FE Jr, Lee KL, Califf RM, Pryor DB. Exercise Treadmill Score for Predicting Prognosis in Coronary Artery Disease. *Ann Intern Med.* 1987;106:793–800.

8. Mark DB, Lauer MS. Exercise Capacity: The Prognostic Variable That Does Not Get Enough Respect. *Circulation.* 2003;108:1534–1535.

9. Morris CK, Myers J, Froelicher VF, Kawaguchi T, Ueshima K, Hideg A. Nomogram Based on Metabolic Equivalents and Age for Assessing Aerobic Exercise Capacity in Men. *J Am Coll Cardiol.* 1993;22:175–182.

10. Mahler DA, Froelicher VF, Houston Miller N, York TD. *ACSM Guidelines for Exercise Testing and Prescription*, 7th ed. Baltimore, MD: William & Wilkins; 2006.

11. McNeer JF, Margolis JR, Lee KL, et al. The Role of the Exercise Test in the Evaluation of Patients for Ischemic Heart Disease. *Circulation.* 1978;57:64–70.

12. Abraham RD, Freedman SB, Dunn RF, et al. Prediction of Multivessel Coronary Artery Disease and Prognosis Early After Acute Myocardial Infarction by Exercise Electrocardiography and Thallium-201 Myocardial Perfusion Scanning. *Am J Cardiol.* 1986;58:423–427.

10 Graded Exercise Testing

Clinton A. Brawner, MS, RCEP

CONTENTS

For many clinicians, an exercise stress test offers diagnostic and prognostic information. Foremost is the assessment of chest pain and repolarization changes in the electrocardiogram (ECG) suggestive of myocardial ischemia. However, other data collected during an exercise stress test provide useful prognostic information and are helpful in guiding return to work, developing an exercise prescription, and managing the patient during exercise training. This chapter focuses on the procedures necessary to insure that the exercise stress test yields information useful for guiding exercise training in cardiac rehabilitation or at home.

BACKGROUND

An exercise stress test, also known as a graded exercise test (GXT), provides important information on the patient beginning an exercise-training program. The primary reasons for a GXT are risk stratification, development of an exercise prescription, and to quantify functional capacity. The GXT provides information related to the presence of ischemia or arrhythmias, heart rate and blood pressure response during exercise, exercise-related symptoms or limitations, and exercise tolerance or

From: *Contemporary Cardiology: Cardiac Rehabilitation*
Edited by: W. E. Kraus and S. J. Keteyian © Humana Press Inc., Totowa, NJ

functional capacity. Together this information is useful when developing the exercise prescription and managing the patient during exercise training.

The GXT performed for an exercise-training program should be sign- or symptom-limited. Optimally, the GXT will continue until the patient reaches his/her maximal effort. The test should not be terminated at a predefined target heart rate or work rate. Recommended end points that should be considered prior to the patient reaching a maximal effort are summarized in Table 1.

Table 1
Graded Exercise Test End Points

Absolute end points

- Signs of severe fatigue
- Patient request*
- Sustained ventricular tachycardia
- Moderate to severe angina
- Signs of poor perfusion: moderate to severe dizziness, near-syncope, confusion, ataxia, cold or clammy skin
- Technical difficulties in monitoring ECG or BP
- Drop in systolic BP despite increasing work rate in the presence of other signs of ischemia or worsening arrhythmia
- New onset atrial fibrillation
- Supraventricular tachycardia
- Third degree atrioventricular heart block
- ST elevation (> 1 mm) in leads without diagnostic Q-waves (other than V1 or aVR)
- ST depression (> 2 mm) with normal resting ECG and patient not taking digoxin
- Systolic BP > 250 mmHg or diastolic BP > 115 mmHg
- Heart rate within 10 beats of ICD threshold

Relative end points

- Drop in systolic BP with two consecutive increases in work rate in the absence of other signs of ischemia or worsening arrhythmia
- Worsening ventricular ectopy, especially if it exceeds 30% of complexes
- ST depression > 2 mm with abnormal resting ECG or patient taking digoxin
- New onset bundle branch block, especially if indistinguishable from ventricular tachycardia
- Dyspnea and wheezing
- Severe claudication

BP, blood pressure; ECG, electrocardiogram; ICD, implanted cardiac defibrillator.
*Due to anxiety, some patients may prematurely request to stop. In these patients, it is important to provide reassurance and encouragement.
Modified and adapted from *ACSM's Guidelines for Exercise Testing and Prescription (1)* and *ACC/AHA 2002 Guideline Update for Exercise Testing (2)*.

The importance of a symptom-limited *maximal exercise* test cannot be overemphasized. Specifically, if an exercise test is stopped when a patient reaches a predetermined heart rate or work rate, or before symptom-limited maximum, it will result in a lower peak heart rate. As a result, the exercise-training target heart rate developed from this peak heart rate will be lower than if the patient achieved their true maximum heart rate. Thus, while following this target heart rate the patient will train at an exercise intensity that does not provide optimal benefits. Furthermore, some patients might not remain engaged with their exercise program at this low intensity because it feels too easy. Last, hemodynamic information (e.g., heart rate and blood pressure) derived from a non exercise stress test (e.g., Adenosine or Dobutamine stress test) is not useful for developing an exercise prescription.

In some patients, the baseline ECG precludes clinically meaningful assessment of repolarization changes related to ischemia. Examples include patients with left bundle branch block, atrial fibrillation, pacemakers, and cardiac transplant. When assessing the presence of ischemia in these patients, a GXT with imaging (e.g., echocardiography or nuclear imaging) is recommended *(2)*. However, in the absence of suspected ischemia, a GXT with ECG alone provides useful information to establish an exercise prescription and guide the patient during an exercise-training program.

TIMING OF THE GXT

A symptom-limited maximal GXT can be safely performed 2 weeks after an uncomplicated acute myocardial infarction *(1)*. A similar time period can be used for patients who have had a percutaneous coronary intervention or coronary artery bypass surgery. For patients who have had surgery involving a sternotomy, allowing additional time before the GXT may allow for continued resolution of pain and healing of the sternum. Peak exercise capacity (as measured by peak VO_2) is lower in patients entering cardiac rehabilitation after coronary artery bypass surgery and may be due to postoperative discomfort *(3)*.

Although a GXT provides useful information, it may not be necessary for all patients participating in cardiac rehabilitation. McConnell et al. *(4)* reported that patients completing 12 weeks of cardiac rehabilitation can be safely progressed and demonstrate similar improvements in caloric expenditure, independent of whether they have a GXT prior to starting the program. However, current guidelines support testing prior to starting cardiac rehabilitation in most patients *(2)*. Despite this, it is not uncommon for patients to begin phase II cardiac rehabilitation without a recent GXT. In a survey by Andreuzzi et al. *(5)*, 60% of phase II cardiac rehabilitation programs do not require a GXT prior to program entry.

Scheduling the GXT to occur some time during a patient's stay in cardiac rehabilitation may be helpful in situations where obtaining the GXT may delay the patient's ability to start the program. Delayed scheduling of the GXT may also be helpful for patients with very low functional capacity *(1)*, inexperience with exercise, or anxiety to exercise. These patients may be able to provide a better effort during a GXT after having participated in several visits in cardiac rehabilitation to "practice" exercising.

REPEATING THE GXT

In select patients, the GXT may need to be repeated. If a patient experiences new or worsening symptoms during exercise training, they should be re-evaluated by their physician and a repeat GXT considered. Also, if a patient's beta-adrenergic blocking agent is decreased or discontinued, it would be appropriate to repeat the GXT to re-assess their heart rate response and the presence of ischemia. Conversely, if a patient's beta-blocker is increased, repeating the GXT is not as important because new ischemia will not be a concern. However, they will not be able to reach their target heart rate range and instead should guide exercise intensity using perceived exertion.

In isolated patients, the prescribed target heart rate may not seem to be a "good fit." These patients typically report very low ratings of perceived exertion while exercising within or above their target heart rate range, and some may even be comfortably exercising at or above their peak heart rate. It is possible that these patients did not truly undergo a maximal GXT at program entry. Repeating the GXT in these patients is especially important if they plan to return to a physically demanding job or leisure activity. However, before repeating a GXT in these patients, it should be confirmed that they are taking their medications as prescribed and that they understand the perceived exertion scale.

PRE-TEST CONSIDERATIONS

Pre-test recommendations and patient instructions have been published (2) and are summarized in Table 2. Because the purpose of the GXT performed in conjunction with an exercise-training program is to establish an exercise prescription, it is important that conditions during the GXT are similar to those experienced by the patient during exercise training. Most important among these are the timing of medications and the time of day.

Patients should take their medications as prescribed by their physician 3–10 hours prior to the GXT. Most important among these are beta-adrenergic blocking agents and long-acting nitrates. If a patient forgets to take either of these medications, consider rescheduling the test. The absence of the beta-blocker will result in an accentuated heart rate response and a resultant target heart rate range that will not mimic conditions when the beta-blocker is taken. Also, the absence of the beta-blocker or nitrate may result in exercise being limited by ischemia or chest pain, which will limit peak heart rate and the assessment of functional capacity.

PROTOCOL SELECTION

The Bruce protocol is the most frequently used treadmill protocol (6). Work rate during the first stage is estimated at 4.6 metabolic equivalents (METs) and increases by 2.5–3.0 METs with each 3-min stage. The peak MET level of patients entering cardiac rehabilitation is 4–6 METs (3) and is even lower in patients with heart failure. On the basis of this information, the Bruce protocol is often not the protocol of choice for patients entering cardiac rehabilitation because they are only able to complete 1–2 stages (< 6 min) of this protocol. An appropriately selected protocol should result in an exercise test duration of ≈ 10 min (7). This provides time to assess heart rate and blood pressure response, as well as functional capacity. Therefore, a treadmill protocol with a lower starting MET level and increments of ≈ 2 METs per stage

Table 2
Pre-Test Patient Instructions and Planning

Patient instructions

- Take medications as prescribed and at least 3 h prior to test
- Avoid the following for at least 3 h prior to test
  o Caffeine and alcohol
  o Tobacco use
  o Large meal
- Avoid using skin lotion on chest and abdomen
- Do not exercise for 24 h prior to test
- Wear comfortable clothes suitable for exercise. Do not wear shoes with heels

Pre-test planning

- Schedule the test at a similar time of day as exercise training will be performed
- If a 6-min walk test is scheduled on the same day, it should occur at least 1 h before or after the test
- Consider rescheduling the test if the beta-adrenergic blocking agent or long-acting nitrate is not taken
- Do not perform the test if the patient has clinical changes that would limit their ability to provide a maximal exertion, such as resolving upper respiratory tract infection or an exacerbation of gout or arthritis.

Adapted from *ACC/AHA 2002 Guideline Update for Exercise Testing (2).*

should be considered in these patients. Examples are the Balke or Naughton protocols. Although the Modified Bruce protocol starts at an appropriate work rate (estimated 2.3 METs), beginning with stage 3 (1.7 mph and 10% grade), it then assumes the same work rate profile as the standard Bruce protocol and, therefore, is not a protocol of choice.

When possible, a GXT should be performed on a treadmill because it usually results in higher physiologic responses than tests performed using a leg or an arm ergometer. Compared with leg ergometry, treadmill exercise results in a higher measured peak VO_2 (10–15%) and peak heart rate (5–20%) *(6)*. Some patient who present with obesity, arthritis, or other comorbidities may be unable to adequately perform treadmill exercise and may need to be tested using an alternate exercise mode. When using a leg ergometer, the protocol should begin at 0–10 watts and increase by 10 watts per min or 20–30 watts per 2–3-min stage.

Arm ergometry is an alternative for patients who cannot perform leg exercise. Peak VO_2 during arm ergometry is 20–30% lower than that during leg ergometry, due to the smaller muscle mass recruited. During submaximal exercise at the same power output, heart rate and blood pressure are higher, whereas stroke volume and VO_2 are lower during arm (compared with leg) ergometry *(8)*.

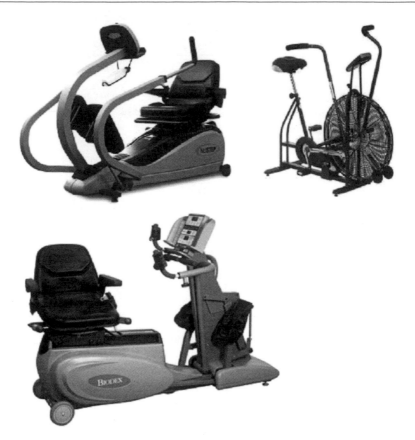

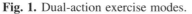

Fig. 1. Dual-action exercise modes.

Traditionally, GXTs have involved treadmill or ergometry (arm or leg) exercise. The treadmill is not an option for all patients, and regional muscle fatigue prematurely limits many patients during arm or leg ergometry. Alternatives to these traditional exercise modes are dual-action devices that utilize both the arms and legs (Fig. 1). These devices represent useful alternatives for patients who might not be able to provide sufficient effort during treadmill, arm, or leg exercise. However, little data are available comparing exercise responses with these modes to treadmill or leg ergometry.

PREPARING FOR THE GXT

Prior to starting the GXT, a medical history and informed consent should be obtained. It is important to assess the patient's physical activity history and symptoms they may be experiencing. Confirm that medications were taken as directed and that there is no clinical condition that indicates that the test should not be performed.

The patient should be prepped with electrode placement modified to monitor the ECG during exercise (9). Baseline ECG, vital signs, and symptoms should be assessed prior to starting the test in both supine and upright (seated or standing) positions. If the patient is able to walk without physical discomfort or limitation, then a treadmill protocol should be selected. Otherwise another exercise mode should be considered.

During a GXT, patients should be continuously monitored with an ECG. At regular intervals during the test, it is important to obtain a 12-lead ECG and assess blood pressure and the patient's rating of perceived exertion using a validated scale *(1)*. Measuring blood pressure via the auscultatory technique using the first and fifth Korotkoff sounds with a mercury sphygmomanometer remains the "gold standard." Regardless of whether the blood pressure is obtained manually or with an automated device, attention must be given to proper cuff size, stethoscope placement, and insuring that the observer is properly trained *(10)*.

CONDUCTING THE GXT

When using a treadmill, it is important to evaluate how the patient is walking. Instruct them as needed to improve walking mechanics. Patients should be encouraged to use the handrail only to maintain their balance. If comfortable, they should be allowed to walk without holding the handrail or holding it with only one arm. If the patient demonstrates difficulty walking and may benefit from additional instruction, consider stopping the protocol to allow for this. Optimally this decision should be made within the first 1–2 min of exercise. If this occurs, the protocol should be restarted from stage 1.

Continuously encourage the patient to exercise as long as possible to reach his/her maximum. During the test, regularly provide positive encouragement and avoid phrases that ask whether they are tired or ready to stop. At regular intervals during the test inquire about symptoms and record as present.

Some patients may feel they need to stop early into the protocol. It is important to re-assure them when appropriate. It can be helpful to ask them why they feel they need to stop. Many times these patients can be encouraged to continue to exercise well beyond the point where they initially felt they needed to stop. Again, encourage the patient to continue as long as they can. Obtain an ECG, blood pressure, and rating of perceived exertion as close to the end of the test as possible (before or immediately after).

When present, it is important to identify the heart rate, blood pressure, work rate, and signs or symptoms at the ischemic threshold. This information is useful in guiding the patient during exercise training. The point during exercise when systolic blood pressure declines or there is a significant increased frequency or complexity of ventricular arrhythmias (ventricular couplets or triplets) should also be noted *(1)*.

HEART RATE AND BLOOD PRESSURE RESPONSE
TO A GXT

Among patients with heart disease, with or without beta-adrenergic blockade therapy, heart rate increases with increasing work rate, however the peak response is reduced compared to those without the disease *(11)*. Furthermore, heart rate response is significantly lower in patients with, versus those without, beta-blocker therapy. Traditional equations to predict maximum heart rate (e.g., 220-Age) over predict and should not be used in patients with heart disease. However, maximum heart rate can be reasonably predicted using population-specific equations *(12)*; but as discussed previously, this should not be used as a reason to stop the test.

Systolic blood pressure progressively increases during a GXT from rest through peak exercise, whereas diastolic blood pressure does not change or decreases. An increase in systolic blood pressure of 10 mmHg per 1 MET increase in work rate can be expected.

Systolic blood pressure that does not rise with increasing work rate may be a sign of myocardial ischemia and/or left ventricular dysfunction *(1)*.

FUNCTIONAL CAPACITY

The analysis of expired air (oxygen consumption, VO_2) obtained during the GXT to quantify functional capacity is typically not completed during routine exercise testing associated with entry into cardiac rehabilitation. Fortunately, nomograms and mathematical formulae exist to estimate VO_2 using the exercise time for a given protocol or based on the highest work rate achieved. Most ECG/treadmill controllers calculate peak work rate and report it in METs; however, these methods can overestimate measured VO_2 by up to 30%. A large part of this discrepancy is due to the patient holding the treadmill's handrail for support.

PACEMAKERS AND IMPLANTED CARDIAC DEFIBRILLATORS

The GXT is useful and can be performed safely in patients with a pacemaker and/or implanted cardiac defibrillator (ICD). Information regarding chronotropic response during exercise in a patient with a rate-responsive pacemaker can be used to develop an exercise-training target heart rate range (Chap. 15). It is important to point out that some patients may reach their programmed upper rate, yet are able to continue to exercise to higher work rates. In this situation the heart rate will either not increase above the upper rate or it will increase due to the underlying intrinsic (non paced) rhythm. In either case the GXT can be continued to maximum exertion as long as systolic blood pressure is maintained and other indications to stop the test do not present (Table 1). The patient's cardiologist or electrophysiologist should be notified of the finding so they can consider increasing the upper rate setting. If the upper rate on the pacemaker is increased it may be useful to repeat the GXT. If the pacemaker is not reprogrammed then their blood pressure should be closely monitored during the initial exercise sessions to be sure it is maintained during exercise.

In patients with an ICD, the arrhythmia detection rate at which the ICD fires should be identified before the GXT is started *(13)*. In the absence of other reasons for stopping the test, the GXT should be stopped when the heart rate is 10 beats below the ICD fire rate.

SUPERVISION AND SAFETY

According to the American Heart Association *(9)*, trained personnel who are knowledgeable in exercise physiology should conduct the GXT. It is important to have a strong understanding of normal and abnormal responses to exercise in order to recognize and prevent adverse events. Training should include testing of a wide range of patient populations. Exercise physiologists, nurses, physician assistants, or physicians can be trained to administer exercise tests. They should also be trained in advanced cardiopulmonary resuscitation.

When performed by properly trained persons, a GXT is considered safe. Myocardial infarction or cardiac death occurs during 5 of 100,000 tests in patients without coronary artery disease and up to 10 per 10,000 tests in patients with coronary artery disease *(9)*. A properly trained physician should ensure that testing personnel are competent and oversee test interpretation. The American College of Cardiology and the American

Heart Association recommend that new physicians participate in at least 50 tests to insure adequate competence *(14)*. The degree of direct physician supervision during a GXT may vary depending on the clinical status of the patients being tested and the training and experience of the exercise physiologist or nurse supervising the test.

REFERENCES

1. American College of Sports Medicine. *ACSM Guidelines for Exercise Testing and Prescription*, 7th ed. Philadelphia, PA: Lippincott Williams & Wilkins; 2005.
2. Balady GJ, Bricker JT, Chaitman BR et al. ACC/AHA 2002 Guideline Update for Exercise Testing: A Report of the American College of Cardiology/American Heart Association Task Force on Practice Guidelines (Committee on Exercise Testing); 2002. Available at http://www.acc.org/clinical/guidelines/exercise/dirIndex.htm
3. Ades PA, Savage PD, Brawner CA et al. Aerobic Capacity in Patients Entering Cardiac Rehabilitation. Circulation. 2006;113:2706–2712.
4. McConnell TR, Klinger TA, Gardner JK, Laubach CA, Herman CE, Hauck CA. Cardiac Rehabilitation Without Exercise Tests for Post-Myocardial Infarction and Post-Bypass Surgery Patients. *J Cardiopulm Rehabil*. 1998;18:458–463.
5. Andreuzzi RA, Franklin BA, Gordon NF, Haskell WL. National Survey of Exercise Practices in Outpatient Cardiac Rehabilitation Programs. *Med Sci Sports Exerc*. 2004;34(Suppl 5):S181.
6. Myers J, Froelicher VF. Optimizing the Exercise Test for Pharmacological Investigations. *Circulation*. 1990;82:1839–1846.
7. Fleg JL, Pina IL, Balady GJ et al. Assessment of Functional Capacity in Clinical and Research Applications: An Advisory from the Committee on Exercise, Rehabilitation, and Prevention, Council on Clinical Cardiology, American Heart Association. *Circulation*. 2000;102:1591–1597.
8. Keteyian SJ, Marks CRC, Brawner CA, Levine AB, Kataoka T, Levine TB. Responses to Arm Exercise in Patients with Compensated Heart Failure. *J Cardiopulm Rehabil*. 1996;16:366–371.
9. Fletcher GF, GJ Balady, Amsterdam EA et al. Exercise Standards for Testing and Training: A Statement for Healthcare Professionals from the American Heart Association. *Circulation*. 2001;104:1694–1740.
10. Pickering TG, Hall JE, Appel LJ et al. Recommendations for Blood Pressure Measurement in Humans and Experimental Animals Part 1: Blood Pressure Measurement in Humans. *Hypertension*. 2005;45:142–161.
11. Bruce RA, Fisher LD, Cooper MN et al. Separation of Effects of Cardiovascular Disease and Age on Ventricular Function with Maximal Exercise. *Am J Cardiol*. 1974;34:757–763.
12. Brawner CA, Ehrman JK, Schairer JR, Cao JJ, Keteyian SJ. Predicting Maximum Heart Rate Among Patients with Coronary Heart Disease Receiving β-Adrenergic Blockade Therapy. *Am Heart J*. 2004;148:910–914.
13. Stevenson WG, Chaitman BR, Ellenbogen KA et al. Clinical Assessment and Management of Patients with Implanted Cardioverter-Defibrillators Presenting to Nonelectrophysiologists. *Circulation*. 2004;110:3866–3869.
14. Rodgers GP, Ayanian JZ, Balady G et al. ACC/AHA Clinical Competence Statement on Stress Testing: A Report of the American College of Cardiology/American Heart Association/American College of Physicians–American Society of Internal Medicine Task Force on Clinical Competence. *J Am Coll Cardiol*. 2000;36:1441–1453.

11

The Use of Cardiopulmonary Exercise Testing in Cardiac Rehabilitation: A Primer and Case Analysis

Paul Chase, MEd, RCEP®, CPFT, and Daniel Bensimhon, MD

CONTENTS

INTRODUCTION

Although cardiopulmonary exercise (CPX) testing remains the gold standard for assessing a patient's physiologic response to exercise, it is not routinely used in the cardiac rehabilitation (CR) setting. In fact, in their summary statement on exercise testing, the American College of Cardiology and American Heart Association have given CPX testing a Class IIb (usefulness or efficacy is less well established by evidence or opinion) indication for the determination of the intensity for exercise training as part of comprehensive CR *(1)*.

Nevertheless, when used in the appropriate settings, CPX testing can play a vital role in maximizing the potential benefit of CR in selected patients. The aim of this chapter is to provide a background on CPX testing techniques and interpretation and to help the practitioner identify CR scenarios in which CPX testing may serve as a useful adjunct to standard exercise testing.

CPX TESTING OVERVIEW

By using gas exchange analysis, CPX testing allows for the simultaneous study of cellular, cardiovascular, and ventilatory responses to exercise. As illustrated in Fig. 1

From: *Contemporary Cardiology: Cardiac Rehabilitation*
Edited by: W. E. Kraus and S. J. Keteyian © Humana Press Inc., Totowa, NJ

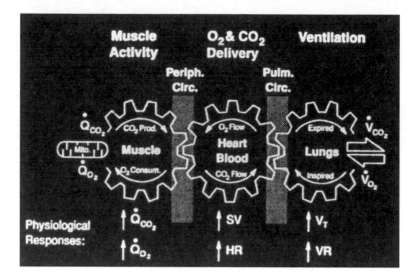

Fig. 1. Schematic of gas exchange mechanisms coupling cellular to pulmonary respiration during exercise *(4)*.

by Wasserman, exercise involves a complex series of steps by which oxygen is brought in by the respiratory system, delivered to working muscles by the circulatory system, and then turned into ATP to fuel work by the cellular apparatus within the muscles. Waste products from this process (predominantly CO_2) are then transported away from the muscles in a similar fashion. In combination with a general knowledge of exercise physiology, CPX testing can provide powerful insights into the etiology of a patient's exercise intolerance and help tailor the rehabilitation program to best suit his or her needs.

CARDIOPULMONARY EXERCISE-TESTING EQUIPMENT

The Ergometer

Cardiopulmonary exercise (CPX) testing can be performed on any type of exercise equipment that allows for a controlled, graded increase in the workload. Typically, testing is performed on a standard cycle ergometer or treadmill but can also be performed on an upper body ergometer for those who are unable to cycle or walk. Although each modality – bike and treadmill – has its proponents, neither should be considered superior as each has its advantages and disadvantages (Table 1). Many exercise-testing laboratories prefer a cycle ergometer as it takes up less space, is accessible to a wider group of patients, and permits a clearer assessment of workload – the workload is essentially weight independent. In contrast, other laboratories (including ours) favor a treadmill, as this is more akin to the daily activities patients will be performing. To ensure proper use, ergometers should be calibrated at least every 6 months using standard protocols or by a trained service representative.

Table 1
Relative Advantages of Treadmill Versus Cycle Ergometer
for Cardiopulmonary Exercise (CPX) Testing (2)

	Cycle	Treadmill
VO_2 max	Lower	Higher
Work rate measurement	Yes	No
Blood gas collection	Easier	More difficult
Noise and artifacts	Less	More
Safety	Safer	Less safe?
Weight bearing in obese	Less	More
Degree of leg muscle training	Less	More
More appropriate for	Patients	Active normal subjects

VO_2 max, maximal oxygen uptake.

The Metabolic Cart

Although a mass spectrometer remains the gold standard for gas exchange analysis, most laboratories now use commercially manufactured metabolic cart systems that contain both a flow meter device and gas cells to measure expired CO_2 and O_2 during exercise using either a breath-by-breath or mixing chamber format. Although each type of system has its advantages and disadvantages, these are beyond the scope of this chapter, and it should suffice to say that for general testing purposes either format is acceptable. Commonly used systems are made by several manufacturers [MedGraphics, Viasys (Sensormedics), and Parvomedics], although many other quality carts exist. For complete testing, the CPX cart should also be able to perform resting spirometry to measure FEV_1 and FVC, although it need not be able to measure lung volumes or diffusion capacity. With the expired gas data in hand, the metabolic cart is then able to use algorithms to back calculate values for inspired CO_2 and O_2 and display these in tabular format along with values for ventilation (Ve) or the amount of air being moved over a given time.

Although most of the hands-on CR staff can be trained to operate a metabolic cart and run an uncomplicated CPX test, there are many nuances to testing and numerous sources for potential error. Thus, we strongly advocate that CPX testing be done by an exercise physiologist who has been well trained in the modality and can troubleshoot the cart and make adjustments quickly. CPX training courses are available. [For more information go to the Medgraphics education website (3).]

Mouthpieces versus Masks for Collection of Expired Gases

Although several manufacturers have begun to promote the use of a facemask to serve as a scientifically equivalent – and more comfortable – alternative to a mouthpiece for collection of expired gases, it is our experience that these have not proven to be equivalent interfaces between the subject and cart. Even with various sizes of masks available, the range of variability in facial structure remains far greater and thus the use of a mask predisposes testing to a gas leak, which will falsely lower measured Ve and gas consumption values. As a result, we recommend the use of a mouthpiece for all testing unless the subject absolutely cannot tolerate it after multiple attempts with various-sized mouthpieces.

CPX TESTING PROTOCOLS

The same principles that guide the choice of an exercise protocol for standard graded exercise testing (GXT) should guide those for CPX testing (see chapter 10 on GXT). In general, a protocol should be chosen which leads to volitional fatigue in 8–10 min. If the protocol is too difficult and does not provide an adequate warm-up or the ramp between workloads is too steep, the patient may be overwhelmed and stop well before a maximum effort is given or equilibrium is attained. Conversely, if the workload starts too low or the ramp is too slow, the patient may stop prematurely due to boredom or lack of muscular endurance prior to reaching their maximal aerobic effort. For young, otherwise healthy individuals, a standard Bruce protocol remains the test of choice on the treadmill, whereas a 30W/min ramp protocol is often used on the bicycle. For older individuals or those with advanced heart disease [i.e., congestive heart failure (CHF)], a modified Naughton protocol (Table 2) that increases the workload 1 metabolic equivalent (MET) every 2 min is often the test of choice on the treadmill, and a 10W/min ramp is used on the bike.

INTERPRETING CPX TESTS

Test Reports

Data from a standard CPX test usually come in two or three parts. All reports should include a time-down or tabular data sheet showing values for preselected parameters [i.e., rate of O_2 consumption (VO_2), rate of CO_2 production (VCO_2), Ve, and respiratory exchange ratio (RER)] over various time averages. We recommend having the data formatted in 15–20-s intervals to allow for smoothing of the breath-by-breath data without too much averaging. Important parameters that should be captured on the time-down sheet include, but are not limited to, the workload (speed/grade for treadmill; watts for bicycle), absolute VO_2 (l/min), relative VO_2 (ml/kg/min), VCO_2 (l/min), Ve (BTPS), the RER or respiratory quotient (RQ), and end tidal CO_2 (if available).

Graphic displays of test results are also helpful. Most commercial systems have a standard set of graphs that they produce with each test. However, almost all allow the user to specify which graphs are created. The use and interpretation of these graphs are beyond the scope of this chapter; for more information consult *Principles of Exercise Testing and Interpretation (4)*.

Finally, many commercial metabolic carts generate a summary report of test data including both graphical depiction of exercise data and a computerized interpretation.

Table 2
Modified Naughton Exercise-Testing Stages

Stage	Rest	1	2	3	4	5	6	7	8	9	10
Time (min)	0	2	4	6	8	10	12	14	16	18	20
Speed (mph)	0	1.0	1.5	2.0	2.0	2.0	3.0	3.0	3.0	3.0	3.4
Slope (%)	0	0	0	3.5	7.0	10.5	7.5	10.0	12.5	15.0	14.0
METs	1.2	2.3	3.3	4.5	5.5	6.5	7.5	8.5	9.5	10.5	11.5

METs, metabolic equivalents.

Although the graphical reports are essential for test interpretation, we discourage the use of the computerized written summary report as test data can often be highly variable, and accurate interpretation is best done by trained personnel looking directly at the test data.

Important CPX Test Parameters

As with any standard exercise test, overall exercise time, clinical symptoms, electrocardiogram (ECG) changes, and the heart rate (HR) and BP response to exercise remain crucial variables during CPX testing. However, CPX testing offers other information that can add to the clinical assessment. A few of the most important and commonly used variables are as follows:

(i) VO_2 – Peak VO_2 or O_2 consumption. This is typically the most sought after variable as it provides an objective measure of peak exercise tolerance. In selected cardiac patients (i.e., those with LV dysfunction or heart failure), peak VO_2 has strong prognostic abilities. It must be pointed out that although prediction equations and charts exist to estimate peak VO_2 or peak METs from work rate on a treadmill or bike, these equations are based on the supposition that VO_2 increases linearly with increasing work rate. This is often not the case in patients with cardiovascular disease or obesity, and the use of these prediction equations should be avoided in CR *(4, p. 84)*.

When selecting the peak VO_2, many laboratories favor averaging the two or three of the 15- or 20-s average values obtained over the last minute of exercise. However, others feel that unless a true VO_2 plateau is reached, the single highest (nonaberrant) value should be counted as the peak measured VO_2. It is not uncommon for the VO_2 to peak in the early (first 30 s of recovery), as ventilatory responses naturally lag the cellular activity *(5)*.

Although we favor using the absolute VO_2 (l/min) over the relative VO_2 (ml/kg/min) as the former reading is not confounded by obesity, the relative VO_2 has become the more commonly used parameter. It is important to remember that many obese people will have a normal or supra-normal absolute O_2 consumption; however, when their absolute O_2 consumption is divided by their body weight, the relative VO_2 may be quite low compared with age, height, and gender-derived norms, essentially a fit person hiding in a large body. If your laboratory chooses to report relative VO_2 as a measure of overall fitness, the percentage predicted VO_2 calculated should be also reported. Standard formulas to calculate predicted VO_2 based on age, height, weight, and gender for "healthy" sedentary adults are available in *Principles of Exercise Testing and Interpretation (4)*.

When Interpreting VO_2, General Convention is as Follows:

- 80% predicted VO_2 = normal functional capacities
- 60–80% predicted VO_2 = mildly reduced functional capacity
- 40–60% predicted VO_2 = moderately reduced functional capacity
- <40% predicted VO_2 = severely reduced functional capacity

(ii) **Respiratory exchange ratio or respiratory quotient**. By providing an objective assessment of effort, the RER or RQ is perhaps the biggest factor that puts CPX testing ahead of standard exercise testing for use in CR. Calculated by dividing the amount of CO_2 produced by the amount of O_2 consumed, the RER indicates the predominant fuel being used for exercise and thus provides an independent measure of exercise intensity. An RER 0.7 indicates that fat is the predominant fuel source for activity and suggests a low workload. As the RER approaches 1.0, it signifies a switch to predominantly glucose being used as a fuel source and suggests an increasing but not maximum effort. At values greater than 1.0, the RER indicates increasing levels of lactate production and an increasing anaerobic and more difficult workload. An RER ≥ 1.10 is generally accepted as a maximal effort, although motivated individuals can often exceed 1.20 or 1.30.

(iii) **Ve/MVV**. The ventilation/maximum voluntary ventilation ratio also known as the dyspnea index or its derivative, the breathing reserve (1 – Ve/MVV), provides important information as to the nature of a subject's exercise limitation. Once exercise Ve approaches 50% of the measured MVV, dyspnea will occur. At 80%, dyspnea will be severe and exercise will usually end within 1 min due to a ventilatory limitation. Typically, during maximum exercise, subjects will be limited by their circulatory system and not their Ve (Ve/MVV < 70% at peak); however, a ventilatory limit is often seen in patients with significant intrinsic lung disease or morbid obesity. Occasionally, exceptionally fit subjects can also reach a ventilatory limit, but this is quite rare. The MVV should be determined by a 12-s spirometry on the day of the test (or from recent pulmonary function tests) and not be estimated from prediction equations. As a rough check, the MVV should approximate 35–40 times the measured FEV_1 unless a significant component of respiratory muscle fatigue is present.

(iv) **Ventilatory (anaerobic) threshold**. The anaerobic threshold is the work rate or VO_2 at which lactate begins to accumulate in exercising muscles. This cellular phenomenon is reflected by changes in Ve as VCO_2 exceeds VO_2 due to the production of excess CO_2 created by the bicarbonate buffering of lactic acid in the blood. Graphically, this inflection point is known as the ventilatory threshold (VT) or ventilatory anaerobic threshold (VAT) and can be determined by plotting VCO_2 versus VO_2, Ve/VCO_2 versus Ve/VO_2, or the RER over time. The most accepted way of determining the VT has been deemed the V-slope method ATS/ACCP and consists of plotting the VCO_2 (ml/min) for each time point (usually in 15- or 20-s averages) on the y-axis versus the VO_2 (ml/min) and looking for the point at which the slope of the line becomes more steep *(6)*. (Most commercial carts will plot this graph automatically.) The VO_2 corresponding to the inflection point is considered the VT and can be an important measure in guiding exercise prescription as will be discussed in a subsequent section. In normal subjects, the VT should typically fall between 40 and 70% of the *predicted* peak VO_2 and can improve significantly with appropriate training.

(v) **O_2 pulse**. The O_2 pulse is calculated as the VO_2/HR and serves as a surrogate for stroke volume, although it also takes into account the ability of skeletal muscles to extract O_2 from the blood. Most commercially available metabolic carts include age and gender reference values for O_2 pulse. The presence of a low-flattened O_2 pulse on a CPX test should arise suspicion for underlying heart failure or other circulatory limitations (i.e., myocardial ischemia).

(vi) Ve-VCO$_2$ slope. The ratio comparing the rate of increase in exercise Ve to the rate of increase in CO$_2$ production is an indicator of ventilatory efficiency and the amount of dead space. In patients with conditions such as advanced heart failure, intrinsic lung disease, pulmonary hypertension, and chronic pulmonary emboli, there can be significant Ve perfusion mismatching and up-regulated ergo- and chemoreceptors leading to an elevated Ve–VCO$_2$ slope. Several studies have shown that an elevated Ve-VCO$_2$ slope (≥ 34) portends a worse prognosis in patients with both systolic and diastolic heart failure and should be the cause for intensification of management (7,8).

USING CPX TESTING IN CR: CASE EXAMPLES

Although standard exercise testing is usually sufficient to determine the appropriate exercise intensity for participants in CR, there are instances where a standard exercise prescription based on the heart reserve formula may appear too easy or too stringent for a patient, and this is when CPX testing with gas exchange analysis can be used to determine a more appropriate exercise prescription or alter therapy.

When CPX Testing might be a more Appropriate than Standard Exercise Testing for Exercise Prescription or Evaluation

- HR-based exercise seems too hard. Subject potentially working over VT. Can be common in patients with advanced HF who have low VTs.
- HR-based exercise seems too easy. Subject potentially did not give maximum effort on entry exercise test, and HR prescription is artificially low
- Description of perceived exertion/symptoms does not match patient appearance, i.e., patient reports an RPE of 19 but is able to talk during exercise or subject reports RPE of 10 but appears to be giving near maximal effort
- Measuring impact of comorbid conditions, i.e., chronic obstructive pulmonary disease (COPD) or identifying other causes of exercise intolerance
- To quantitatively measure impact of a specific therapy on exercise capacity

---

The following three cases illustrate how CPX testing results can be used to modify exercise prescription successfully.

Case #1: Heart Rate Reserve-Based Exercise Prescription Appears too Easy

A 58-year-old man who recently had a large anterior myocardial infarct complicated by a ventricular fibrillation arrest requiring defibrillation and emergent stenting of his left anterior descending has been referred to CR. The patient, who was previously healthy and active, now has severe left ventricular dysfunction with an ejection fraction of 20% and a left bundle-branch block. Prior to enrollment he exercised for 4 min on a standard Bruce protocol and stopped due to shortness of breath. Peak Borg RPE was 15/20. Resting HR was 85 beats/min (bpm); peak HR was 122 bpm. Using the heart rate reserve (HRR) method, the patient was given a training range 107–111 bpm (60–70% HRR). The patient has now been exercising for 3 weeks, and both the patient and the rehab staff feel that the workload is inappropriately low for him; however, his physician has been reluctant to allow him to exercise above 70% of his HRR.

A CPX test is ordered. The patient exercises for 10:30 on a modified Naughton protocol. Resting HR is 78 bpm. Peak is 128. Exercise is again stopped due to dyspnea. Peak VO_2 is 18.9 ml/kg/min (62% predicted). Peak RER is 1.01. Peak RPE is 14/20. VAT was reached at 16.2 ml/kg/min (53% of maximum predicted VO_2). Peak Ve/MVV ratio is 49% suggesting ventilatory reserve remained. Ve–VCO_2 slope was 30 suggesting a relatively normal ventilatory efficiency. There were occasional premature ventricular contractions (PVCs) but no arrhythmias. Exercise ECG was uninterpretable for ST-T wave changes due to the left bundle-branch block. On the basis of this test, the 60–70% HRR training range would be 108–113 bpm. Alternatively, a rest HR+20-bpm prescription would give a training range of 98–103.

After reviewing the CPX test, it appears that the patient stopped short of a true maximum aerobic or ventilatory effort as the RER is well below 1.10 and the peak Ve/MVV is well under 80. It should be noted that although an RER of 1.10 is traditionally accepted as an indicator of a maximum effort, a significant amount of patients – especially those with advanced heart failure – may not be able to attain this threshold despite a true maximal effort. However, the normal VT and "lowish" peak RPE (should be at least 17–18 with true max effort) suggest that the patient may have stopped a bit prematurely, perhaps due to a reasonable fear of pushing himself too hard. The results of the CPX test were reviewed with the patient and the referring physician. Both were reassured regarding the safety of exercise, and the HR prescription was increased to a range of 115–125 bpm, which the patient was able to tolerate comfortably and appeared more appropriate.

Case #2: Patient's Symptoms or Exercise Intolerance Appear More Severe than Expected from Clinical Data

A 52-year-old woman was referred to CR for chronic angina. She is an ex-heavy smoker (stopped 10 years ago) who experienced an acute inferior myocardial infarction 6 years ago, which was treated with stenting of her right coronary artery. She did well until the past few months when she began to notice decreased exercise tolerance and chest pain and has been having difficulty completing her normal 3-mile walk. She underwent an exercise nuclear study during which she walked for 5:30 on a standard Bruce protocol and stopped due to chest pain and shortness of breath. Resting HR was 68. Peak HR was 109 (65% of age-predicted maximum). There were no significant ST-T wave changes on the exercise ECG, although the peak HR was inadequate. Imaging revealed an ejection fraction (EF) 57% with a previous inferior infarction but no inducible ischemia. Owing to continued chest discomfort and exercise intolerance, the patient was referred to cardiac catheterization, which showed a patent right coronary artery (RCA) stent with minimal nonobstructive coronary disease elsewhere. Right heart catheterization revealed normal pressures and cardiac output. This was followed by a chest CT scan that ruled out pulmonary embolus. Patient was presumed to have microvascular coronary disease and thus referred to cardiac rehab. During the first few weeks of rehabilitation, the patient appeared markedly dyspneic and experienced chest tightness on starting exercise, which occasionally improved after warming up; however, the patient was unable to get HR much over 100 bpm. Pool exercises were recommended, but the patient was unable to tolerate due to severe dyspnea. A CPX test was ordered to further evaluate the cause of patient's dyspnea and chest pain.

Patient walked 9:20 on a modified Naughton protocol. Stopped due to severe dyspnea and chest discomfort. Patient noticed to have end-exercise wheezing. Peak HR was 106. Peak VO_2 was 18.2 ml/kg/min (74% predicted). Peak RER was 0.99 suggesting a submaximal aerobic effort, although peak RPE was 19/20. There were no ECG changes. The O_2 pulse and VT were normal. Peak Ve was 48 l/min with a peak respiratory rate 54 breaths/min. Resting spirometry was normal with FEV_1 1.95 l (82% predicted), FVC 2.36 (82% predicted), FEV_1/FVC 83%, and MVV 78 l/min. However, immediate (< 30 s) postexercise spirometry revealed a marked reduction (27%) in the patient's FEV_1 from rest at 1.43 l. Thus, peak MVV was recalculated using the formula $FEV_1 \times 40$ to give a peak MVV of 57 l/min and an Ve_1/MVV of 84% suggesting a pulmonary/ventilatory limitation related to exercise-induced bronchospasm. The patient was referred to a pulmonologist and started on inhalers with a marked improvement in her exercise capacity and relief of her chest discomfort. She completed 12 weeks of a combined cardiac/pulmonary rehab program.

Case #3: Heart Rate-Based Exercise Prescription Appears too Difficult for Patient

A 69-year-old obese man with an ischemic cardiomyopathy was referred for CR after his second coronary artery bypass surgery. He was markedly debilitated and had a left ventricular EF of 15%. Given his debility, an entrance exercise test was deferred, and he was given a training HR of resting HR (87 bpm)+20–25 bpm for a training range of 107–112. However, he was unable to achieve this HR comfortably. A CPX test was ordered to assess patient's functional capacity and ability to exercise. Resting HR was 84 bpm. The patient walked for 4:45 on a modified Naughton protocol. Peak VO_2 was 13.4 ml/kg/min (58% of predicted maximum). Peak HR was 127 (84% of age-predicted maximum). Exercise was stopped due to fatigue. There was no chest pain or significant ECG changes. Peak RER was 1.18 suggesting a maximal effort. Peak RPE was 18/20. The O_2 pulse was flattened suggesting a circulatory limitation. The VT was low and reached at 6.7 ml/kg/min (29% of predicted peak VO_2). The HR at VT was 99 bpm.

Using a traditional HRR method to calculate an exercise prescription for 60–70% of max HRR, the training range was determined to be 110–114 bpm, which the patient had already proven he could not tolerate. In looking at the results of the CPX test, it was noted that the patient's ventilatory anaerobic threshold was quite low as can be seen in deconditioned patients and those with advanced heart failure. At that point, two options were considered. (1) Using a HR prescription based on the patient's HR at VT (typically we use a training range from HR at VT-10 bpm as the lower training range up to HR at VT – 5 beats/min) or (2) using an RPE -based prescription. Although we have had success with both in our program, the RPE-based prescription tends to allow patients to increase their exercise heart rates naturally as their fitness improves.

Thus, the patient was given a training range based on RPE of 12–14. The patient was then allowed to resume exercise. Using RPE 12–14, exercise heart rates ranged from 94 to 100, which fell just below and ranged up to the patient's ventilatory threshold. After 12 weeks of rehab, the patient's exercise tolerance improved markedly. CPX testing was repeated revealing a nearly 20% increase in peak VO_2 as well as his VT, and the patient was then able to be transitioned back to a standard HRR prescription.

REFERENCES

1. Gibbons RJ, Balady GJ, Bricker JT, et al. ACC/AHA 2002 Guideline Update for Exercise Testing: A Report of the American College of Cardiology/American Heart Association Task Force on Practice Guidelines (Committee on Exercise Testing); 2002. Available at http://www.acc.org/clinical/guidelines/exercise/dirIndex.htm
2. ATS/ACCP. Statement on Cardiopulmonary Exercise Testing. *Am J Respir Crit Care Med.* 2003;167(2):232.
3. Medgraphics. Available at http://www.medgraphics.com/education.html
4. Wasserman K, Hansen JE, Sue DY, et al. *Principles of Exercise Testing and Interpretation*, 4th ed. Philadelphia, PA: Lippincott Williams & Williams; 2005.
5. Cohen-Solal A, Czitrom D, Geneves M, Gourgon R. Delayed Attainment of Peak Oxygen Consumption After the End of Exercise in Patients with Chronic Heart Failure. *Int J Cardiol.* 1997;60(1):23–29.
6. Beaver WL, Wasserman K, Whipp BJ. A New Method for Detecting the Anaerobic Threshold by Gas Exchange. *J Appl Physiol.* 1986;60:2020–2027.
7. Chua TP, Ponikowski P, Harrington D, et al. Clinical Correlates and Prognostic Significance of the Ventilatory Response to Exercise in Chronic Heart Failure. *J Am Coll Cardiol.* 1997;29(7):1585–1590.
8. Robbins M, Francis G, Pashkow FJ, et al. Ventilatory and Heart Rate Responses to Exercise: Better Predictors of Heart Failure Mortality than Peak Oxygen Consumption. *Circulation.* 1999;100(24):2411–2417.

12 Role of the 6-Minute Walk Test in Cardiac Rehabilitation

Vera Bittner, MD, MSPH

BACKGROUND

Exercise testing is a key component of the initial patient assessment performed when a patient enrolls in a cardiac rehabilitation program, and change in functional capacity has become a common clinical outcome in cardiac rehabilitation programs (1). Traditionally, exercise testing has been conducted on a treadmill or bicycle ergometer using graded intensity protocols designed to determine maximal exercise capacity. Maximal exercise testing has been extensively validated for diagnosis, prognostication, and exercise prescription, all of which are discussed in detail elsewhere in this book. However, such testing requires specialized facilities, equipment, and personnel and is associated with considerable cost, which may or may not be covered by third-party payers in the cardiac rehabilitation setting.

Submaximal exercise testing using the 6-min walk test is now used by many cardiac rehabilitation programs both for initial assessment and to document functional outcomes after completion of the cardiac rehabilitation program. The 6-min walk test was originally described by Guyatt et al. (2). It is simple to conduct, has excellent patient acceptance because exercise levels during the test closely resemble usual patient activities, and costs of administration are low. Reference equations for expected walk performance exist for middle-aged and older adults (3,4). The 6-min walk has been widely used in the research setting in patients with cardiovascular and pulmonary disease as a measure of functional capacity, as a marker for disease severity and prognosis,

From: *Contemporary Cardiology: Cardiac Rehabilitation*
Edited by: W. E. Kraus and S. J. Keteyian © Humana Press Inc., Totowa, NJ

and as an outcome measure in clinical trials testing medical and surgical/procedural therapies *(5)*. Data collected in the cardiac rehabilitation setting are more limited *(6–8)*. This chapter will describe how to conduct 6-min walk testing, how to effectively use the data in the cardiac rehabilitation setting [largely based on the experiences at the University of Alabama at Birmingham (UAB)], and highlights gaps in the research literature that warrant further study.

HOW TO CONDUCT A 6-MIN WALK

Table 1 summarizes the 6-min walk protocol that has been used at the UAB Hospital Cardiopulmonary Rehabilitation Program since 1996; the current data collection sheet is reproduced in Fig. 1. The walk tests are conducted by cardiac rehabilitation professionals when a patient enters the program and again at graduation. Presence of a physician is not required, but all testers are trained in advanced cardiac life support, and resuscitation equipment is immediately available. Studies have shown that the instructions provided to the patient at the beginning of the walk, the length of the walking track, the use of encouragement, the provision of a time frame (by calling out to the patient at the 2-min and 4-min time points), and positioning of the tester (walking with the patient versus being stationary in one area of the track) can all significantly influence distance walked *(5)*. Although there is no single best walk test protocol, standardization of walk test administration within a cardiac rehabilitation program is critically important, if valid data are to be obtained. Each tester should be carefully trained to perform the testing, and review of procedures and retraining as necessary should be done at regular intervals. Standardization of protocols across programs would be desirable to permit pooled data analyses and between program comparisons. Data obtained during the 6-min walk test together with many demographic and clinical variables can be prospectively recorded in a clinical outcome database and patient information tracked from time of enrollment through the completion of the cardiac rehabilitation program. This database can be used for report generation, program assessment, quality improvement initiatives, and, if approved by an Institutional Review Board, for research purposes.

The data collection sheet used in the UAB program is depicted in Fig. 1. Based on the prognostic groups in the Studies of Left Ventricular Dysfunction (SOLVD) Registry Substudy, walk distances are stratified into four levels, where Level 1 represents the shortest walk distances and poorest prognosis, and Level 4 represents the longest walk distances and best prognosis *(9)*. In the UAB program, 24% of patients perform at Level 1 during their baseline test, 23% at Level 2, 26% at Level 3, and 27% at Level 4 (unpublished data based on an interim analysis in January 2006). Although we believe that this classification helps us to risk-stratify patients, it is important to realize that the relationship between 6-min walk distance and long-term mortality or hospitalization has not been validated in a cardiac rehabilitation population. In addition to the distance walked, ratings of perceived exertion (RPE) and presence and severity of angina and dyspnea are recorded. Blood pressure and heart rate are measured before and after testing. Monitoring of oxygen saturation during testing is not mandatory, but because many patients have concomitant heart and lung diseases and elevated pulmonary arterial pressures, such monitoring occasionally documents oxygen desaturation during the walk, at times severe enough to warrant the prescription of supplemental oxygen during

Table 1
Six-Minute Walk Test Protocol

Purpose

To provide a simple, inexpensive, and noninvasive method for assessing a cardiac or pulmonary patient's functional capacity.

Equipment

1. Level walking surface that is at least 100 ft in length and free from obstruction. Mark walking surface at 10-ft intervals.
2. Chair available at 50-ft distance.
3. Stopwatch.
4. Six-minute walk documentation form
5. Stethoscope and sphygmomanometer.
6. If patient's clinical status requires: telemetry monitor, pulse oximetry, supplemental portable oxygen.

Exclusion criteria

Persons with musculoskeletal problems that significantly limit walking such as paralysis, pain, and other problems that would contribute to suboptimal walking performance; uncontrolled angina or hypertension, recent history of cardiac dysrhythmia or myocardial infarction, and other significant medical conditions that might be worsened by physical exertion.

Procedure

1. Resting vital signs are recorded before walk: blood pressure, heart rate, and pulse oximetry (if indicated).
2. The walks should be carried out in an area with minimal traffic that is at least 100 ft in length.
3. The following instructions are given to participants:
   "The purpose of this test is to find out how far you can walk in 6 minutes. You will start from this point (indicate marker at one end of the course) and follow the path until the 6-minute period is complete. If you need to stop during this time, please do but remain where you are until you can go again. I will tell you the time every two minutes and when to stop when the 6 minutes are up. When I say 'stop', please stand right were you are." (Subjects are then asked to repeat their understanding of the instructions).
4. During the walk, the following words of encouragement are provided at 30-s intervals: "keep up the good work" or "you're doing fine".
5. Staff member may walk behind (*but not with*) the patient so as not to influence the subject's pace.
6. Participants are told when 2, 4, and 6 min (Stop) have elapsed.
7. The distance walked is measured and recorded to the nearest foot. If patient had to stop and rest, the duration of the rest time is recorded.
8. Immediately following completion of the walk test, participants are asked to rate their level of exertion (Borg Scale) and indicate what symptoms (if any) limited their walking according to the angina and/or dyspnea scale.
9. Immediately following completion of the walk test, staff member will assess and record patient's blood pressure, heart rate, and pulse oximetry (if indicated).
10. Staff member who administered the test will sign and date the form.

The 6 Minute Walk in Cardiac Rehabilitation
21

UAB *HOSPITAL*

Cardio-Pulmonary Rehabilitation

Six-Minute Walk Test

Keyplate

Resting Vital Signs: Heart Rate _____ Systolic BP _____ Diastolic BP _____ Pulse Oximetry _____

Mark number of laps made: _____

Total distance completed: _____ feet

Level I (<984 ft) _____   Level II (985–1229 ft) _____

Level III (1230 – 1476 ft) _____   Level IV (>1477 ft) _____

Number of times stopped: _____   Duration of rest times _____

End of walk test:

Heart Rate _____   Systolic BP _____   Diastolic BP _____   Pulse Oximetry _____

EXERTION SCALE		ANGINA SCALE		DYSPNEA SCALE	
6					
7	Very, Very Light				
8		0	No Angina	0	No Dyspnea
9	Very Light				
10					
11	Fairly Light	1	Light, barely noticeable	1	Mild, noticeable
12					
13	Somewhat Hard				
14		2	Moderate, bothersome	2	Mild, some difficulty
15	Hard				
16					
17	Very Hard	3	Severe, very uncomfortable	3	Moderate difficulty, can continue
18					
19	Very, Very Hard				
20		4	Most severe pain ever experienced	4	Moderate difficulty, cannot continue

Fall Risk Assessment (if any risk factor is observed or reported, document on problem list)

_____Unsteady gait/dizziness/imbalance
_____Impaired memory or judgment
_____Weakness
_____History of falls
_____Uses ambulatory assistance (e.g. cane, walker, w/c)

Test administered by: _____   Date: _____

Fig. 1. Six-minute walk data form. The figure depicts the data form used in our program to record all relevant 6-min walk data at entry to the program and at program completion.

exercise in the cardiac rehabilitation program and during activities of daily living. The cardiac rehabilitation professional also makes careful note of gait abnormalities or balance problems that mandate modification of the exercise prescription.

DETERMINANTS OF WALK PERFORMANCE

Age, gender, height, and body mass determine walk performance in healthy populations *(3–5)*. In the UAB cardiac rehabilitation program, walk performance is worse in older compared with that in younger individuals, in women compared with that in men, and in non-White patients compared with that in White patients. Baseline walk performance in the UAB program stratified by gender and ethnic group (non-Whites are predominantly African American) is summarized in Table 2 (unpublished data based on an interim analysis in January 2006). Walk performance also correlates with the American Association of Cardiovascular and Pulmonary Rehabilitation (AACVPR) risk stratification for events (a composite measure that takes into account left ventricular function, dysrhythmias, severity of underlying disease, symptoms of ischemia, and functional capacity and hemodynamic response as assessed by maximal exercise testing when available), history of sedentary lifestyle as determined by the cardiac rehabilitation professional, patient self-reported physical activity levels, and physical function as determined by the SF-36 questionnaire *(7)*. Also, we previously found that diabetes was an independent correlate of poorer walking performance unpublished data, and there was no relationship between distance walked and admitting diagnosis, left ventricular ejection fraction or body mass index. In a multivariate linear regression model with baseline walk distance as the dependent variable, age (standardized regression coefficient beta $= -0.33$, $p = 0.0014$) and self-reported level of physical function (standardized beta $= 0.51$, $p < 0.0001$) were strong independent predictors of performance, whereas RPE was only weakly, albeit significantly correlated (adjusted R^2 for the model: 0.53, $p < 0.0001$) *(7)*. Hamilton and Haennel observed similar age and gender differences in a Canadian cardiac rehabilitation population *(6)*. Note that walk distances were substantially higher in the Canadian population (mean $\pm$ SD 1680 $\pm$ 367 ft) compared with the UAB population (mean $\pm$ SD 1221 $\pm$ 398 ft), suggesting that each cardiac rehabilitation setting should establish its own typical ranges of distances walked.

Several studies have assessed the correlation between distance walked and maximal exercise capacity with variable results, likely due to the types of patients tested: the two tests tend to correlate best in populations with low functional capacity and worst in those with high functional capacity. Data in the cardiac rehabilitation setting are limited. In the Canadian cardiac rehabilitation population cited above, 6-min walk performance and metabolic equivalents (METs) achieved on a symptom-limited graded exercise test correlated with an $r = 0.687$ ($p < 0.001$) with maximum METs accounting for 47% of the variance in distance walked *(6)*. In a recent interim analysis of 471 patients with ischemic heart disease who completed the UAB program, the mean and median RPE during the walk were both approximately 11 with a standard deviation of 2 and a range from 6 to 18; 150 patients (32%) reported an RPE of 13 or greater, and 24 patients (5%) reported an RPE of 15 or greater (unpublished data). Although we

Table 2
Baseline Walk Distances Among Patients with Ischemic Heart Disease in the UAB Cardiac Rehabilitation Program

	White males (n = 562)	White females (n = 177)	Non-White males (n = 195)	Non-White females (n = 176)
Mean $\pm$ SD (ft)	1351 $\pm$ 361	1163 $\pm$ 380	1172 $\pm$ 372	915 $\pm$ 348
Median (ft)	1382	1206	1206	946
Minimum (ft)	120	117	125	80
Maximum (ft)	2322	2064	2040	1632

do not have maximal exercise test data in our population, the RPE analysis suggests that the 6-min walk test is more than a "submaximal" exercise test in a substantial proportion of patients enrolling in cardiac rehabilitation.

At program completion, patients tend to report fewer symptoms than at program entry (7). Most patients improve their walk distance, although some do not. Among the 471 UAB patients cited above, 82% increased their walk distance. Overall, median walk distance at baseline was 1303 ft and improved 202 ft (range: −367 to +1674 ft). A British cardiac rehabilitation program reported an improvement in 6-min walk distance from 1032 ± 249 to 1238 ± 258 ft over 6 weeks of training (two exercise sessions per week) but did not indicate what proportion of their patients improved (8). Although baseline walk distance tends to be the strongest predictor of distance walked at program graduation, several other correlates of change in walked distance are important. In a multivariate analysis published several years ago, age was inversely related to percent change in walking distance, whereas male gender, higher clinical risk score, percent change in exercise intensity over the course of the cardiac rehabilitation program, improvement in the chronotropic response during the walk, symptoms during the follow-up walk, and self-reported relative change in physical activity level all independently predicted greater improvement in walking distance (adjusted $R^2 =$ 0.44, $p < 0.0001$) (7). It is unclear whether the lower degree of improvement among women and older patients is a function of gender and age or relates to a more conservative exercise prescription in these patients who are not accustomed to exercising on treadmills and bicycles and have lower activity levels at home.

WHAT ELSE TO DO WITH THE DATA

Potential uses of the 6-min walk data are summarized in Table 3. Assessment of functional capacity at program entry, assessment of symptoms and oxygenation, and outcome assessment at the program level have already been described above. Results of the entry and graduation walk are reported to the referring physician; thus, providing outcome assessment at the individual level is important as well. Recently, we have begun to calculate "% predicted walk distance" based on the reference equations of Enright et al., thus providing an external "benchmark" for our walk test results (3,10). Mean walk distance improved from 74% of what was predicted for age, gender, height, and weight at program entry to 88% at program completion. Expressing walk test results relative to those achieved by a similar healthy adult may provide patients and clinicians with a better understanding of the benefits achieved during participation in cardiac rehabilitation.

Distance walked provides prognostic information beyond the AACVPR risk assessment, and we make a point to monitor poor performers more closely during exercise. Poor performance on the entry 6-min walk test is also an independent predictor of dropout from cardiac rehabilitation, in patients who drop out for medical reasons as well as among those who drop out for nonmedical reasons (11). Although we have not found an intervention that will "prevent" dropout, we try to provide extra encouragement to those with poor walk distances (i.e., those in Level 1) and follow up immediately by telephone when they miss an exercise session.

Table 3
Potential Uses of the 6-Min Walk Test in Cardiac Rehabilitation

- Assessment of functional capacity
- Identification of gait abnormalities and balance problems
- Assessment of symptoms and relative perceived exertion
- Detection of oxygen desaturation or hemodynamic compromise with exercise
- Prognostication/risk assessment
- Identification of individuals at risk for drop out from the cardiac rehabilitation program
- Exercise prescription
- Outcomes assessment
  - Individual
  - Program

The 6-min walk test data also guide our initial exercise prescription by making use of the American College of Sports Medicine (ACSM) Walking Equation *(12)*, which specifies that approximately 0.1 ml of oxygen is needed for transporting each kilogram of body mass a horizontal distance of 1 m, that is, 0.1 ml/kg/min. This equation tends to be most accurate for speeds of 50–100 m/min (1.9–3.7 mph) *(12)*. An example of such a calculation that converts 6-min walk distance into walking speed and a MET level in cardiac rehabilitation is summarized in Table 4. The walking speed and MET level are used to tailor the initial phase of exercise to closely match the patient's current level of function. The exercise plan is updated at least weekly as exercise tolerance improves over the course of the supervised exercise sessions.

Table 4
Example of Using 6-Min Walk Data for Exercise Prescription

- **Distance measured**: the patient walked 1292 ft in 6 min.
- **Calculate walking speed**
  - Convert feet to meters: as 1 m = 3.281 ft; 1292 ft translates into 1292 ft/3.281 = 393.8 m.
  - Calculate speed in m/min: 393.8 m/6 min = 65.6 m/min [corresponds to 2.4 mph (1 mph = 26.8 m/min; thus 65.6 m/min/26.8 = 2.4 mph) which can be used to set treadmill speed]
- **Calculate metabolic value for walking without grade**
  - 1 MET = 3.5 ml/kg/min
  - 0.1 is the constant for converting m/min to ml/kg/min
  - Estimated oxygen consumption: VO_2 = 3.5 ml/kg/min + 65.6 m/min × 0.1 = (3.5 + 6.56) ml/kg/min = 10.06 ml/kg/min
  - MET level achieved: 10.06 ml/kg/min/3.5 = 2.9 METs
  - Metabolic value can be used for exercise prescription on apparatus other than treadmill

MET, metabolic equivalent.

SOME CAVEATS

Like all exercise testing, performance by a given patient is dependent not only on the patient's capacity to exercise but also on his/her motivation. There is no objective measure to determine whether a patient did his/her best during a given walk, and some "noise" is expected when conducting serial walks. Investigators have also described a learning effect when a patient performs 6-min walk testing on multiple occasions, but the extent of the learning effect and determinants of its extent remain controversial *(5,13)*. Performance of multiple walks at baseline and at follow-up has been advocated by some investigators and may be appropriate in clinical trial settings when greater precision of measurement before and after an intervention is critical. Repeated testing is generally not feasible in day-to-day clinical practice, as some patients are too ill at entry into cardiac rehabilitation programs to perform multiple consecutive tests on the same day, and transportation logistics may preclude serial testing on consecutive days before cardiac rehabilitation enrollment and at program graduation.

Distance covered during the 6 min of testing is a function of stride length and frequency. Because neither can be increased beyond a certain point without changing from walking to running, the 6-min walk has a built-in "ceiling effect" and is thus not a good measure of functional capacity in healthy, fit individuals. In contemporary cardiac rehabilitation settings where patient populations are older, often sedentary, and have a high comorbidity burden, this limitation is generally not a major concern. It is clear, however, that the 6-min walk test when conducted serially as an outcome measure tends to be most sensitive to improvement among those with shorter walking distances at baseline and least sensitive among those who performed very well at baseline *(7)*.

SUMMARY AND FUTURE RESEARCH DIRECTIONS

The 6-min walk is a safe and practical tool for outcome assessment in cardiac rehabilitation. It is well accepted by patients and staff, does not require specialized equipment (unless one chooses to supplement the testing with oximetry), and is less costly than standard maximal exercise testing. The test provides valid and reproducible data provided that a standardized protocol is used consistently. Such standardization is feasible in a busy clinical cardiac rehabilitation program. Performance on the baseline 6-min walk can be used for initial exercise prescription when data from maximal exercise testing are not available or when maximal exercise testing is contraindicated. Increases in self-reported physical activity level and improved functional capacity through exercise training are reflected in better walk performance at graduation from cardiac rehabilitation.

Further research is needed to ascertain in greater detail determinants and correlates of baseline walk performance and changes in walk performance after participation in cardiac rehabilitation. The impact of age, gender, ethnicity, and diabetes in particular also deserves further exploration. Once we understand what drives differences in walk performance, we can attempt to develop targeted interventions to optimize outcomes in all subgroups. It is unknown whether baseline walk distances in a cardiac rehabilitation population correlate with long-term mortality and morbidity, and we also do not know whether improvements in 6-min walk distances achieved in cardiac rehabilitation are sustained long-term or whether such improvements correlate with improvements in morbidity and mortality. Such analyses will be difficult to accomplish in single-site investigations, and multicenter collaborations should thus be encouraged.

ACKNOWLEDGMENT

I acknowledge and thank Bonnie Sanderson, PhD, RN, manager of the UAB Hospital Cardiopulmonary Rehabilitation program, and the Cardiopulmonary Rehabilitation staff, Chris Schumann, MA, RCEP, Jenny Breland, RN, Nicole Williams, RN, and Kelly Saunders, BA, for their dedicated efforts in patient care, data collection, and maintenance of data integrity that permits ongoing patient and program outcome assessment. Special credit goes to Chris Schumann, MA, RCEP, who developed the exercise prescription using 6-min walk test data. I also acknowledge and thank Steve Duncan, data analyst, for developing and maintaining our departmental database, Cardiopulmonary Outcomes: Prospective Evaluation (COPE).

REFERENCES

1. American Association of Cardiovascular and Pulmonary Rehabilitation. *Guidelines for Cardiac Rehabilitation and Secondary Prevention Programs*, 4th ed., Williams MA (ed.). Champagne, IL: Human Kinetics; 2004.
2. Guyatt GH, Sullivan MJ, Thompson PJ, Fallen EL, Pugsley SO, Taylor DW, Berman LB. The 6-Minute Walk: A New Measure of Exercise Capacity in Patients with Chronic Heart Failure. *Can Med Assoc J.* 1985;132:919–923.
3. Enright PL, Sherrill DL. Reference Equations for the Six Minute Walk in Healthy Adults. *Am J Respir Crit Care Med.* 1998;158:1384–1387.
4. Gibbons WJ, Fruchter N, Sloan S, Levy RD. Reference Values for a Multiple Repetition 6-Minute Walk Test in Healthy Adults Older than 20 Years. *J Cardiopulm Rehabil.* 2001;21:87–93.
5. American Thoracic Society. ATS Statement: Guidelines for the Six-Minute Walk Test. *Am J Respir Crit Care Med.* 2002;166:111–117.
6. Hamilton DM, Haennel RG. Validity and Reliability of the 6-Minute Walk Test in a Cardiac Rehabilitation Population. *J Cardiopulm Rehabil.* 2000;20:156–164.
7. Bittner V, Sanderson B, Breland J, Adams C, Schumann C. Assessing Functional Capacity as an Outcome in Cardiac Rehabilitation: Role of the 6-Minute Walk Test. *Clin Exerc Physiol.* 2000;21:19–26.
8. Wright DJ, Khan KM, Gossage EM, Saltissi S. Assessment of a Low-Intensity Cardiac Rehabilitation Programme Using the Six Minute Walk Test. *Clin Rehabil.* 2001;15:119–124.
9. Bittner V, Weiner DH, Yusuf S, et al. for the SOLVD Investigators. Prediction of Mortality and Morbidity with a 6-Minute Walk Test in Patients with Left Ventricular Dysfunction. *JAMA.* 1993;270:1702–1707.
10. Sanderson BK, Bittner V. Practical interpretation of 6-minute walk data using healthy adult reference equations. *J Cardiopulm Rehabil.* 2006;26:167–171.
11. Sanderson BK, Phillips MM, Gerald L, Fish L, DiLillo V, Bittner V. Factors Associated with the Failure of Patients to Complete Cardiac Rehabilitation for Medical or Non-Medical Reasons. *J Cardiopulm Rehabil.* 2003;23:281–289.
12. American College of Sports Medicine. *ACSM's Guidelines for Exercise Testing and Prescription*, 7th ed. Philadelphia, PA: Lippincott Williams & Wilkins; 2006:288.
13. Wu G, Sanderson BK, Bittner V. The 6 Min Walk Test: Is the Learning Effect Sustained Over Time? *Am Heart J.* 2003;146:129–133.

13

Cardiac Rehabilitation: Statins and the Rationale for Implementation of Lipid-Lowering Therapy

Ryan Neal and Christie Ballantyne

CONTENTS

From: *Contemporary Cardiology: Cardiac Rehabilitation*
Edited by: W. E. Kraus and S. J. Keteyian © Humana Press Inc., Totowa, NJ

CORONARY HEART DISEASE AND SECONDARY PREVENTION

Coronary heart disease (CHD) remains the leading cause of death in the United States. Although there has been an overall decline in mortality from acute coronary events, the prevalence of CHD continues to rise, largely due to the aging population and improved survival after myocardial infarction (post-MI). This increase has led to more patients at risk for recurrent ischemic events and subsequent death.

According to the American Heart Association (1), within 1 year of an MI, 25% of men and 38% of women will die of heart disease. Within the following 6 years of such an event, 18–34% of patients will suffer another MI, approximately 6% will have sudden death, 22–46% will develop congestive heart failure, and 8–11% will have a stroke (1). The total economic burden of cardiovascular disease will exceeds $300 billion in the United States annually this year alone (1). Although there is a growing body of evidence that lifestyle modification and pharmacological therapies can reduce recurrent events, numerous studies have carefully documented that clinicians are not following the available guidelines for secondary prevention to achieve appropriate outcomes. Current evidence clearly indicates that both secondary prevention and cardiac rehabilitation programs are effective systems for improving risk reduction (2). When combined, these two systems can offer the synergistic effect of achieving multiple goals for risk factor modification.

SECONDARY PREVENTION AND THE TREATMENT GAP

Secondary prevention is defined as an intervention or treatment that reduces the risk of recurrence, progression, or mortality in a person known to have cardiovascular disease. Multiple studies have documented the benefit of secondary prevention of CHD with lipid-lowering therapy (LLT) (3), hypertension control (4), smoking cessation (5), physical exercise (6), weight management (6), antiplatelet therapy (5), beta-blocker therapy (5), and angiotensin-converting enzyme (ACE)-inhibitor therapy (6) as single interventions as well as combined or comprehensive interventions. The implementation of LLT alone has the ability to reduce coronary events such as recurrent MI, angina pectoris, and coronary mortality by 25–42% (7). In addition, medical compliance with aspirin therapy has been shown to have a risk reduction benefit of 20–30%, beta-blocker therapy 20–35%, and ACE-inhibitor therapy 22–25% (5).

Despite these well-defined benefits in risk reduction, the data from the Can Rapid Risk Stratification of Unstable Angina Patients Suppress Adverse Outcomes With Early Implementation of the American College of Cardiology/American Heart Association Guidelines (CRUSADE) Quality Improvement Initiative trial found only 58% of patients admitted with acute coronary syndrome (ACS) had their low-density lipoprotein cholesterol (LDL-C) tested, and of those tested and appropriate for LLT, more than 30% were not treated with LLT (8). The definition of the treatment gap is the difference in the percent of patients eligible for a specific treatment and the percent of patients actually receiving that treatment. The estimated treatment gap for CHD patients, according to National Registry of Myocardial Infarction (9) and the Quality Assurance Program (10) data, is 66% for outpatient office practices and 68–80% for hospital discharges. Barriers to implementing risk factor modification guidelines for patients with CHD are several: (i) problem-focused physician visits, (ii) lack of systems to implement protocols or guidelines, (iii) time constraints and lack of incentives (including reimbursement), (iv) lack of knowledge and training on the benefits, and (v) lack of specialist–generalist communication. As a result, a large percentage of the patients with CHD are therefore undertreated and are at unnecessary risk for preventable cardiovascular events.

CARDIAC REHABILITATION

As outlined elsewhere in this volume, cardiac rehabilitation combines supervised prescriptive exercise training with CHD risk factor modification principles in patients with established CHD. Patients with the diagnosis of CHD, post-MI, coronary artery bypass surgery, post-percutaneous angioplasty, and other past cardiovascular surgeries including valve surgery and cardiac transplantation are eligible for referral to cardiac rehabilitation programs. The American Heart Association Medical/Scientific Position Statement on Cardiac Rehabilitation Programs (11) states that cardiac rehabilitation efforts targeted at exercise, lipid management, hypertension control, and smoking cessation can reduce cardiovascular mortality (12), improve functional capacity (13), attenuate myocardial ischemia (14), retard the progression of atherosclerosis (15), and reduce the risk for further coronary events (16). Therefore, cardiac rehabilitation is the standard of care and should be integrated into the overall treatment plan of patients with CHD.

RISK FACTOR MODIFICATION IN CARDIAC REHABILITATION

The concept of combining comprehensive risk factor modification with cardiac rehabilitation has been assessed in previous trials such as the Stanford Coronary Risk Intervention Project (SCRIP) (6). In this study, researchers evaluated the effects of intensive multiple risk factor reduction on coronary atherosclerosis over a 4-year period and found significant improvements in lipid profiles, body weight, and dietary compliance as well as decreased progression of coronary atherosclerosis. This study revealed that combining comprehensive secondary prevention guidelines with a standardized approach to cardiac rehabilitation could improve the effectiveness of implementing evidence-based risk factor modification standards.

DYSLIPIDEMIA AND THE RISK OF CHD

Dyslipidemia remains one of the major risk factors for CHD. The origin of the lipid hypothesis began with Virchow (17), who along with other scientists of his time observed the deposition of cholesterol within atherosclerotic plaques. Much later, the development of fractional assays allowed clinicians to identify and measure plasma cholesterol in humans. This discovery sparked desire to determine whether there was a link between plasma cholesterol in humans and the development of atherosclerotic plaques. Basic science researchers first established this relationship between cholesterol and atherosclerosis in animal models (18,19). This finding then led to a great interest in determining the role of cholesterol in humans, which led to the delineation of the cholesterol pathway, mechanisms involved in lipid deposition, and the discovery of the LDL receptor pathway (20). These discoveries and others opened the door to the practice of treating dyslipidemia and reducing CHD risk.

OBSERVATIONAL DATA FOR CHOLESTEROL AND THE RISK OF CHD

Multiple observational studies, such as The Framingham Heart Study *(21)* and the Multiple Risk Factor Intervention Trial (MRFIT) screenees *(22)*, began to solidify a direct relationship between patients with elevated cholesterol levels and the development of CHD. Moreover, these trials established a directly proportional relationship between total cholesterol (TC) and LDL-C to CHD.

These observational studies led to the development of randomized clinical trials (RCTs) to test the reverse hypothesis of whether lowering cholesterol in patients with elevated cholesterol levels reduces the risk of CHD. The earliest trials involved lifestyle modifications, such as diet, exercise, and weight loss, directed at lowering cholesterol and reducing the risk of CHD *(23)*. Soon thereafter, RCTs with pharmacologic LLTs began to confirm the hypothesis that lowering TC and LDL-C lowered the risk of cardiovascular morbidity and mortality *(24)*. As the wealth of clinical evidence mounted in support of lowering cholesterol to reduce the risk of cardiovascular disease, and as basic science evidence grew surrounding the understanding of LDL as the principal lipoprotein involved in the development of atherosclerosis, LDL-C emerged as the primary target for cholesterol lowering.

CHOLESTEROL METABOLISM AND STATINS

The world of treating dyslipidemia was revolutionized when a better understanding of cholesterol metabolism was established surrounding the role of HMG-CoA reductase and the LDL receptor pathway. Statins were developed as competitive inhibitors of HMG-CoA reductase. The inhibition of HMG-CoA reductase with statins blocked the formation of mevalonate, the rate-limiting step in cholesterol synthesis. This inhibition leads to an up-regulation of LDL receptors and at high doses decreases the hepatic production of very lowdensity lipoprotein (VLDL), which results in the lowering of plasma levels of TC, LDL-C, and VLDL-C. Subsequently, numerous clinical trials have now documented the benefits of statins on lowering LDL-C and reducing cardiovascular events.

EVIDENCE-BASED DATA FOR STATIN THERAPY

During the past two decades, numerous RCTs have established the riskreduction benefit of statin therapy. The combined RCTs represent nearly 100,000 patients. The majority of these trials achieved statistical significance for the reduction of cardiovascular events and CHD mortality *(25)*. There have been several clinical trials designed to determine whether statins offered a primary prevention benefit for reducing the risk of CHD. These trials, based on their appearance in the literature, are as follows: (i) the West of Scotland Coronary Prevention Study (WOSCOPS) *(26)*, (ii) the Air Force/Texas Coronary Atherosclerosis Prevention Study (AFCAPS/TexCAPS) *(27)*, (iii) the Anglo-Scandinavian Cardiac Outcomes Trial–Lipid Lowering Arm (ASCOT-LLA) *(28)*, and (iv) the Collaborative Atorvastatin Diabetes Study (CARDS) *(29)*. Several trials were also designed to test the benefit of the risk reduction of statins in both primary and secondary prevention of CHD. These trials are as follows: (i) the Heart Protection Study (HPS) *(30)*, (ii) the PROspective Study of Pravastatin in the

Elderly at Risk (PROSPER) *(31)*, and (iii) the Antihypertensive and Lipid-Lowering Treatment to Prevent Heart Attack Trial–Lipid-Lowering Trial (ALLHAT-LLT) *(32)*. In addition, multiple clinical trials were also designed to determine the risk reduction benefit of statins in patients with known CHD. They include (i) the Scandinavian Simvastatin Survival Study (4S) *(7)*, (ii) the Cholesterol and Recurrent Events (CARE) trial *(33)*, (iii) the Long-Term Intervention with Pravastatin in Ischaemic Disease (LIPID) trial *(34)*, and (iv) the Myocardial Ischemia Reduction with Aggressive Cholesterol Lowering (MIRACL) trial *(35)*. More recently, statin-versus-statin trials have emerged in the literature to determine whether more aggressive lowering of LDL-C, particularly in high-risk patients, can further improve clinical outcomes. Clinical trials such as the Pravastatin or Atorvastatin Evaluation and Infection Therapy–Thrombolysis in Myocardial Infarction 22 (PROVE IT) trial *(36)*, Treating to New Targets (TNT) trial *(37)*, A to Z trial *(38)*, and the Incremental Decrease in End Points Through Aggressive Lipid Lowering (IDEAL) study *(39)* were designed to determine whether more aggressive lowering of LDL-C with higher-dose statins offered greater risk reduction benefits.

RECENT CLINICAL TRIALS AND THE ADULT TREATMENT PANEL III GUIDELINES: NEW RECOMMENDATIONS AND TREATING TO GOAL

In 2001, the National Cholesterol Education Program (NCEP) released the Adult Treatment Panel III (ATP III) guidelines on the management of hyperlipidemia *(40)*. These guidelines were based on the clinical trial data prior to 2001. The RCTs prior to 2001 consistently showed that lowering LDL-C with statins was beneficial in reducing cardiovascular morbidity and mortality. Therefore, the LDL-C level is the primary goal of therapy. At the time of ATP III, the optimal goal for LDL-C was determined to be less than 100 mg/dl. This goal was the target for patients categorized as high-risk, such as CHD or CHD risk equivalent patients (Table 1). The rationale behind this goal was based on several facts: (i) there was a consistent log-linear relationship between LDL-C levels and CHD risk reduction in epidemiological studies; (ii) at the time of publication, this was the lowest LDL-C level supported by the available RCTs; and (iii) this was an achievable goal for high-risk patients based on the standard doses of available therapies *(40)*. However, after the 2001 ATP III guidelines were published, newer clinical trials were released that appeared to support the rationale that lowering LDL-C beyond < 100 mg/dl might result in further risk reduction benefit.

THE IMPLICATIONS OF NEW CLINICAL TRIALS

The clinical trials published after ATP III in 2001 offered new insights into lowering LDL-C levels in higher-risk patients. Studies such as the HPS, ASCOT-LLA, CARDS, PROVE IT, TNT, and IDEAL all showed further risk reduction benefit with treating to lower LDL-C levels in higher-risk patients. Prior to these clinical trials, it was well established that lowering LDL-C to the goal of less than 100 mg/dl significantly reduced the risk of CHD events; however, what was less certain was the continued benefit of further LDL-C lowering significantly beyond this goal.

Several different hypotheses were proposed in an attempt to define the likely relationship between further LDL-C lowering and CHD risk. The first hypothesis

Table 1
Adult Treatment Panel III Guidelines: LDL-C Goals and Cut-Points for Drug Therapy *(40)*

| Risk category | LDL-C (mg/dl) | | |
	Goal	*Initiation level for TLC*	*Consideration level for drug therapy*
CHD or CHD risk equivalents (10-year risk > 20%)	< 100	≥ 100	≥ 130 (100–129: drug optional)
2+ risk factors (10-year risk ≤ 20%)	< 130	≥ 130	10-year risk 10–20%: ≥ 130 10-year risk < 10%: ≥ 160
0–1 risk factor	< 160	≥ 160	≥ 190 (160–189: LDL-C-lowering drug optional)

CHD, coronary heart disease; LDL-C, low-density lipoprotein cholesterol; TLC, therapeutic lifestyle changes.

suggested that the goal of less than 100 mg/dl was the optimal LDL-C goal and that lowering LDL-C significantly beyond this goal would not result in additional risk reduction benefit. This was described as the "threshold effect." The second hypothesis proposed that lowering the LDL-C beyond the goal of less than 100 mg/dl would result in only a modest benefit but not of the same magnitude as seen with previous studies. This was described as the hypothesis of "diminishing returns." And finally, third hypothesis that stated that lowering LDL-C well beyond the goal of less than 100 mg/dl would continue resulting in a proportional risk reduction benefit. This was termed "lower is better."

NEWER STATIN TRIALS ESTABLISH THAT LOWER LDL-C LEVELS ARE ASSOCIATED WITH LOWER CHD RISK IN HIGH-RISK PATIENTS

In HPS, more than 20,000 high-risk patients were randomized to receive simvastatin 40 mg versus placebo. In this study, simvastatin demonstrated a 17% reduction in cardiovascular death ($p < 0.0001$) and a 24% reduction in major cardiovascular events ($p < 0.0001$) *(30)*. This benefit was seen irrespective of the baseline LDL-C level. Moreover, the 3400 high-risk patients in HPS that had an LDL-C level at baseline of less than 100 mg/dl, achieved a similar risk reduction benefit as those patients with baseline LDL-C level greater than 130 mg/dl. These data established a foundation for treating high-risk patients who already have a baseline LDL-C of less than 100 mg/dl with statin therapy.

The PROVE IT trial later established the clinical benefit of more aggressive LDL-C lowering in high-risk patients with ACS *(36)*. In this trial, more than 4000 patients with ACS were randomized to receive either atorvastatin 80 mg (intensive therapy) or pravastatin 40 mg (moderate therapy). Although the moderate-dose therapy group on pravastatin achieved the optimal LDL-C goal of less than 100 mg/dl (95 mg/dl), the intensive therapy group on atorvastatin achieved an LDL-C goal well below the optimal level of less than 100 mg/dl (62 mg/dl). On the basis of this greater lowering of LDL-C, the intensive therapy group reduced the risk of cardiovascular events by 16% over the moderate therapy group ($p = 0.005$). These data begin to establish the benefit of LDL-C lowering less than 70 mg/dl to be of benefit in the very high risk patient.

THE "OPTIMAL" VERSUS "OPTIONAL" LDL-C LEVEL

Data from the more recent RCTs, which represented higher risk patients and more aggressive LDL-C goals, were the basis for the addendum to ATP III published in 2004 *(3)*. Evidence from these RCTs suggests that lower LDL-C levels offer continued risk reduction benefit, especially in high risk and very high risk patients. This addendum offered an *optional* LDL-C level that was lower than the previous *optimal* LDL-C level. The new optional LDL-C level of less than 70 mg/dl was determined to be a reasonable target LDL-C for the "very high risk" patient. In addition, a new *optional* goal of less than 100 mg/dl was added to the guidelines for moderately high-risk patients (Table 2).

This addendum to the ATP III guidelines had thereby established a new risk group of patients called "very high risk." This new risk group is assigned the optional LDL-C goal of < 70 mg/dl. The "very high risk" group of patients are those who have established CHD plus one of the following: (i) diabetes mellitus; (ii) severe or poorly controlled risk factors; (iii) the presence of multiple risk factors, such as the metabolic syndrome; or (iv) ACS *(3)* (Table 1).

Table 2
Updated Adult Treatment Panel III Recommendations: LDL-C Cut-Points

Risk category	LDL-C (mg/dl)		
	Goal	Initiation level for TLC	Consideration level for drug therapy
Very high risk: CHD + other risk factors (10-year risk > 20%)	< 100 (optional: < 70)	≥ 100	≥ 100 (< 100: consider drug options)
High risk: CHD or CHD risk equivalents (10-year risk > 20%)	< 100	≥ 100	≥ 100 (< 100: consider drug options)
Moderately high risk: 2+ risk factors (10-year risk 10–20%)	< 130 (optional: < 100)	≥ 130	≥ 130 (100–129: consider drug options)
Moderate risk: 2+ risk factors (10-year risk < 10%)	< 130	≥ 130	≥ 160
Lower risk: 0–1 risk factor (10-year risk < 10%)	< 160	≥ 160	≥ 190 (160–189: drug optional)

CHD, coronary heart disease; LDL-C, low-density lipoprotein cholesterol; TLC, therapeutic lifestyle changes.

Therefore, with the addition of new evidence-based data and new LDL-C goals, the guidelines were modified to include the optional LDL-C goal of less than 70 mg/dl *(3)*. The *optimal* LDL-C for high risk patients remains less than 100 mg/dl. However, for very high risk patients, although the LDL-C goal of less than 100 mg/dl is strongly recommended as the minimal target, the *optional* LDL-C goal of less than 70 mg/dl is considered a reasonable therapeutic option. For moderately high risk patients, the LDL-C goal is less than 130 mg/dl; however, a therapeutic goal of less than 100 mg/dl is a reasonable option (Table 2). All patients with lifestyle risk factors are candidates for therapeutic lifestyle changes (TLC). When drug therapy is implemented, a minimum of 30–40% reduction in LDL-C is recommended for moderately high risk and high risk patients *(3)* (Table 3). Cardiac rehabilitation offers the ideal settings to implement TLC and achieve the current LDL-C goals for high risk and very high risk patients. A simpler approach is to treat all patients with CHD to an optional LDL-C goal of < 70 mg/dl as recommended in the American Heart Association/American College of Cardiology (AHA/ACC) guidelines for secondary prevention *(5)*.

THE ABILITY TO ACHIEVE NEW LDL-C GOALS

An analysis of the National Health and Nutrition Examination Survey III (NHANES III) evaluated LDL-C levels from approximately 6800 adults *(41)*. On the basis of an estimated number of adults with CHD, it was determined that the mean LDL-C in this population of patients was 132.8 mg/dl. More importantly, it was determined that only 16.6% of individuals with CHD achieved an LDL-C of less than 100 mg/dl and only 11.1% were on LLT. This information correlates with other data regarding implementation of LLT in CHD patients *(9,10)*. Even though more recent statistical data show the percentages have improved *(42)*, there continues to be a significant number of high-risk CHD patients who do not achieve either the optimal or the optional goal for LDL-C.

Therefore, to achieve these new and more aggressive guidelines, clinicians must incorporate more aggressive treatment practices and utilize more effective secondary prevention protocols and programs such as cardiac rehabilitation. Recommendations regarding pharmacologic options for attaining LDL-C goals in CHD patients are as follows: (i) use a highly efficacious statin at appropriate dose as first-line therapy; (ii) the intensity of therapy should be sufficient to achieve at least 30–40% reduction

Table 3
Drug Dose to Achieve LDL-C Reduction 30–40% *(3)*

Drug	Dose (mg/day)	LDL-C reduction (%)
Atorvastatin	10	39
Lovastatin	40	31
Pravastatin	40	34
Simvastatin	20–40	35–41
Fluvastatin	40–80	25–35
Rosuvastatin	5–10	39–45

LDL-C, low-density lipoprotein cholesterol.

Table 4
Drug Dose to Achieve LDL-C Reduction ≥ 50%

Drug	Dose (mg/day)	LDL-C reduction (%)
Ezetimibe/simvastatin (44)	10/20*–10/80[†]	52–60
Rosuvastatin (45)	20–40[†]	52–55
Atorvastatin (46)	80[†]	51–54

LDL-C, low-density lipoprotein cholesterol.
* Recommended usual starting dose.
[†] Not recommended as usual starting dose per US Food and Drug Administration (FDA) package insert.

in LDL-C; and (iii) earlier consideration for combination lipid-drug therapy (3,43). For many high-risk patients in cardiac rehabilitation programs, an LDL-C goal of < 70 mg/dl is desirable and will frequently require ≥ 50% LDL-C reduction (Table 4).

TREATMENT OPTIONS

Therapeutic lifestyle changes

ATP III recommends a systematic approach to TLC to reduce the risk of CHD. TLC should be emphasized for all patients at risk for CHD, regardless of whether they qualify for drug therapy. TLC should be initiated if the LDL-C level is above the recommended goal. If the patient is at moderately high risk or above, LLT should be initiated at the same time as TLC. Evidence-based recommendations for TLC target four goals: (i) reduced intake of saturated fat and cholesterol, (ii) dietary and therapeutic options for enhancing LDL-C lowering, (iii) weight reduction [body mass index (BMI) 18.5–24.9 kg/m^2 and/or waist circumference less than 88 cm for women and 102 cm for men), and (iv) increased regular physical exercise (40). Unfortunately, TLC alone frequently does not allow high-risk patients to achieve LDL-C targets.

Statin Monotherapy

Statin therapy has become the mainstay of treating dyslipidemia, particularly in the setting of CHD and in patients at risk for CHD. However, there remain several challenges facing clinicians trying to treat high-risk CHD patients to appropriate targets. Although less than 50% of patients achieve their LDL-C goal with the initial dose of statin therapy, 75% of patients remain on their initial dose after 1 year (47). Therefore, many patients, specifically those who are at the highest risk of disease and requiring the lowest goals for LDL-C, are often left undertreated. This undertreatment of CHD patients, also known as the "treatment gap," has led to a need to develop protocols (such as "Get with the Guidelines") and enhance programs (such as cardiac rehabilitation) designed to improve both the implementation of appropriate risk reduction therapy in CHD patients and the achievement of appropriate therapeutic goals for CHD patients.

The NCEP ATP III guidelines recommend statins as the first line of pharmacotherapy for the following reasons: (i) statins are the most effective therapies for lowering LDL-C; (ii) statins have demonstrated the greatest risk reduction benefit in CHD patients; and (iii) statins have a reasonable safety profile (40). The revised ATP III guidelines recommend that therapy should be initiated with statins that have the ability to lower LDL-C by at least 30–40% *(3)* (Table 3). However, to reach an LDL-C of < 70 mg/dl, many patients will require ≥ 50% LDL-C lowering.

The ACC/AHA/National Heart, Lung and Blood Institute (NHLBI) published a public advisory statement regarding the safety of statins *(48)*. Regarding liver function, the advisory states that statin therapy appears to increase liver transaminases in 0.5–2.0% of patients. In patients with elevated transaminases, the liver function test should be repeated, and if transaminases are still elevated > 3 times the upper limit of normal, the statin should be stopped. In addition, the ACC/AHA/NHLBI advisory board has also given recommendations regarding muscle toxicity. The advisory board states that statins carry a small but definite risk of myopathy of less than 1.0%. The board further goes on to state that although nonspecific muscle aches and joint pains are common, these symptoms are rarely associated with significant increases of creatine kinase (CK). While statins rarely cause a true myopathy (muscle pains or weakness with a CK levels > 10 × upper limit of normal [ULN] or clinical rhabdomyolysis (muscle pain or weakness with CK levels > 10 × ULN and kidney involvement), when these clinical conditions such myositis do occur, statins patients should be discontinued from statins.

Other Lipid-Lowering Therapy

In addition to statins, other lipid-lowering agents have the ability to treat dyslipidemia. These therapies include niacin, fibrates, bile acid resins, and ezetimibe.

Niacin lowers LDL-C by reducing the synthesis of VLDL. Niacin appears to improve dyslipidemia by several mechanisms: (i) decreasing the release of free fatty acids by adipose tissue; (ii) enhancing VLDL catabolism and clearance of chylomicron triglyceride (TG) from the plasma by activation of lipoprotein lipase; (iii) decreases the synthesis of apolipoprotein B-100; (iv) enhancing the shift in LDL particle size from small, dense LDL to large, buoyant LDL; and (v) enhancing the structure and function of high-density lipoprotein cholesterol (HDL-C) by decreasing the catabolism of apolipoprotein A-I *(49,50)*. Niacin decreases LDL-C by 15–25%, increases HDL-C by 15–30%, and decreases TG by 25–35% *(40)*.

Fibric acid derivatives in the form of fibrates can reduce TG and raise HDL-C by activation of peroxisome proliferator activated receptor-α (PPAR-α) *(51)*. This activation increases the activity of lipoprotein lipase and thereby enhances lipolysis and clearance of TG-rich lipoproteins. Fibrates also alter the LDL particle size from small, dense LDL to large, buoyant LDL through significant TG lowering. Activation of PPAR-α also appears to enhance the production of apolipoprotien A-I and increases HDL-C. Fibrates increase HDL-C by 5–15% and decrease TG by 25–40% *(40)*. Fibrates can either increase or decrease LDL-C, depending on baseline TG.

Bile acid sequestrants (BAS) bind cholesterol in the form of bile acids in the intestines. This bile acid complex is excreted in the feces and therefore decreases the amount of bile acid reabsorption *(52)*. The result is a decrease in the amount of bile acids returning to the liver through enterohepatic circulation. This in turn creates an increased conversion of cholesterol to bile acids in the liver. Therefore, BAS cause a decrease in the intrahepatic cholesterol pool, which results in an increase in hepatic LDL receptors and enhanced clearance of LDL-C from the plasma. BAS decrease LDL-C by 20–30%, increase HDL-C by 5%, and increase TG by 10% *(40)*.

Because of the potential increase in TG, BAS are relatively contraindicated in severe hypertriglyceridemia.

Ezetimibe is a cholesterol absorption inhibitor. Ezetimibe acts in the brush border of the small intestin. Ezetimibe appears to localize in the small intestine and inhibit absorption of cholesteryl esters (CE) from entering into the circulation through chylomicrons *(53)*. This decrease in CE absorption causes a decrease in intrahepatic cholesterol, which results in an up-regulation of LDL receptors and subsequently a decrease in plasma LDL-C. In a pooled analysis of 1719 patients with primary hypercholesterolemia, ezetimibe monotherapy decreased LDL-C by 19%, increased HDL-C by 3%, and lowered TG by 8% compared with placebo *(54)*. Ezetimibe provides an incremental 25% reduction in LDL-C when added to a statin *(55)*.

Combination Therapy

As evidence-based medicine continues to support lower LDL-C goals, combination therapy will become more common and even necessary in many high-risk CHD patients. The rationale behind combination therapy involves both the ability to more effectively lower LDL-C and the ability to better manage more complex lipid abnormalities than with statin monotherapy. The ability to improve the HDL-C/TG axis has been shown to improve cardiovascular outcomes in patients near goal for LDL-C *(56)*. Effective combinations are generally statin-based combinations. Effective combination therapies for lowering LDL-C are statin plus ezetimibe and statin plus BAS *(3)*. Combinations that improve mixed dyslipidemia are (i) statin plus fenofibrate, (ii) statin plus nicotinic acid, and (iii) statin plus fish oil *(57)*.

Omega-3 Fatty Acids

Omega-3 fatty acids may add a unique benefit as a therapeutic agent for patients with CHD. Omega-3 fatty acids have been shown to both lower high TGs *(58)* and reduce the risk of cardiovascular events in CHD patients *(59)*. The omega-3 fatty acids believed to be of benefit in cardiovascular disease are eicosapentaenoic acid (EPA) and docosahexaenoic acid (DHA), both derived from marine sources. Omega-3 fatty acids have the ability to lower high TG by 15–45% when used at higher doses of 3–6 g/day *(60)*. In addition, there is modest evidence that omega-3 fatty acids lower the risk for cardiovascular events, in particular sudden cardiac death, when used at lower doses of 1–2 g/day. The GISSI-Prevenzione Trial (post-MI) showed a 21% reduction in all-cause mortality and a 45% reduction in sudden death in the omega-3 fatty acid treated group versus placebo ($p < 0.01$) *(59)*. These benefits are the rationale behind using omega-3 fatty acids in CHD patients. The most common therapeutic utilization would be in combination with statins.

CHD AND THE TREATMENT OF DYSLIPIDEMIA

Evidence-based medicine strongly supports lowering LDL-C to reduce the risk of CHD. TLC and pharmacotherapy remain the mainstay of treatment for improving LDL-C levels. Statins have emerged as the treatment of choice to both lower LDL-C and reduce the risk of CHD. Therefore, LDL-C is the primary target of intervention to reduce CHD risk. Based on the most recent data, the ideal LDL-C for risk reduction may be well below 100 mg/dl. As such, the latest recommendations according to the ATP III addendum suggest lower LDL-C targets for patients. In patients at "very high risk," the optional LDL-C goal is less than 70 mg/dl, and it may be reasonable, and a simpler approach, to treat all CHD patients to LDL-C less than 70 mg/dl, as recommended in the AHA/ACC guidelines for secondary prevention (5). In patients at "high risk," the optimal LDL-C goal remains less than 100 mg/dl. In patients considered to be at "moderately high risk," an LDL-C goal of less than 130 mg/dl is recommended, with an optional LDL-C goal of less than 100 mg/dl.

TLC remains an essential modality in the management of CHD patients. TLC probably reduces the risk of CHD by means other than just lowering LDL-C. Supervised exercise associated with cardiac rehabilitation has been shown to improve multiple cardiovascular and hemodynamic parameters beyond LDL-C lowering and without LLT (5).

Statins reduce morbidity and mortality in patients with known CHD, with or without elevated LDL-C levels. Aggressive LDL-C lowering with statins reduces recurrent ischemic events in patients with ACS (36). In one meta-analysis of 25 studies enrolling 69,511 patients with CHD, statins reduced the risk of CHD mortality or nonfatal MI by 25% and had an absolute risk reduction for these events of 3.8% [number needed to treat (NNT) = 26] (61). Statins also lowered all-cause mortality by 16% and yielded an absolute risk reduction for all-cause mortality of 1.8% (NNT = 56), while lowering CHD mortality by 23%, with an absolute risk reduction of 1.4% (NNT = 71) (61).

LIPID-LOWERING THERAPY IN CARDIAC REHABILITATION

Cardiac rehabilitation is uniquely positioned to play a vital role in optimizing secondary prevention. Cardiac rehabilitation creates a bridge between inpatient management of CHD and outpatient follow-up. It allows optimization of all CHD risk factors through TLC recommendations (nutrition management, supervised exercise therapy, and psychosocial management) and pharmacotherapy goals. The newer guidelines for achieving "optimal" and "optional" LDL-C goals in high-risk (CHD and CHD risk equivalent) patients and very high risk (CHD plus other specified risk factors) patients will require more intensive lipid lowering, which can be achieved by the use of higher efficacy statins and combination therapies.

REFERENCES

1. American Heart Association Statistics Committee, Stroke Statistics Subcommittee. Heart Disease and Stroke Statistics—2006 Update. *Circulation*. 2006;113:e85–e151.
2. Wenger NK, Froelicher ES, Smith LK, et al. Cardiac Rehabilitation as Secondary Prevention. *Clin Pract Guidel Quick Ref Guide Clin*. 1995:1–23.
3. Grundy SM, Cleeman JI, Bairey Merz CN, et al. Implications of Recent Clinical Trials for the National Cholesterol Education Program Adult Treatment Panel III Guidelines. *Circulation*. 2004;110:227–239.
4. Chobanian AV, Bakris GL, Black HR, et al. The Seventh Report of the Joint National Committee on Prevention, Detection, Evaluation, and Treatment of High Blood Pressure: The JNC 7 Report. *JAMA*. 2003;289:2560–2572.

5. Smith SC Jr, Allen J, Blair SN, et al. AHA/ACC Guidelines for Secondary Prevention for Patients with Coronary and Other Atherosclerotic Vascular Disease: 2006 Update: Endorsed by the National Heart, Lung, and Blood Institute. *Circulation*. 2006;113:2363–2372.

6. Haskell WL, Alderman EL, Fair JM, et al. Effects of Intensive Multiple Risk Factor Reduction on Coronary Atherosclerosis and Clinical Cardiac Events in Men and Women with Coronary Artery Disease: The Stanford Coronary Risk Intervention Project (SCRIP). *Circulation*. 1994;89:975–990.

7. Scandinavian Simvastatin Survival Study Group. Randomised Trial of Cholesterol Lowering in 4444 Patients with Coronary Heart Disease: The Scandinavian Simvastatin Survival Study (4S). *Lancet*. 1994;344:1383–1389.

8. Foody JM, Roe MT, Chen AY, et al. Lipid Management in Patients with Unstable Angina Pectoris and Non-ST-Segment Elevation Acute Myocardial Infarction (from CRUSADE). *Am J Cardiol*. 2005;95:483–485.

9. Fonarow GC, French WJ, Parsons LS, Sun H, Malmgren JA, for the National Registry of Myocardial Infarction 3 Participants. Use of Lipid-Lowering Medications at Discharge in Patients with Acute Myocardial Infarction: Data from the National Registry of Myocardial Infarction 3. *Circulation*. 2001;103:38–44.

10. Sueta CA, Chowdhury M, Boccuzzi SJ, et al. Analysis of the Degree of Undertreatment of Hyperlipidemia and Congestive Heart Failure Secondary to Coronary Artery Disease. *Am J Cardiol*. 1999;83:1303–1307.

11. Leon AS, Franklin BA, Costa F, et al. Cardiac Rehabilitation and Secondary Prevention of Coronary Heart Disease: An American Heart Association Scientific Statement from the Council on Clinical Cardiology (Subcommittee on Exercise, Cardiac Rehabilitation, and Prevention) and the Council on Nutrition, Physical Activity, and Metabolism (Subcommittee on Physical Activity), in Collaboration with the American Association of Cardiovascular and Pulmonary Rehabilitation. *Circulation*. 2005;111:369–376.

12. O'Connor GT, Buring JE, Yusuf S, et al. An Overview of Randomized Trials of Rehabilitation with Exercise after Myocardial Infarction. *Circulation*. 1989;80:234–244.

13. Balady GJ, Jette D, Scheer J, Downing J. Changes in Exercise Capacity Following Cardiac Rehabilitation in Patients Stratified According to Age and Gender: Results of the Massachusetts Association of Cardiovascular and Pulmonary Rehabilitation Multicenter Database. *J Cardiopulm Rehabil*. 1996;16:38–46.

14. Hambrecht R, Niebauer J, Marburger C, et al. Various Intensities of Leisure Time Physical Activity in Patients with Coronary Artery Disease: Effects on Cardiorespiratory Fitness and Progression of Coronary Atherosclerotic Lesions. *J Am Coll Cardiol*. 1993;22:468–477.

15. Schuler G, Hambrecht R, Schlierf G, et al. Regular Physical Exercise and Low-Fat Diet: Effects on Progression of Coronary Artery Disease. *Circulation*. 1992;86:1–11.

16. Paffenbarger RS Jr, Hyde RT, Wing AL, Lee IM, Jung DL, Kampert JB. The Association of Changes in Physical-Activity Level and Other Lifestyle Characteristics with Mortality Among Men. *N Engl J Med*. 1993;328:538–545.

17. Virchow R. *Die Cellulär Pathologie*. Berlin: August Hirschwald; 1858.

18. Steiner A, Kendall FE. Atherosclerosis and Arteriosclerosis in Dogs Following Ingestion of Cholesterol and Thiouracil. *Arch Pathol*. 1946;42:433–444.

19. Watanabe Y, Ito T, Shiomi M. The Effect of Selective Breeding on the Development of Coronary Atherosclerosis in WHHL Rabbits: An Animal Model for Familial Hypercholesterolemia. *Atherosclerosis*. 1985;56:71–79.

20. Brown MS, Goldstein JL. A Receptor-Mediated Pathway for Cholesterol Homeostasis. *Science*. 1986;232:34–47.

21. Anderson KM, Castelli WP, Levy D. Cholesterol and Mortality: 30 Years of Follow-up from the Framingham Study. *JAMA*. 1987;257:2176–2180.

22. Neaton JD, Blackburn H, Jacobs D, et al. Serum Cholesterol Level and Mortality Findings for Men Screened in the Multiple Risk Factor Intervention Trial. *Arch Intern Med.* 1992;152:1490–1500.
23. Research Committee. Low-Fat Diet in Myocardial Infarction: A Controlled Trial. *Lancet.* 1965;2:501–504.
24. Lipid Research Clinics Program. The Lipid Research Clinics Coronary Primary Prevention Trial results. I. Reduction in Incidence of Coronary Heart Disease. *JAMA.* 1984;251:351–364.
25. Cholesterol Treatment Trialists' (CTT) Collaboration. Efficacy and Safety of Cholesterol-Lowering Treatment: Prospective Meta-Analysis of Data from 90,056 Participants in 14 Randomised Trials of Statins. *Lancet.* 2005;366:1267–1278.
26. Shepherd J, Cobbe SM, Ford I, et al. Prevention of Coronary Heart Disease with Pravastatin in Men with Hypercholesterolemia. *N Engl J Med.* 1995;333:1301–1307.
27. Downs JR, Clearfield M, Weis S, et al. Primary Prevention of Acute Coronary Events with Lovastatin in Men and Women with Average Cholesterol Levels: Results of AFCAPS/TexCAPS. *JAMA.* 1998;279:1615–1622.
28. Sever PS, Dahlof B, Poulter NR, et al. Prevention of Coronary and Stroke Events with Atorvastatin in Hypertensive Patients who have Average or Lower-than-average Cholesterol Concentrations, in the Anglo-Scandinavian Cardiac Outcomes Trial–Lipid Lowering Arm (ASCOT-LLA): A Multicentre Randomised Controlled Trial. *Lancet.* 2003;361:1149–1158.
29. Colhoun HM, Betteridge DJ, Durrington PN, et al. Primary Prevention of Cardiovascular Disease with Atorvastatin in Type 2 Diabetes in the Collaborative Atorvastatin Diabetes Study (CARDS): Multicentre Randomised Placebo-Controlled Trial. *Lancet.* 2004;364:685–696.
30. Heart Protection Study Collaborative Group. MRC/BHF Heart Protection Study of Cholesterol Lowering with Simvastatin in 20 536 High-Risk Individuals: A Randomised Placebo-Controlled Trial. *Lancet.* 2002;360:7–22.
31. Shepherd J, Blauw GJ, Murphy MB, et al. Pravastatin in Elderly Individuals At Risk of Vascular Disease (PROSPER): A Randomised Controlled Trial. *Lancet.* 2002;360:1623–1630.
32. ALLHAT Officers and Coordinators for the ALLHAT Collaborative Research Group. Major Outcomes in Moderately Hypercholesterolemic, Hypertensive Patients Randomized to Pravastatin vs Usual Care: The Antihypertensive and Lipid-Lowering Treatment to Prevent Heart Attack Trial (ALLHAT-LLT). *JAMA.* 2002;288:2998–3007.
33. Sacks FM, Pfeffer MA, Moye LA, et al. The Effect of Pravastatin on Coronary Events after Myocardial Infarction in Patients with Average Cholesterol Levels. *N Engl J Med.* 1996;335:1001–1009.
34. Long-Term Intervention with Pravastatin in Ischaemic Disease (LIPID) Study Group. Prevention of Cardiovascular Events and Death with Pravastatin in Patients with Coronary Heart Disease and a Broad Range of Initial Cholesterol Levels. *N Engl J Med.* 1998;339:1349–1357.
35. Schwartz GG, Olsson AG, Ezekowitz MD, et al. Effects of Atorvastatin on Early Recurrent Ischemic Events in Acute Coronary Syndromes: The MIRACL Study: A Randomized Controlled Trial. *JAMA.* 2001;285:1711–1718.
36. Cannon CP, Braunwald E, McCabe CH, et al. Comparison of Intensive and Moderate Lipid Lowering with Statins after Acute Coronary Syndromes. *N Engl J Med.* 2004;350:1495–1504.
37. LaRosa JC, Grundy SM, Waters DD, et al. Intensive Lipid Lowering with Atorvastatin in Patients with Stable Coronary Disease. *N Engl J Med.* 2005;352:1425–1435.
38. De Lemos JA, Blazing MA, Wiviott SD, et al. Early Intensive vs a Delayed Conservative Simvastatin Strategy in Patients with Acute Coronary Syndromes: Phase Z of the A to Z Trial. *JAMA.* 2004;292:1307–1316.
39. Pedersen TR, Faergeman O, Kastelein JJ, et al. High-Dose Atorvastatin vs Usual-Dose Simvastatin for Secondary Prevention after Myocardial Infarction: The IDEAL Study: A Randomized Controlled Trial. *JAMA.* 2005;294:2437–2445.

40. Expert Panel on Detection, Evaluation, and Treatment of High Blood Cholesterol in Adults. Executive Summary of the Third Report of the National Cholesterol Education Program (NCEP) Expert Panel on Detection, Evaluation, and Treatment of High Blood Cholesterol in Adults (Adult Treatment Panel III). *JAMA.* 2001;285:2486–2497.

41. Jacobson TA, Griffiths GG, Varas C, Gause D, Sung JC, Ballantyne CM. Impact of Evidence-Based "Clinical Judgment" on the Number of American Adults Requiring Lipid-Lowering Therapy Based on Updated NHANES III Data. *Arch Intern Med.* 2000;160:1361–1369.

42. Muntner P, DeSalvo KB, Wildman RP, Raggi P, He J, Whelton PK. Trends in the Prevalence, Awareness, Treatment, and Control of Cardiovascular Disease Risk Factors Among Noninstitutionalized Patients with a History of Myocardial Infarction and Stroke. *Am J Epidemiol.* 2006;163:913–920.

43. McKenney JM. Optimizing LDL-C Lowering with Statins. *Am J Ther.* 2004;11:54–59.

44. Goldberg AC, Sapre A, Liu J, Capece R, Mitchel YB. Efficacy and Safety of Ezetimibe Coadministered with Simvastatin in Patients with Primary Hypercholesterolemia: A Randomized, Double-Blind, Placebo-Controlled Trial. *Mayo Clin Proc.* 2004;79:620–629.

45. Jones PH, Davidson MH, Stein EA, et al. Comparison of the Efficacy and Safety of Rosuvastatin Versus Atorvastatin, Simvastatin, and Pravastatin Across Doses (STELLAR* Trial). *Am J Cardiol.* 2003;92:152–160.

46. Jones P, Kafonek S, Laurora I, Hunninghake D. Comparative Dose Efficacy Study of Atorvastatin Versus Simvastatin, Pravastatin, Lovastatin, and Fluvastatin in Patients with Hypercholesterolemia (The CURVES Study). *Am J Cardiol.* 1998;81:582–587.

47. Andrews TC, Ballantyne CM, Hsia JA, Kramer JH. Achieving and Maintaining National Cholesterol Education Program Low-Density Lipoprotein Cholesterol Goals with Five Statins. *Am J Med.* 2001;111:185–191.

48. Pasternak RC, Smith SC Jr, Bairey-Merz CN, Grundy SM, Cleeman JI, Lenfant C. ACC/AHA/NHLBI Clinical Advisory on the Use and Safety of Statins. *J Am Coll Cardiol.* 2002;40:567–572.

49. Jin FY, Kamanna VS, Kashyap ML. Niacin Decreases Removal of High-Density Lipoprotein Apolipoprotein A-I but Not Cholesterol Ester by Hep G2 Cells. Implication for Reverse Cholesterol Transport. *Arterioscler Thromb Vasc Biol.* 1997;17:2020–2028.

50. Jin FY, Kamanna VS, Kashyap ML. Niacin Accelerates Intracellular ApoB Degradation by Inhibiting Triacylglycerol Synthesis in Human Hepatoblastoma (HepG2) Cells. *Arterioscler Thromb Vasc Biol.* 1999;19:1051–1059.

51. Staels B, Dallongeville J, Auwerx J, Schoonjans K, Leitersdorf E, Fruchart JC. Mechanism of Action of Fibrates on Lipid and Lipoprotein Metabolism. *Circulation.* 1998;98:2088–2093.

52. Grundy SM, Ahrens EH Jr, Salen G. Interruption of the Enterohepatic Circulation of Bile Acids in Man: Comparative Effects of Cholestyramine and Ileal Exclusion on Cholesterol Metabolism. *J Lab Clin Med.* 1971;78:94–121.

53. Sudhop T, Lutjohann D, Kodal A, et al. Inhibition of Intestinal Cholesterol Absorption by Ezetimibe in Humans. *Circulation.* 2002;106:1943–1948.

54. Knopp RH, Dujovne CA, Le Beaut A, Lipka LJ, Suresh R, Veltri EP. Evaluation of the Efficacy, Safety, and Tolerability of Ezetimibe in Primary Hypercholesterolaemia: A Pooled Analysis from Two Controlled Phase III Clinical Studies. *Int J Clin Pract.* 2003;57:363–368.

55. Gagné C, Bays HE, Weiss SR, et al. Efficacy and Safety of Ezetimibe Added to Ongoing Statin Therapy for Treatment of Patients with Primary Hypercholesterolemia. *Am J Cardiol.* 2002;90:1084–1091.

56. Rubins HB, Robins SJ, Collins D, et al. Gemfibrozil for the Secondary Prevention of Coronary Heart Disease in Men with Low Levels of High-Density Lipoprotein Cholesterol. *N Engl J Med.* 1999;341:410–418.

57. Jones PH. Statins as the Cornerstone of Drug Therapy for Dyslipidemia: Monotherapy and Combination Therapy Options. *Am Heart J.* 2004;148:S9–13.

58. Harris WS. Fish Oil Supplementation: Evidence for Health Benefits. *Cleve Clin J Med.* 2004;71:208–210, 212, 215–218.
59. GISSI-Prevenzione Investigators. Dietary Supplementation with n-3 Polyunsaturated Fatty Acids and Vitamin E after Myocardial Infarction: Results of the GISSI-Prevenzione Trial. *Lancet.* 1999;354:447–455.
60. Pownall HJ, Brauchi D, Kilinc C, et al. Correlation of Serum Triglyceride and Its Reduction by Omega-3 Fatty Acids with Lipid Transfer Activity and the Neutral Lipid Compositions of High-Density and Low-Density Lipoproteins. *Atherosclerosis.* 1999;143:285–297.
61. Wilt TJ, Bloomfield HE, MacDonald R, et al. Effectiveness of Statin Therapy in Adults with Coronary Heart Disease. *Arch Intern Med.* 2004;164:1427–1436.

14 Treating to Goal: Diabetes and Hypertension

Neil F. Gordon, MD, PhD, MPH

CONTENTS

Diabetes is one of the most common chronic diseases in the United States and one of the major public health issues facing the world in the twenty-first century. The human toll of diabetes can be gauged not only by medical statistics, which show it to be the leading cause of end-stage renal disease and new cases of visual loss in persons under the age of 65 years and a major cause of macrovascular disease, but also by the quantity of health care resources consumed. Moreover, whereas the prevalence of type 1 diabetes is increasing slowly, the prevalence of type 2 diabetes is increasing explosively (1).

According to the most recent NHANES survey (1999–2000), 31% of adult Americans have prehypertension [i.e., systolic blood pressure (BP) of 120–139 mmHg and/or diastolic BP of 80–89 mmHg] and another 27% have hypertension (i.e., systolic BP ≥ 140 mmHg and/or diastolic BP ≥ 90 mmHg and/or use of antihypertensive medication) (2). Recent data further indicate that the prevalence of hypertension is increasing and that control rates among those with hypertension remain low (3,4).

In this chapter, the classification, diagnosis, complications, and, especially, medical management of diabetes and hypertension are briefly reviewed.

DIABETES MELLITUS

Diabetes Classification and Diagnosis

In 1997, the American Diabetes Association (ADA) revised their classification and diagnostic criteria (5). The revised classification includes four major clinical classes of diabetes, namely:

- Type 1 diabetes (results from beta-cell destruction, usually leading to absolute insulin deficiency).

From: *Contemporary Cardiology: Cardiac Rehabilitation*
Edited by: W. E. Kraus and S. J. Keteyian © Humana Press Inc., Totowa, NJ

- Type 2 diabetes (results from a progressive insulin secretory defect on the background of insulin resistance).
- Other specific types of diabetes mellitus due to other causes, e.g., genetic defects in beta-cell function, genetic defects in insulin action, diseases of the exocrine pancreas (such as cystic fibrosis), and drug or chemical induced (such as in the treatment of acquired immunodeficiency syndrome or after organ transplantation).
- Gestational diabetes mellitus (diagnosed during pregnancy).

For the clinician and patient, it is less important to label the particular type of diabetes than it is to understand the pathogenesis of the hyperglycemia and to manage it effectively *(5)*.

The vast majority of cases of diabetes fall into two broad etiopathogenetic categories, namely, type 1 diabetes and type 2 diabetes. Generally, people with type 1 diabetes present with acute symptoms of diabetes and marked hyperglycemia. Type 2 diabetes (90–95% of individuals with diabetes) is far more prevalent than type 1 diabetes (5–10% of individuals with diabetes) but frequently goes undiagnosed for many years because the hyperglycemia develops gradually and, at earlier stages, is often not severe enough for the patient to notice any of the classic symptoms of diabetes. Unfortunately, this relatively symptom-free undiagnosed period of diabetes is not benign – approximately 20% of newly diagnosed patients with type 2 diabetes already have evidence of chronic complications *(1)*.

Criteria for the diagnosis of diabetes in nonpregnant adults are shown in Table 1. Hyperglycemia not sufficient to meet the diagnostic criteria for diabetes is categorized as impaired fasting glucose (fasting plasma glucose = 100 to 125 mg/dl) or impaired glucose tolerance (2-h plasma glucose = 140–199 mg/dl), and both of these conditions have been officially termed "prediabetes" *(5,6)*.

Complications of Diabetes

Acute, potentially life-threatening consequences of untreated or poorly managed diabetes are hyperglycemia with ketoacidosis or nonketotic hyperosmolar syndrome. Ketoacidosis seldom occurs spontaneously in persons with type 2 diabetes; when

Table 1
Criteria for the Diagnosis of Diabetes Mellitus

1. Symptoms of diabetes plus casual plasma glucose concentration ≥ 200 mg/dl. Casual is defined as any time of day without regard to time since last meal. The classic symptoms of diabetes include polyuria, polydipsia, and unexplained weight loss.

Or

2. Fasting plasma glucose ≥ 126 mg/dl. Fasting is defined as no caloric intake for at least 8 h.

Or

3. Two-hour postload plasma glucose ≥ 200 mg/dl during an oral glucose tolerance test. The test should be performed as described by the World Health Organization, using a glucose load containing the equivalent of 75-g anhydrous glucose dissolved in water.

In the absence of unequivocal hyperglycemia, these criteria should be confirmed by repeat testing on a different day. The third measure (oral glucose tolerance test) is not recommended for routine clinical use *(5)*.

seen, it usually arises in association with the stress of another illness such as acute infection. Hypoglycemia is most likely to occur in patients with diabetes who receive treatment with insulin and, to a lesser degree, insulin secretagogues (i.e., sulfonylureas or meglitinides).

Some of the major long-term complications of diabetes include retinopathy with potential loss of vision; nephropathy leading to renal failure; peripheral neuropathy with risk of foot ulcers, amputation, and Charcot joints; and autonomic neuropathy causing gastrointestinal, genitourinary, and cardiovascular symptoms and sexual dysfunction. Most importantly, a large body of epidemiological and pathological data document that both type 1 and type 2 diabetes are independent risk factors for atherosclerotic cardiovascular disease in both men and women (7).

Medical Management of Diabetes

A cardinal feature in preventing the complications of diabetes is early diagnosis and management. People with diabetes should receive medical care from a physician-coordinated team including (but not limited to) physicians, nurses, dietitians, exercise physiologists, and mental health professionals with expertise and special interest in diabetes. The treatment plan should recognize diabetes self-management education as an integral component of care. Although glycemic control is fundamental to the management of diabetes, it must be emphasized that diabetes care is complex and requires that many issues (beyond glycemic control) be addressed. In this respect, a large body of evidence exists, which supports a range of interventions to improve diabetes outcomes. The standards of medical care for patients with diabetes, as recommended by the ADA (6), can be summarized as follows (Table 2).

Recommended glycemic goals for nonpregnant individuals are summarized in Table 2. Hemoglobin A1c (A1C) testing should be performed at least two times a year in patients who are meeting treatment goals (and who have stable glycemic control) and quarterly in patients whose therapy has changed or who are not meeting glycemic goals. The management plan (i.e., lifestyle intervention and insulin therapy/oral antidiabetic medications) should be developed or adjusted to achieve normal or near-normal glycemia with an A1C test goal of < 7% *for patients in general* and as close to normal (< 6%) as possible without significant hypoglycemia *for the individual patient*. The patient should be instructed in self-monitoring of blood glucose, and the patient's technique and ability to use data to adjust therapy should be routinely evaluated.

People with diabetes should receive individualized medical nutrition therapy (MNT) as needed to achieve treatment goals, preferably provided by a registered dietitian familiar with the components of MNT (8). A program of regular physical activity, adapted to the presence of complications, is recommended for all patients with diabetes who are capable of participating (6,9) – see chap. 19 for exercise-specific guidelines. In addition to MNT and regular physical activity, cigarette smokers should receive smoking cessation counseling and other forms of treatment as a routine component of diabetes care.

A target BP goal of < 130/80 mmHg is recommended. BP should be measured at every routine diabetes visit. Patients with a systolic BP of 130–139 mmHg or a diastolic BP of 80–89 mmHg should be given lifestyle/behavioral therapy alone for a maximum of 3 months and then, if targets are not achieved, in addition, be treated

Table 2
Summary of Recommendations for Adults with Diabetes

Glycemic control	
A1C	$< 7.0\%^*$
Preprandial capillary plasma glucose	90–130 mg/dl
Peak postprandial capillary plasma glucose[†]	< 180 mg/dl
Blood pressure	$< 130/80$ mmHg
Lipids[‡]	
LDL	< 100 mg/dl
Triglycerides	< 150 mg/dl
HDL	> 40 mg/dl[§]

Key concepts in setting glycemic goals

- A1C is the primary target for glycemic control
- Goals should be individualized
- Certain populations (children, pregnant women, and elderly) require special considerations
- More stringent glycemic goals (i.e., a normal A1C, $< 6\%$) may further reduce complications at the cost of increased risk of hypoglycemia
- Less intensive glycemic goals may be indicated in patients with severe or frequent hypoglycemia
- Postprandial glucose may be targeted if A1C goals are not met despite reaching preprandial glucose goals

A1C, hemoglobin A1c; HDL, high-density lipoprotein; LDL, low-density lipoprotein.

[*] Referenced to a nondiabetic range of 4.0–6.0% using a Diabetes Control and Complications Trial (DCCT)-based assay.

[†] Postprandial glucose measurements should be made 1–2 h after the beginning of the meal, generally peak levels in patients with diabetes.

[‡] Current guidelines suggest that in patients with triglycerides ≥ 200 mg/dl, the "non-HDL cholesterol" (total cholesterol minus HDL) be utilized. The goal is < 130 mg/dl.

[§] For women, it has been suggested that the HDL goal be increased by 10 mg/dl (8).

pharmacologically. Patients with hypertension (systolic BP ≥ 140 mmHg or diastolic BP ≥ 90 mmHg) should receive drug therapy in addition to lifestyle/behavioral therapy.

In hypertensive patients with microalbuminuria or clinical albuminuria/nephropathy, an angiotensin-converting enzyme (ACE) inhibitor or angiotensin-receptor blocker (ARB) should be used. Initial drug therapy for hypertensive patients should be with a drug class demonstrated to reduce cardiovascular events in patients with diabetes (i.e., ACE inhibitors, ARBs, beta-blockers, diuretics, and calcium channel blockers).

Low-density lipoprotein (LDL) cholesterol should be lowered to < 100 mg/dl as the primary goal of therapy for adults; an LDL goal of < 70 mg/dl is a therapeutic option for patients with diabetes with cardiovascular disease. Triglycerides should be lowered to < 150 mg/dl and high-density lipoprotein (HDL) cholesterol raised to > 40 mg/dl in men and > 50 mg/dl in women. Lifestyle modification focusing on the reduction of saturated fat and cholesterol intake, weight loss (if indicated), and increased physical activity has been shown to improve the lipid profile in patients with diabetes and is recommended for all patients. For those diabetic patients with cardiovascular disease or over the age of 40 years, statin therapy to achieve an LDL cholesterol reduction of 30–40% regardless of baseline LDL cholesterol levels is recommended. For those diabetic patients under the age of 40 years without cardiovascular disease but at increased risk due to other cardiovascular risk factors who do not achieve lipid goals with lifestyle modification alone, the addition of statin therapy is also appropriate. Lowering triglycerides and/or increasing HDL cholesterol with a fibrate or niacin should be considered in diabetic patients with elevated triglycerides and/or low HDL cholesterol.

Aspirin therapy (75–162 mg/day) is recommended as a secondary prevention strategy in those with diabetes and a history of cardiovascular disease. Aspirin therapy (75–162 mg/day) is recommended as a primary prevention strategy in those with type 1 or type 2 diabetes at increased cardiovascular risk (including those who are > 40 years of age). Aspirin therapy should also be considered for primary prevention in patients between the age of 30 and 40 years with diabetes, particularly in the presence of other cardiovascular risk factors. Combination therapy using other antiplatelet agents such as clopidogrel in addition to aspirin should be considered in certain specific subsets of patients with diabetes with cardiovascular disease.

In asymptomatic patients without documented cardiovascular disease, a risk factor evaluation should be considered to stratify patients by 10-year risk, and risk factors should be treated accordingly. The screening of asymptomatic patients with cardiac stress testing remains controversial. Candidates for a screening exercise stress test include those with a history of peripheral or carotid occlusive disease and those with a sedentary lifestyle who are > 35 years of age and plan to begin a vigorous exercise program. Candidates for a diagnostic exercise test include those with typical or atypical cardiac symptoms and those with an abnormal resting electrocardiogram. Patients with an abnormal exercise test and patients unable to perform an exercise test require additional or alternative testing. Stress nuclear perfusion imaging and stress echocardiography are considered to be valuable next-level diagnostic procedures.

In patients > 55 years of age, with or without hypertension but with cardiovascular disease or another cardiovascular risk factor (e.g., dyslipidemia, microalbuminuria, or smoking), an ACE inhibitor (if not contraindicated) should be considered to reduce the risk of cardiovascular events. In patients with a prior myocardial infarction or in patients undergoing major surgery, beta-blockers should be considered to reduce mortality. In patients with treated heart failure, metformin use is contraindicated. The thiazolidinediones are associated with fluid retention, and their use can be complicated by the development of heart failure. Caution in prescribing thiazolidinediones in the setting of known heart failure or other heart diseases, as well as in patients with pre-existing edema or concurrent insulin therapy, is required.

An annual test for the presence of microalbuminuria should be performed in type 1 diabetic patients who have had diabetes ≥ 5 years and all type 2 diabetic patients starting at diagnosis. Serum creatinine should be measured at least annually for the estimation of glomerular filtration rate in all adults with diabetes regardless of the degree of urine albumin excretion. The serum creatinine alone should not be used as a measure of kidney function but instead used to estimate glomerular filtration rate and stage the level of chronic kidney disease. To reduce the risk and/or slow the progression of nephropathy, we should optimize both glucose and BP control. In the treatment of microalbuminuria/macroalbuminuria/nephropathy, either ACE inhibitors or ARBs should be used (except during pregnancy). With the onset of overt nephropathy, dietary protein intake should be restricted to ≤ 0.8 g/kg body weight/day (approximately 10% of daily calories); further restriction may be useful in selected patients.

A comprehensive foot examination should be performed annually on patients with diabetes to identify risk factors predictive of ulcers and amputations. Patients' feet should be visually inspected at each routine visit. All patients, especially those with risk factors or prior lower-extremity complications, should be educated about the risk and prevention of foot problems and self-care behavior reinforced. A multidisciplinary approach is recommended for persons with foot ulcers and high-risk feet, especially those with a history of prior ulcer or amputation. Patients with significant claudication or a positive ankle–brachial index should be referred for further vascular assessment and exercise training, medications, and surgical options considered.

Patients with type 1 diabetes should have an initial dilated and comprehensive eye examination by an ophthalmologist or optometrist within 3–5 years after the onset of diabetes. Patients with type 2 diabetes should have an initial dilated and comprehensive eye examination by an ophthalmologist or optometrist shortly after the diagnosis of diabetes. Subsequent examinations for type 1 and type 2 diabetic patients should be repeated annually. Patients with any level of macular edema, severe nonproliferative diabetic retinopathy, or any proliferative diabetic retinopathy should be promptly referred to an ophthalmologist who is knowledgeable and experienced in the management and treatment of diabetic retinopathy. Laser therapy can reduce the risk of vision loss in patients with high-risk characteristics.

All patients should be screened for distal symmetric polyneuropathy at diagnosis and at least annually thereafter, using simple clinical tests. Once the diagnosis of distal symmetric polyneuropathy is established, special foot care is appropriate for insensate feet to decrease the risk of amputation. Screening for autonomic neuropathy should be instituted at diagnosis of type 2 diabetes and 5 years after the diagnosis of type 1 diabetes. A wide variety of medications may be considered for the relief of specific symptoms related to neuropathy (including tricyclic drugs, anticonvulsants, and duloxitene for the management of neuropathic pain; metoclopramide for gastroparesis; and various medications for bladder and erectile dysfunction).

An influenza vaccine should be provided annually to all adult diabetic patients. In addition, adults with diabetes should receive at least one lifetime pneumococcal vaccine. A one-time revaccination is recommended for individuals > 64 years of age previously immunized when they were < 65 years of age if the vaccine was administered > 5 years ago.

HYPERTENSION

Hypertension Classification and Diagnosis

An accurate BP reading is the most important part of the classification and diagnosis of hypertension. Table 3 provides The Joint National Committee on Prevention, Detection, Evaluation, and Treatment of High Blood Pressure (JNC 7) classification of BP for adults aged 18 years or older *(10)*. The JNC 7 classification is based on the mean of two or more properly measured seated BP readings on each of two or more office visits.

Table 3
Classification and Management of Blood Pressure for Adults*

| BP classification | SBP mmHg* | DPB mmHg* | Lifestyle modification | Initial drug therapy | |
				Without compelling indication	With compelling indications[†]
Normal	< 120	And < 80	Encourage		
Prehypertension	120–139	Or 80–89	Yes	No antihypertensive drug indicated.	Drug(s) for compelling indications.[‡]
Stage 1 hypertension	140–159	Or 90–99	Yes	Antihypertensive drug(s) indicated.	Drug(s) for compelling indications.[‡] Other antihypertensive drugs, as needed.
Stage 2 hypertension	≥ 160	Or ≥ 100	Yes	Antihypertensive drug(s) indicated. Two-drug combination for most.[†]	

DBP, diastolic blood pressure; SBP, systolic blood pressure.

* Treatment determined by highest BP category.

[†] Initial combined therapy should be used cautiously in those at risk for orthostatic hypotension.

[‡] Compelling indications include heart failure, postmyocardial infarction, high coronary artery disease risk, diabetes, chronic kidney disease, and recurrent stroke prevention. Treat patients with chronic kidney disease or diabetes to BP goal of < 130/80 mmHg (10).

In addition to BP determination, evaluation of patients with hypertension has three primary objectives, namely, to assess lifestyle and identify other cardiovascular risk factors or concomitant disorders that may impact prognosis and help guide therapy, to reveal identifiable causes of hypertension, and to assess the presence or absence of cardiovascular disease and target organ damage. The medical history, physical examination, routine laboratory tests, and other diagnostic procedures are needed to obtain the required information (10).

In more than 95% of cases, the etiology of hypertension is unknown, and it is called primary, essential, or idiopathic hypertension. Secondary hypertension is hypertension with a known cause. Identifiable causes of hypertension include sleep apnea, drug-induced or drug-related causes, chronic kidney disease, primary aldosteronism, renovascular disease, chronic steroid therapy and Cushing syndrome, pheochromocytoma, coarctation of the aorta, and thyroid or parathyroid disease (10).

Complications of Hypertension

Chronic hypertension produces target organ damage to the heart, brain, kidneys, peripheral vasculature, and eyes. Fortunately, the major clinical trials of antihypertensive therapy have demonstrated multiple benefits, including a 35–40% reduction in the incidence of stroke, 20–25% reduction in myocardial infarction, and more than 50% reduction in heart failure *(11)*.

The relationship between BP and risk for cardiovascular events is continuous, consistent, and independent of other cardiovascular risk factors. For individuals 40–70 years of age, each increment of 20 mmHg in systolic BP or 10 mmHg in diastolic BP doubles the risk of cardiovascular disease across the entire BP range from 115/75 to 185/115 mmHg. Although both systolic and diastolic BP are important, in persons older than 50 years, systolic BP is a much more important cardiovascular disease risk factor than diastolic BP *(10)*.

Medical Management of Hypertension

The goals of antihypertensive therapy are to control BP and to reduce cardiovascular and renal morbidity and mortality by the least intrusive means possible. This may be achieved through lifestyle modification alone or in combination with pharmacologic treatment (Table 3). Individuals with a systolic BP of 120–139 mmHg and/or a diastolic BP of 80–89 mmHg should be considered as "prehypertensive" and also require lifestyle intervention.

The BP goal is < 130/80 mmHg in patients with hypertension with diabetes or chronic kidney disease and < 140/90 mmHg in other patients with hypertension. Because most patients with hypertension, especially those older than 50 years, will reach the diastolic BP goal once systolic BP is at the goal level, JNC 7 recommends that the primary focus be on achieving the systolic BP goal. Fig. 1 depicts the algorithm recommended by JNC 7 for the treatment of hypertension. Therapeutic lifestyle changes and pharmacologic interventions advocated by JNC 7 and the American Heart Association can be briefly summarized as follows *(10,12)*.

LIFESTYLE MODIFICATIONS

Regular aerobic physical activity, such as brisk walking, should be performed for at least 30 min/day on most days of the week – see chap. 16 for exercise-specific guidelines. Overweight or obese persons should receive guidance on weight loss, with the goal ideally being to attain a body mass index < 25 kg/m^2; for nonoverweight persons, a desirable body mass index of 18.5–24.9 kg/m^2 should be maintained. Salt intake should be lowered as much as possible, ideally to approximately 65 mmol/day (corresponding to 1.5 g/day of sodium or 3.8 g/day of salt).

With the assistance of a dietician (if feasible), a diet rich in fruits and vegetables (8–10 servings/day), rich in low-fat dairy products (2–3 servings/day), and reduced in saturated fat and cholesterol should be recommended. Potassium intake should be increased to 120 mmol/day (4.7 g/day), which is also the level provided in Dietary Approaches to Stop Hypertension (DASH)-type diets. For those who drink alcohol, consumption should be limited to no more than 2 drinks/day in most men and 1 drink/day in women and lighter-weight persons. For overall cardiovascular risk reduction, cigarette smokers should quit smoking.

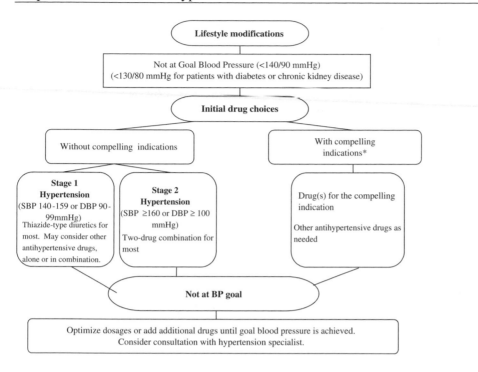

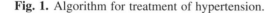

DBP, diastolic blood pressure; SBP, systolic blood pressure.
*Compelling indications include heart failure, postmyocardial infarction, high coronary heart disease risk, diabetes, chronic kidney disease, and recurrent stroke prevention. Treat patients with chronic kidney disease or diabetes to a goal of <130/80 mmHg(10).

Fig. 1. Algorithm for treatment of hypertension.

Pharmacologic Treatment

Most patients with hypertension who require drug therapy in addition to lifestyle modification will require two or more antihypertensive medications to achieve goal BP. If BP is > 20/10 mmHg above the goal, consideration should be given to initiating antihypertensive therapy with two agents, one of which should usually be a thiazide-type diuretic. Thiazide-type diuretics should be used in drug treatment for most patients with uncomplicated hypertension, either alone or combined with drugs from other classes. Certain high-risk conditions are compelling indications for the initial use of other antihypertensive drug classes. Compelling indications include heart failure (diuretics, beta-blockers, ACE inhibitors/ARBs, and aldosterone antagonists), postmyocardial infarction (beta-blockers, ACE inhibitors/ARBs, and aldosterone antagonists), patients at high risk for coronary artery disease (diuretics, beta-blockers, ACE inhibitors/ARBs, and calcium channel blockers), diabetes (diuretics, beta-blockers, ACE inhibitors/ARBs, and calcium channel blockers), chronic kidney disease (ACE inhibitors/ARBs), and recurrent stroke prevention (diuretics and ACE inhibitors/ARBs).

After initiation of drug therapy, most patients should return for follow-up and adjustment of medications at approximately monthly intervals until the BP goal is reached. More frequent follow-up may be needed for patients with stage 2 hypertension or with complicating comorbid conditions. Serum potassium and creatinine should be monitored at least 1–2 times per year. Follow-up visits can usually be at 3–6-month intervals once BP is at goal and stable.

Other cardiovascular risk factors (such as serum lipids and lipoproteins and diabetes) should be treated to their respective goals. Other evidence-based cardio-protective drugs should be initiated, if clinically indicated. Low-dose aspirin therapy for cardiovascular risk reduction should only be considered when BP is controlled, because the risk of hemorrhagic stroke is increased in patients with uncontrolled hypertension.

SUMMARY

Current evidence provides a strong rationale for the long-term aggressive control of multiple cardiovascular disease risk factors as an essential strategy to normalize endothelial function; halt or reverse the progression of atherosclerosis; prevent the instability, rupture, and thrombosis of atherosclerotic plaques; and reduce mortality, recurrent hospitalization, and the ongoing cost of medical care. In this chapter, the classification, diagnosis, complications, and, especially, medical management of two of the major cardiovascular disease risk factors, namely, diabetes and hypertension, are briefly reviewed.

REFERENCES

1. American Diabetes Association. *Therapy for Diabetes Mellitus and Related Disorders*, HE Lebovitz (ed.). Alexandria, VA: American Diabetes Association; 1998.
2. Wang Y, Wang QJ. The Prevalence of Prehypertension and Hypertension Among U.S. Adults According to the New Joint National Committee Guidelines: New Challenges of the Old Problem. *Arch Intern Med*. 2004;164:2126–2134.
3. Fields LE, Burt VL, Cutler JA, Hughes J, Roccella EJ, Sorlie P. The Burden of Adult Hypertension in the United States 1999 to 2000: A Rising Tide. *Hypertension*. 2004;44: 398–404.
4. Hajjar I, Kotchen TA. Trends in Prevalence, Awareness, Treatment, and Control of Hypertension in the United States, 1988–2000. *JAMA*. 2003;290:199–206.
5. American Diabetes Association. Diagnosis and Classification of Diabetes Mellitus. *Diabetes Care*. 2006;29(Suppl 1):S43–S48.
6. American Diabetes Association Standards of Medical Care in Diabetes–2006. *Diabetes Care*. 2006;9(Suppl 1):S4–S42.
7. Grundy SM, Benjamin IJ, Burke GL, Chait A, Eckel RH, Howard BV, Mitch W, Smith SC, Sowers JR. Diabetes and Cardiovascular Disease: A Statement for Healthcare Professionals from the American Heart Association. *Circulation*. 1999;100:1134–1146.
8. American Diabetes Association. Nutrition Recommendations and Interventions for Diabetes. *Diabetes Care*. 2007;30:S48–S65.
9. American Diabetes Association. Diabetes Mellitus and Exercise (Position Statement). *Diabetes Care*. 2000;23(Suppl 1):S50–S54.
10. Chobanian AV, Bakris GL, Black HR, et al. The Seventh Report of the Joint National Committee on Prevention, Detection, Evaluation, and Treatment of High Blood Pressure. The JNC 7 Report. *JAMA*. 2003;289:2560–2572.

11. Neal B, MacMahon S, Chapman N. Effects of ACE Inhibitors, Calcium Antagonists, and Other Blood Pressure-Lowering Drugs. *Lancet*. 2000;356:1955–1964.

12. Appel LJ, Brands MW, Daniels SR, Karanja N, Elmer PJ, Sacks FM. Dietary Approaches to Prevent and Treat Hypertension: A Scientific Statement from the American Heart Association. *Circulation*. 2006;47:296–308.

15 Exercise in Patients with Cardiovascular Disease

John R. Schairer, DO, FACC, and Steven J. Keteyian, PhD

CONTENTS

INTRODUCTION

Today, physical activity is seen as a behavior that generally has beneficial effects on exercise capacity and many of the physiologic processes involved in the development of, as well as, primary prevention of coronary artery disease. Current public health recommendations state that all people over 2 years of age should accumulate 30 min of moderate-intensity endurance-type physical activity on most (preferably all) days of the week (1). Additionally, the American College of Sports Medicine recommends that at least two sessions each week incorporate resistance or strength training involving the major muscle groups (2). For the past 25 years, exercise has also been recommended for patients with heart disease.

Despite these benefits, the prevalence of no leisure-time physical activity in the U.S. is approximately 24% and another 55% of Americans engage in exercise on an irregular basis (3,4). Individuals with chronic illnesses such as myocardial infarction (MI), heart failure, and stroke have rates of no leisure-time physical activity that approach 50% (4), and only 30% of patients eligible for cardiac rehabilitation actually are referred to formal cardiac rehabilitation programs (5). For women and the elderly, the rates of referral to cardiac rehabilitation are even less.

The goals of this chapter are to (i) describe the cardiovascular response during an acute bout of exercise, (ii) describe the cardiovascular response to an exercise-training program and (iii) discuss the nuances of the exercise prescription for patients with specific cardiovascular disease entities.

From: *Contemporary Cardiology: Cardiac Rehabilitation*
Edited by: W. E. Kraus and S. J. Keteyian © Humana Press Inc., Totowa, NJ

PHYSIOLOGIC RESPONSES TO EXERCISE

The physiologic response to exercise varies depending on whether you are describing the physiology of a single or acute bout of exercise, as occurs during an exercise test, or whether you are describing the chronic adaptations that occur in response to repetitive bouts of exercise training, as occurs with cardiac rehabilitation. Also, patients with coronary artery disease may demonstrate a normal or abnormal physiological response to exercise. Common hemodynamic responses to both acute and chronic exercise are discussed below.

Heart Rate

The normal heart rate response during exercise is linear, due to a decrease in vagal tone and an increase in sympathetic tone that allows the patient to achieve a heart rate that is within two standard deviations of an age-predicted maximum. During recovery, vagal tone increases and causes the heart rate to decrease fairly quickly (Fig. 1). The measurement of heart rate at 1 and 2 min is termed heart rate recovery. Failure to achieve predicted maximum heart rate, in the absence of beta-adrenergic blocking agents, is called chronotropic incompetence. Abnormal heart rate recovery is defined as a delayed decrease in heart rate of ≤ 12 beats per minute at 1 min and ≤ 22 beats per minute at 2 min. The presence of either chronotropic incompetence or abnormal heart rate recovery during exercise is partly due to abnormalities of sympathetic and parasympathetic tone and known predictors of higher cardiovascular morbidity and mortality *(6,7)*. With regular exercise training, vagal tone is increased and sympathetic tone is decreased, resulting in a lower resting heart rate and improvement in chronotropic incompetence.

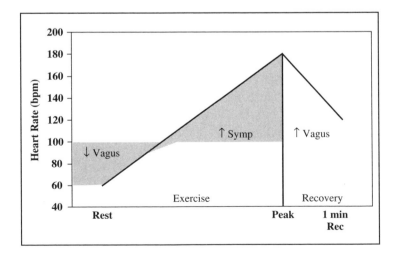

Fig. 1. Neurohumoral and heart rate changes during exercise. ↑= increase tone; ↓= decrease tone.

Blood Pressure

The normal response of systolic blood pressure during incremental exercise is a progressive rise of about 10 ± 2 mmHg/metabolic equivalent (MET), with a possible plateau at peak exercise. Systolic blood pressure during exercise in patients with coronary artery disease may respond normally or it may increase or decrease abnormally. Exertional hypertension during a stress test is defined as a systolic blood pressure of more than 250 mmHg and is a relative indication to stop the test *(8)*. Exertional hypotension is defined as a drop below resting blood pressure or a failure of systolic blood pressure to rise. A decrease of $\geq$ 10 mmHg during an exercise stress test is an indication to stop the test *(8)*. Exertional hypotension may be attributed to left ventricular dysfunction, a large area of exercise-induced ischemia or papillary muscle dysfunction with mitral regurgitation and is associated with an increased risk of cardiac events *(8,9)*.

Because of a reduction in systemic vascular resistance in the metabolically more active skeletal muscles during exercise, diastolic blood pressure usually remains the same or decreases during exercise. Although an increase in diastolic blood pressure of 15 mmHg or more may be associated with covert coronary artery disease, several studies have shown that an exaggerated response of the systolic blood pressure ($>$ 220 mmHg) and/or an abnormal diastolic pressure response (increase of 10 mmHg or $>$ 90 mmHg) is more likely a marker for future hypertension *(10,11)*.

With an exercise-training program one can expect a modest decrease in both the systolic and the diastolic blood pressure. The decrease in blood pressure is greatest in patients with mild-to-moderate hypertension and averages 6 mmHg for systolic blood pressure and 5 mmHg for diastolic blood pressure *(12)*. In 1995, the effectiveness of exercise training as a complement to pharmacologic therapy was demonstrated in adult African-American men with severe hypertension *(13)*.

Cardiac Output and Oxygen Uptake

Compared to rest, typically there is an 8–10-fold increase in oxygen uptake (VO_2) at peak exercise in healthy, active individuals. With exercise training, VO_2 max can be increased approximately 15–30% *(14)*. In patients with coronary artery disease, however, peak VO_2 is reduced 20–35% when compared with age-matched normals *(5, 15)*. The magnitude of reduction in peak VO_2 depends on the severity of the disease and is due to diminished cardiac output and peak blood flow within the peripheral musculature. Exercise cardiac output may be reduced due to chronotropic incompetence or left ventricular impairment from MI, or transient coronary ischemia, resulting in a decrease in both ejection fraction and stroke volume *(14)*.

Today, the benefits and risks of exercise are being studied on a vascular, cellular, and/or neurohumoral level. The acute responses and chronic adaptations to regular exercise are summarized in Table 1. A summary of the effects of a chronic exercise program on cardiovascular risk factors is summarized in Table 2.

Table 1
Physiologic Benefits of Exercise

	Acute	Chronic
Vascular		
Vascular stenosis	No benefit	Partial regression > 2200 kcal/week
Collaterals	No benefit	No benefit
Endothelial Dysfunction	No benefit	Improved (Nitrous oxide ↑)
Capillary flow	No benefit	Increased
Autonomic nervous systems		
Parasympathetic tone	Decreased	Increased
Sympathetic tone	Increased	Decreased
Hemostatic		
Fibrinogen	Increased	Decreased
Factor VII	–	–
Platelet aggregation	Increased	Decreased
Fibrinolytic	Increased	Increased
Viscosity	Increased	Decreased
Inflammation		
C-reactive protein and cytokines	Increased	Decreased

Table 2
Summary of Effects of Exercise on Selected Cardiovascular Risk Factor

Risk factor	Effect
Smoking	±
Lipid abnormalities	
Cholesterol	±
LDL cholesterol	±
HDL	↑ Mild to moderate (10%)
Hypertension	↓ Incidence (especially among White males)
Systolic	↓ Average 6 mmHg
Diastolic	↓ Average 5 mmHg
Obesity	±
Diabetes	
Insulin sensitivity	↑
Onset of type 2 diabetes	Delayed

LDL, low-density lipoprotein; HDL, high-density lipoprotein; ↑, increase; ↓, decrease; ±, little or no effect.

EXERCISE PRESCRIPTION/PROGRAMMING

Coronary Artery Disease

From primary prevention observational studies, we know that exercise, whether measured as physical activity or physical fitness levels, reduces all-cause and

Table 3
Summary of Unique Exercise Prescription Issue Among Patients with Cardiovascular Disease

Illness	Comment
Coronary artery disease	Frequency, duration, and intensity of training should sum to yield a weekly energy expenditure > 1500 kcal/week to impact mortality.
Myocardial infarction	Begin cardiac rehabilitation 1 week after discharge at 50–60% of maximum VO_2.
Angina	Consider prophylactic nitroglycerin 15 min before anticipated exertion if symptoms limit routine activities of daily living or ability to train. Upper heart rate for training should be set at 10 beats below angina or ischemic threshold.
PTCA with or without stent	Can begin cardiac rehabilitation 24–48 h after Percutaneous Coronary Intervention (PCI) if there is no evidence of myocardial damage or hematoma at catheterization site.
CABG	Can begin cardiac rehabilitation 1–2 weeks postoperative. Limited upper body activities to mild intensity and range of motion until 10–12 weeks postoperative to allow healing of sternal wound.
Heart failure	If needed, initially guide exercise intensity at 60% of heart rate reserve and adjust duration to three bouts of 10 min each. Progress to one bout of 30–40 min. Titrate using the rating of perceived exertion scale, set at 11–14.
Cardiac transplant	Guide training intensity using RPE (11–14) rather than heart rate.
Pacemaker, ICD, RCT	Restrict all arm activity for 2 months and vigorous arm activity for an additional month. Set intensity at 50–85% of heart rate reserve or 10–15 beats below ischemic threshold or ICD-activation threshold.
Valvular heart disease	Follow CABG recommendations.

CABG, coronary artery bypass graft; ICD, implantable cardioverter defibrillator; PTCA, percutaneous transluminal coronary angioplasty; RCT, randomized controlled trial; RPE, rated perceived exertion.

cardiovascular mortality *(16–18)*. Paffenbarger et al. *(16)*, in their Harvard Alumni Study, reported that 1500 and 2000 kcal/week of exercise are necessary to reduce all-cause and cardiovascular mortality, respectively, whereas Blair et al. *(17)* reported that only a modest increase in fitness compared with those least fit is necessary to achieve the benefits of reduced mortality from cardiovascular disease. In patients who already have coronary artery disease, higher levels of physical activity may be needed. Hambrecht et al. *(18)* found that a weekly caloric expenditure > 2200 kcal is associated with partial regression of atherosclerosis in patients who already have coronary artery disease.

A meta-analysis published by Taylor et al. *(19)* examined 48 trials that included 8940 patients who had suffered an MI and were randomized to cardiac rehabilitation versus usual care. The meta-analysis found that cardiac rehabilitation reduced all-cause mortality by 20% and cardiovascular mortality by approximately 25%, but there was no reduction in nonfatal MIs.

With regard to safety, the incidence of fatal and nonfatal cardiac events occurring during or shortly after a cardiac rehabilitation exercise session is low. Fatal events occur at a rate of approximately 1/900,000 patient-hours of participation in supervised exercise training, with most events occurring in those patients considered to be at high-risk for cardiac events. The rate of nonfatal MIs during cardiac rehabilitation is approximately 1/250,000 patient-hours *(20)*.

The general principles of the exercise prescription are discussed in chap. 2 and apply to all patients – cardiac and noncardiac. Particularly among patients with coronary artery disease, a low-intensity warm-up helps avoid the occurrence of ST-segment depression, threatening arrhythmias, and transient LV dysfunction *(21)*. The cool down permits return of heart rate and BP to resting values, reduces the likelihood of postexercise hypotension and dizziness, and combats the potential deleterious effects of the postexercise rise in plasma catecholamines *(22)*. Maintaining the heart rate during exercise between 60 and 80% of heart rate reserve maximizes the health benefits while minimizing the risk. Dynamic resistance exercise for upper and lower body is now part of many structured cardiac rehabilitation programs *(8)*. Moderate-intensity dynamic resistance exercise results in improved muscle strength and endurance, both of which are important for the safe return to activities of daily living, preventing falls, engaging in vocational and avocational activities, and maintaining self-independence.

Myocardial Infarction

Cardiac rehabilitation programs generally include three stages: inpatient rehabilitation, outpatient rehabilitation, and maintenance. In-hospital cardiac rehabilitation is often referred to as Phase I. The goals of Phase I are to minimize the deconditioning that occurs as a result of bed rest and to begin a gradual progressive approach to exercise and education about risk factor modification and the lifestyle changes necessary to reduce future mortality and morbidity. Much of the deterioration in exercise tolerance can be countered through simple exposure to orthostatic or gravitational stress (by intermittent sitting or standing) and range of motion exercises. Patients who suffer an MI should resume limited physical activity, as soon as they are free of chest pain and hemodynamically stable.

Patients with an uncomplicated MI can begin outpatient cardiac rehabilitation 1 week after discharge. Outpatient cardiac rehabilitation is often referred to as Phase II. Phase II is a multifaceted program lasting 1–3 months which emphasizes supervised physical activity to improve conditioning and lifestyle changes to modify risk factors such as smoking cessation, weight management, healthy eating, and other factors to reduce future all-cause and cardiac mortality. Maintenance cardiac rehabilitation is referred to as Phase III (and IV) and involves continuation of exercise habits while additional lifestyle changes are encouraged.

The American College of Cardiology (ACC) and American Heart Association (AHA) Guidelines for Management of ST elevation MI (STEMI) (23) recommend that these patients should be encouraged to participate in cardiac rehabilitation/secondary prevention programs, particularly those STEMI patients with multiple modifiable risk factors and/or moderate- to high-risk patients in whom supervised exercise training is warranted. Most cardiac rehabilitation programs train patients at an intensity equivalent to 60–85% of heart rate reserve, 3 nonconsecutive days per week, for 20–40 min of aerobic exercise, with a 5–10-min warm-up and cool-down period. Patients suffering an MI complicated by heart failure should start their training at the lower end of their intensity range (50–60% of VO_2 or heart rate reserve or 11–13 on the ratings of perceived exertion scale) (8). As patients progress, they should be encouraged to exercise at home as well, so that they are exercising most days of the week (walking, jogging, cycling, or other aerobic activity), supplemented by an increase in daily lifestyle activities (e.g., walking breaks at work, gardening, and household work).

Exercise prescription for Patients with Heart Disease

The Surgeon General's recommendation that all people over the age of 2 years should accumulate 30–40 min of moderate-intensity exercise most days of the week is consistent with an energy expenditure of 1000–1,400 kcal/week (1). For patients participating in a maintenance (e.g., Phase III or IV) cardiac rehabilitation following an MI or coronary revascularization, caloric expenditure has been measured at 230–270 kcal per a 45-min rehabilitation session (24). We, also, evaluated total weekly caloric energy expenditure among patients exercising three times per week in a maintenance cardiac rehabilitation program and observed an energy expenditure of 830 kcal for the week, falling short of the thresholds identified by Paffenbarger et al. (1500 kcal) and Hambrecht et al. (2300 kcal) (25). Cardiac rehabilitation patients, however, were more active outside of the program than we previously realized, expending an additional 675 kcal/week in leisure-time physical activity for a total weekly caloric expenditure ≥ 1500 kcal. In fact, 72% of patients exceeded 1000 kcal and 43% exceeded 1500 kcal in total weekly energy expenditure. Thus, more than one-third of patients reached or exceeded the minimum 1500 kcal threshold felt to reduce all-cause mortality in a general population. It is important to note that patients 70 years and older, those with a BMI ≥ 30 and women, regardless of race, were least likely to achieve 1500 kcal/week and represent groups that need to be targeted with additional adherence strategies and supervision. When generating an exercise prescription for patients with heart disease, the amount of energy expenditure during both cardiac rehabilitation and leisure-time physical activity should be taken into consideration. In addition to frequency, intensity, duration, and type of activity, weekly caloric expenditure should be considered as a fifth component of the exercise prescription. Table 4 summarizes the amount and intensity of exercise required to reach specific caloric expenditure goals.

Nontraditional exercise programs have been shown to be effective and safe in selected populations *(19)*. DeBusk et al. *(26)*, as well as others, have reported their experience with medically directed at-home rehabilitation after an uncomplicated MI. A total of 127 male patients were randomized to home training or group training. At 26 weeks, exercise adherence was 72 and 71% for home training and group training, respectively. No training complications occurred in either group. These findings support the concept that medically directed at-home rehabilitation has the potential to increase the availability and decrease the cost of rehabilitating low-risk survivors of acute MI.

Angina and Myocardial Ichemia

Exercise, lifestyle behavior changes, and medical compliance are beneficial for people with stable angina and help reduce symptom occurrence, reduce overall cardiac risk, and prevent/retard progression of atherosclerotic plaques. After routine coronary angiography, Hambrecht et al. *(27)* randomized 101 male patients with stable coronary artery disease to 12 months exercise training (20 min of exercise ergometry per day) or percutaneous coronary intervention (PCI). Exercise training was associated with greater improvement in subsequent functional capacity and higher event-free survival (88% for exercise group versus 70% in the PCI group, $P = 0.023$). To improve one Canadian Society angina class, $6956 was spent in PCI group versus $3429 in the training group. The significantly lower costs occurred as a result of reduced hospitalizations and revascularizations.

It was initially thought that the threshold at which the myocardium becomes ischemic and angina occurs is reproducible and can be estimated by the rate–pressure product (heart rate × systolic blood pressure). So that for a given patient performing a specific activity at the same time of the day, there does appear to be reproducibility in the rate–pressure product at which angina will occur *(8)*. However, work by Garber et al. *(28)* demonstrated that the angina threshold varies with the type of exercise performed.

Table 4
The Amount and Intensity of Exercise Required to Reach Specific Caloric
Expenditure Goals

Calorie expenditure (kcal)	Intensity	Min/day*	Outcome
1000	Moderate	30	Progression
	Vigorous	20	
1400	Moderate	40	Fitness
	Vigorous	30	
1500	Moderate	45	No change in CAD
	Vigorous	30	↓ All-cause mortality
2000	Moderate	60	↓ CV mortality
	Vigorous	40	
2200	Moderate	65	Regression
	Vigorous	45	

CAD, coronary artery disease; CV, cardiovascular.
* Structured exercise plus leisure-time physical activity.

Specifically, they found that the ischemic threshold varied depending on whether one was performing a maximal stress test or a longer submaximal exercise session. In fact, the ischemic threshold occurred at a lower heart rate during sustained submaximal exercise training than during a maximal stress test. Circadian rhythm also effects ischemic threshold. Quyyumi et al. *(29)* showed that ischemic threshold was lower at 1 p.m. than that at 8 a.m. and 9 p.m. Forearm vascular resistance was increased at 8 a.m. and 9 p.m. when compared with that at 1 p.m., suggesting vascular resistance may be one of the mechanisms for variability in anginal threshold.

One goal for patients with angina is to increase the amount of symptom or ischemia-free work or exercise they can perform at a given pressure–rate product *(8)*. Exercise lowers sympathetic tone, improves peripheral muscle oxygen extraction and endothelial function, and reduces platelet aggregation and vascular tone (Table 1). As a result, patients perform routine daily activities at a lower rate–pressure product, thus reducing the amount of angina and fatigue. Therefore, more intense activities are subsequently required to reach the rate–pressure product associated with ischemia (i.e., ischemic threshold) (Fig. 2).

Exercise programming for patients with angina requires that they first recognize and understand their symptoms. They need to identify the nature of their angina (e.g., chest, throat, back, and arm) and understand that there are no clinical benefits derived from exercising with pain. They also need to identify which activities precipitate their angina and modify the situation accordingly. For example, if walking in the cold causes chest discomfort, then they should exercise indoors or consider wearing a scarf or other protective wear over their mouth to warm/humidify inhaled air. Similarly, if carrying out the garbage or walking the dog frequently causes chest pain, they should talk with their doctor about taking sublingual nitroglycerin beforehand.

For patients with exercise-induced ischemia, the upper heart rate limit during exercise should be set 10 or more beats below the heart rate or rate–pressure product at which ischemia was first noticed *(8)*. Myocardial ischemia may manifest itself as angina, ST-depression with or without chest pain, ventricular arrhythmias, or abnormal blood pressure response.

Medications such as beta-blockers, nitrates, and some calcium channel blockers can influence the ischemic threshold. As a result, it is prudent to ensure that patients take their medications at least 2 h before undergoing an exercise test administered for

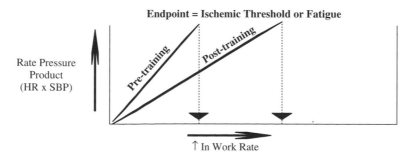

Fig. 2. Regular exercise training attenuates myocardial O_2 demand. During exercise, as estimated by rate–pressure product.

the purpose of establishing the correct exercise training heart rate range. Ideally, the physician would like to repeat the exercise test if a patient's medication or dose is changed, although this is not always realistic due to reimbursement issues.

Revascularization – Coronary Artery Bypass Graft and Percutaneous Coronary Intervention

Patients undergoing coronary revascularization by either angioplasty/stent or coronary artery bypass graft (CABG) surgery are expected to demonstrate an improved exercise response. Signs of ischemia during exercise such as angina, ST-depression, and hemodynamic abnormalities (i.e., chronotropic incompetence and blunted blood pressure response) are often eliminated after revascularization or occur at higher-intensity activities. Additionally, many of the benefits and limitations associated with exercise are the same for patients after revascularization, as they are for patients following an MI.

Recommendations for exercise programming for patients following PCI are generally the same as for other patients with coronary artery disease. However, because most patients undergoing PCI did not experience myocardial damage or extensive surgery, they can sometimes begin cardiac rehabilitation 24–48 h after the procedure *(30)*. ACC/AHA Recommendations for Coronary Artery Bypass Graft Surgery *(31)* state that cardiac rehabilitation should be offered to all eligible patients after CABG. Patients undergoing CABG surgery can begin rehabilitation as early as 1–2 weeks after an uncomplicated surgery; however, upper body exercise should be limited to range of motion and light repetitive or rhythmic type activities such as arm ergometry until 8 weeks after surgery when sternal wound healing has occurred. For many patients, light training with the upper limbs might begin with elastic bands and hand weights, before progressing to resistance-type exercise machines. Physical activities such as golf, bowling, and swimming can place stress on the sternal wound and should be avoided for 12 weeks.

Heart Failure

A hallmark symptom of patients with chronic heart failure is exercise intolerance or dyspnea on exertion. Compared with age-matched healthy normals, peak exercise capacity is reduced approximately 40–50% in patients with heart failure *(32)*. Several mechanisms have been identified to explain the observed exercise intolerance, including a reduction in peak cardiac output (approximately 40%), chronotropic incompetence, and a reduced stroke volume. Also, the ability to increase blood flow to the more metabolically active skeletal muscles during exercise is attenuated, due mostly to both an exaggerated increase in direct sympathetic tone and an attenuated production of endothelium-derived relaxing factor. There are also abnormalities in the skeletal muscle such as a reduction in myosin heavy chain I isoforms, reduced activity of the enzyme-associated aerobic metabolism, and a reduction in fiber size *(32)*.

Current evidence *(32,33)* indicates that moderate exercise is generally safe and results in improvement in quality of life, autonomic balance (i.e., parasympathetic activity), exercise tolerance (peak VO_2, approximately 15–35%), endothelial function, chronotropic responsiveness, and skeletal muscle function. ACC/AHA 2005 CHF Guidelines *(34)* state exercise training should be considered for all stable outpatients with chronic heart failure who are able to participate in the protocols needed to produce physical conditioning.

When compared with apparently healthy people and those with ischemic heart disease and normal ventricular function, there are only a few differences relative to prescribing exercise in patients with New York Heart Association Functional Class II or III heart failure. Specifically, duration of activity may need to be adjusted to allow these patients more opportunity for rest and to progress at their own pace. In fact, some patients may better tolerate discontinuous training involving short bouts of exercise interspersed with bouts of rest (35). The American College of Sports Medicine (8) recommends that patients with a baseline exercise capacity < 3 METs should begin with interval training of 3–5-min duration, two to three times a day to counteract fatigue. Patients with exercise capacity of 3–5 METs can start with 5–10-min sessions one to two times daily. The patient with heart failure should be encouraged to progressively increase exercise duration, as tolerated, until able to tolerate one bout of 30–40 min four to six times per week.

Prior research indicates that different exercise intensities have been used to increase exercise tolerance, yet yielded similar relative gains in cardiovascular fitness (32). On the basis of these data, for the first few exercise sessions, it seems reasonable to guide exercise intensity at 60% of heart rate reserve, titrated based on a patient's subjective feelings of fatigue using the rating of perceived exertion scale of 11–14. In view of conflicting reports about whether there is a further decrease in left ventricular function when patients with chronic heart failure train above ventilatory threshold (VT) (32,36), it seems prudent to set subsequent exercise intensity at 60–70% of heart rate reserve.

Presently, some cardiac rehabilitation programs in the U.S. decide on the use of electrocardiographic (ECG) telemetry monitoring when exercising patients with heart disease, both with and without heart failure, based on a patient's risk for exercise-related events. Although ECG telemetry monitoring during cardiac rehabilitation is common in the U.S., it is important to point out that such an approach is not used in either Canada or Europe. Albeit limited, analysis of safety data from the European Heart Failure Training Group (36) and the EXERT trial (33) suggest that ECG monitoring may not be necessary when exercising patients with stable, chronic heart failure.

Cardiac Transplant

Despite receiving a donor heart with normal systolic function, cardiac transplant recipients continue to experience exercise intolerance after surgery approximately 40–50% below that of age-matched normals. This exercise intolerance is believed to be primarily due to the absence of efferent sympathetic innervation of the myocardium, residual skeletal muscle abnormalities developed prior to transplantation due to heart failure, and decreased skeletal muscle strength (37).

Following surgery, medical management focuses on preventing rejection of the donor heart by suppressing immune system function, while avoiding complicating side effects such as infections, hyperlipidemia, hypertension, osteoporosis, diabetes, certain cancers, and accelerated graft atherosclerosis of the epicardial and intramural coronary arteries. Except for cyclosporine, which may cause an increase in blood pressure at rest and during submaximal exercise, none of the other medications used to control immune system rejection in cardiac transplant recipients appear to influence the physiologic response of these patients during an acute bout of exercise or prevent the development of a safe exercise prescription for aerobic conditioning (37).

Owing to the denervated myocardium in cardiac transplant recipients, many differences in the cardiopulmonary and neuroendocrine response are evident at rest, during exercise and in recovery. These abnormalities include an elevated resting heart rate (often > 90 per min), elevated systolic and diastolic blood pressures at rest due to increased plasma norepinephrine and the immunosuppressive medications (i.e., cyclosporine and prednisone), an attenuated increase in heart rate during submaximal work, a lower peak heart rate and peak stroke volume, a greater rise in plasma norepinephrine during exercise, and a delayed slowing of heart rate in recovery (37). Delayed heart rate in recovery is thought to be due to increased levels of plasma norepinephrine, exerting its positive chronotropic effect in the absence of vagal efferent innervation.

To prescribe exercise and guide exercise intensity in cardiac transplant recipients, it is best to simply disregard all heart rate-based methods because of the abnormal heart rate control in these patients (38). For example, it is common to find persons with cardiac transplant achieving an exercise heart rate during training that not only exceeds 85% of peak but is often equal to or greater than the peak rate attained during their last symptom-limited exercise test. Ratings of perceived exertion between 11 and 14 should be used to guide exercise-training intensity.

Among cardiac transplant patients who undergo exercise training, exercise capacity increases by about 15–40%; resting heart rate is unchanged or decreases slightly; peak heart rate increases; there is little, if any, change in peak stroke volume or cardiac dimensions; and the quality of life is favorably altered (37). In the most comprehensive, prospective, randomized trial to date, Kobashigawa et al. (39) showed a 49% increase in peak VO_2 and a 23 beats per minute increase in peak heart rate.

In addition, these patients can benefit from a systematic program of resistance training, because a leg-strength deficit exists and contributes to the reduced exercise capacity that persists after surgery. Braith and Edwards (40) showed that resistance training improves muscular endurance, but it also partially restores bone mineral density and addresses the skeletal muscle abnormalities (i.e., strength development, lipid content, and fiber size) that commonly occur due to long-term corticosteroid therapy. A progressive resistance training program of 7–10 exercises that focuses on the legs, back, arms, and shoulders is started at least 12 weeks after surgery and performed two times per week should suffice (40).

Pacemakers/Defibrillators

Patients with pacemakers and implantable cardioverter defibrillators (ICDs) should wait 6 weeks following implantation to begin exercise to avoid dislodgement. Today, most patients receive rate-responsive pacemakers that respond to exercise by gradually increasing the rate (referred to as the ramp) until the upper rate of the pacemaker is reached (referred to as the upper rate limit). Both the ramp and the upper rate limit of the pacemaker are adjustable to maximize a patient's exercise performance. ICDs have several programmable parameters for identifying life-threatening arrhythmias. One of these parameters is a threshold heart rate above which the ICD will fire. Obviously, patients with pacemakers and ICDs need to have an exercise prescription that takes into account their age, underlying heart disease, their functional capacity, and their device. Generally, exercise heart rate in these patients should be set at 10 or more beats below the ischemic threshold or ICD-activation threshold *(41)*. Exercise tests performed to evaluate ischemia in patients with pacemakers and/or ICD will require imaging studies during the test because of the abnormal resting ECG.

Valvular Heart Disease

Patients with valvular heart disease are not unlike patients with other types of heart disease, and the basics for exercise programming are the same. Prior to valve surgery, patients with valvular heart disease are frequently limited in physical activity by dyspnea and fatigue similar to patients with congestive heart failure. They are frequently the New York Heart Association (NYHA) class II–IV with a functional work capacity that may be as low as 3–4 METs. For those patients who are not in decompensated heart failure, a regular exercise program is recommended.

After valvular surgery, the exercise component of cardiac rehabilitation is useful in reversing the deconditioning that occurs as a result of bed rest after surgery. Sire *(42)* reported that exercise training increased peak aerobic capacity and decreased the pressure–rate product and the rating of perceived exertion at a fixed workload. After aortic valve replacement, exercise training increased peak aerobic capacity by 38% when compared with no change in similar control patients receiving usual care *(42)*.

CONCLUSION

Since 1972, regular exercise training has become increasingly utilized in patients with a variety of cardiac related problems *(43)*. Exercise training is recommended because of its beneficial effects on symptoms, functional capacity, physiology, mood, and clinical outcomes. Future investigations should be concerned with developing behavioral approaches and techniques to increase a patient's long-term compliance with cardiac rehabilitation strategies. Also, because diastolic function abnormalities are associated with dyspnea and fatigue, two symptoms known to benefit from exercise training, the role of exercise training in treating abnormalities of diastolic function deserves additional study.

REFERENCES

1. US Department of Health and Human Services. *Physical Activities of Health: A Report of the Surgeon General*, Atlanta, GA: US Department of Health and Human Services, Center for Disease Control and Prevention, National Center for Chronic Disease Prevention and Health Promotion; 1996.
2. Pollock ML, Gasser GA, Butcher JD, et al. The Recommended Quantity and Quality of Exercise for Developing and Maintaining Cardiorespiratory and Muscular Fitness, and Flexibility in Adults. *Med Sci Sports Exerc.* 1998;30:975–991.
3. Crespo CJ, Keteyian SJ, Heath GW, et al. Leisure Time Physical Activity Among US Adults. *Arch Intern Med.* 1996;156:93–98.
4. Pate PR, Pratt M, Blair SN, et al. Physical Activity and Public Health: A Recommendation from the Center for Disease Control and Prevention and the American College of Sports Medicine. *JAMA.* 1995;273:402–407.
5. Williams MA, Fleg JL, Aides PA, et al. Secondary Prevention of Coronary Heart Disease in the Elderly (with Emphasis on Patients > or = 75 Years of Age): An American Heart Association

Scientific Statement from the Council on Clinical Cardiology Subcommittee on Exercise, Cardiac Rehabilitation and Prevention. *Circulation*. 2002;105:1735–1743.

6. Ellestad MH, Wan MK. Predictive Implications of Stress Testing: Follow-Up of 2700 Subjects after Maximum Treadmill Stress Testing. *Circulation*. 1975;51:363–369.

7. Cole CR, Blackstone EH, Paskow FJ, et al. Heart-Rate Recovery Immediately after Exercise as a Predictor of Mortality. *N Engl J Med*. 1999;341:1351–1357.

8. American College of Sports Medicine. *ACSM Guidelines for Exercise Testing and Prescription*, 6th ed. Philadelphia, PA: Lippincott Williams and Wilkins; 2000.

9. Irving JB, Bruce RA, DE Rouen TA. Variations in and Significance of Systolic Pressure During Maximal Exercise (Treadmill) Testing: Relation to Severity of Coronary Artery Disease and Cardiac Mortality. *Am J Cardiol*. 1977;39:841–848.

10. Sheps DS, Ernst JC, Briese FW, et al. Exercise-Induced Increase in Diastolic Pressure: Indicator of Severe Coronary Artery Disease. *Am J Cardiol*. 1979;43:708–712.

11. Dlin R, Hanne N, Silverberg DS, et al. Follow-up of Normotensive Men with Exaggerated Blood Pressure Response to Exercise. *Am Heart J*. 1983;106:316–320.

12. American College of Sports Medicine. Position Stand: Exercise and Hypertension. *Med Sci Sports Exerc*. 2004;36:533–553.

13. Kokkinos P, Narayan P, Colleran J, et al. Effects of Regular Exercise on Blood Pressure and Left Ventricular Hypertrophy in African-American Men with Severe Hypertension. *N Engl J Med*. 1995;333:1462–1467.

14. Clausen JP. Circulatory Adjustments to Dynamic Exercise and Effects of Physical Training in Normal Subjects and in Patients with Coronary Artery Disease. In *Exercise and Heart Disease*, EH Sonneblick and M Lesch (eds.). New York: Grune and Stratton; 1977:39–75.

15. ACSM. Position Stand: Exercise for Patients with Coronary Artery Disease. *Med Sci Sports Exerc*. 1994;26:i–v.

16. Paffenbarger RS, Wing AL, Hyde RT. Physical Activity as an Index of Heart Attack Risk in College Alumni. *Am J Epidemiol*. 1978;108:161–175.

17. Blair SN, Kohl HW, Gorgon NF, et al. How Much Physical Activity is Good for Health? *Annu Rev Public Health*. 1992;13:99–126.

18. Hambrecht R, Niebauer J, Marburger C, et al. Various Intensities of Leisure Time Physical Activity in Patients with Coronary Artery Disease: Effects of Cardiorespiratory Fitness and Progression of Coronary Atherosclerotic Lesions. *J Am Coll Cardiol*. 1993;22:468–477.

19. Taylor RS, Brown A, Ebrahim S, et al. Exercise-Based Rehabilitation for Patients with Coronary Artery Disease: Systematic Review and Meta-Analysis of Randomized Controlled Trials. *Am J Med*. 2004;116:682–692.

20. Wenger NK, Froelicher ES, Smith LK, et al. *Cardiac Rehabilitation Clinic Practice Guidelines No. 17*. Rockville, MD: US Department Of Health And Human Services, Public Health Service Agency For Health Care Policy And Research And The National Heart, Lung And Blood Institute, Agency For Health Care Policy And Research Publication No. 96-0672; October 1995.

21. Barnard RJ, Gardner GW, Diaco NV, et al Cardiovascular Responses to Sudden Strenuous Exercise: Heart Rate, Blood Pressure and ECG. *J Appl Physiol*. 1973;34:833–837.

22. Dimsdale JE, Hartly H, Guiney T, et al. Postexercise Peril: Plasma Catecholamines and Exercise. *JAMA*. 1984;251:630–632.

23. Antman EM, Anabe DT, Armstrong PW, et al. ACC/AHA Guidelines for the Management of Patients with ST Elevation Myocardial Infarction. Available at www.acc.org/clinical/guidelines/stemi/index.pdf

24. Schairer JR, Kostelnik T, Proffett SM, et al. Caloric Expenditure During Cardiac Rehabilitation. *J Cardiopulm Rehabil*. 1998;18:290–294.

25. Schairer JR, Keteyian SJ, Ehrman JK, et al. Leisure-Time Physical Activity in Patients in Maintenance Cardiac Rehabilitation. *J Cardiopulm Rehabil*. 2003;23:260–265.
26. DeBusk RF, Haskell WL, Miller NH, et al. Medically Directed At-Home Rehabilitation soon after Clinically Uncomplicated Acute Myocardial Infarction: A New Model for Patient Care. *Am J Cardiol*. 1985;55:251–257.
27. Hambrecht R, Walther C, Mobius-Winkler S, et al. Percutaneous Coronary Angioplasty Compared with Exercise Training in Patients with Stable Coronary Artery Disease. *Circulation*. 2004;109:1371–1378.
28. Garber CE, Carleton RA, Camaione DN, et al. The Threshold for Myocardial Ischemia Varies with Coronary Artery Disease Depending on the Exercise Protocol. *J Am Coll Cardiol*. 1991;17:1256–1262.
29. Quyyumi AA, Panza JA, Diodati JG, et al. Circadian Variation in Ischemic Threshold. *Circulation*. 1992;86:22–28.
30. Schelkun PH. Exercise After Angioplasty: How Much? How Soon? *Phys Sportsmed*. 192;20:199–212.
31. Eagle KA, Guyton RA, Davidoff R, et al. ACC/AHA 2004 Guidelines Update for Coronary Artery Bypass Graft Surgery. Available at http://www.acc.org/clinical/guidelines/cabg/cabg.pdf
32. Keteyian SJ, Spring TJ. Chronic Heart Failure. In *Clinical Exercise Physiology*. Champaign, IL: Human Kinetics; 2003:261–280.
33. McKelvie RS, Teo KK, Roberts R, et al. Effects of Exercise Training in Patients with Heart Failure: The Exercise Prescription Trial (EXERT). *Am Heart J*. 2002;144:23–30.
34. Hunt SA, Abraham WT, Chin MA, et al. ACC/AHA 2005 Guideline Update for the Diagnosis and Management of Chronic Heart Failure in the Adult. Available at www.acc.org/clinical/guielines/failure/index.pdf
35. Meyer K, Samek L, Schwaibold M, et al. Interval Training in Patients with Severe Chronic Heart Failure: Analysis and Recommendations for Exercise Procedures. *Med Sci Sports Exerc*. 1997,29:306–312.
36. European Heart Failure Training Group. Experience from Controlled Trials of Physical Training in Chronic Heart Failure. *Eur Heart J*. 1998;19:466–475.
37. Keteyian SJ, Brawner C. Cardiac Transplant. In *ACSM's Exercise Management for Persons with Chronic Disease and Disabilities*, JL Durstine and GE Moore (eds.). Champaign, IL: Human Kinetics; 2003:70–75.
38. Keteyian SJ, Ehrman J, Fedel F, Rhoads K. Heart Rate-Perceived Exertion Relationship During Exercise in Orthotopic Heart Transplant Patients. *J Cardiopulm Rehabil*. 1990;10:287–293.
39. Kobashigawa JA, Leaf DA, Lee N, et al. A Controlled Trial of Exercise Rehabilitation after Heart Transplantation. *N Engl J Med*. 1999;34:272–277.
40. Braith RW, Edwards DG. Exercise Following Heart Transplantation. *Sports Med*. 2000;30:171–192.
41. Sears SF, Kovacs AH, Conti JB, et al. Expanding the Scope of Practice for Cardiac Rehabilitation: Managing Patients with Implantable Cardioverter Defibrillators. *J Cardiopulm Rehabil*. 2004;24:209–215.
42. Sire S. Physical Training and Occupational Rehabilitation after Aortic Valve Replacement. *Eur Heart J*. 1987;8:1215–1220.
43. Pollock ML, Schmidt DH. p. xvii Heart Disease and Rehabilitation. John Wiley and Sons. New York, 1979.

16 Exercise as a Therapeutic Intervention for Hypertension

Dalynn T. Badenhop, PhD, and Javier Jurado, MD

CONTENTS

Increasing levels of physical activity, together with reduced sodium intake, weight loss, and limited alcohol consumption are therapeutic lifestyle changes known to effectively reduce blood pressure *(1)*. Data from the Coronary Artery Risk Development in Young Adults (CARDIA) study support the fact that cardiovascular fitness is inversely related to the development of hypertension, diabetes, the metabolic syndrome, and hypercholesterolemia *(2)*. Dynamic aerobic training, in particular, has been shown to lower conventional and daytime blood pressure readings among hypertensive patients *(3)*. In general, exercise provides a substantial benefit for patients with both hypertension and cardiovascular disease and reduces the 10-year cardiovascular risk by 25% *(4)*. From a clinical standpoint, a reduction of as little as 3 mmHg in average population systolic blood pressure (SBP) has been estimated to reduce coronary heart disease by 5–9%, stroke by 8–14%, and all-cause mortality by 4%. Two other advantages of exercise as a therapeutic intervention are its positive effect on multiple cardiovascular disease risk factors and the fact that moderate exercise is low risk and has very few contraindications for most people.

MECHANISMS OF BLOOD PRESSURE RESPONSE TO EXERCISE

Exercise has been shown to have both an acute and a chronic effect on blood pressure. The typical blood pressure response to an acute bout of aerobic exercise is a gradual increase in SBP and a gradual decrease or no change in diastolic blood pressure (DBP). Shown in Fig. 1 are the systemic blood pressures (A) and systemic

From: *Contemporary Cardiology: Cardiac Rehabilitation*
Edited by: W. E. Kraus and S. J. Keteyian © Humana Press Inc., Totowa, NJ

vascular resistance (B) responses at rest and during dynamic exercise. Systolic and diastolic pressures at rest average around 125 and 80 mmHg, respectively, with a mean pressure of about 95 mmHg. Systemic vascular resistance in humans can be calculated from the relationship:

$$\text{Systemic vascular resistance } (R) = \frac{\text{mean pressure } (P_{\text{mean}})}{\text{cardiac output } (Q)}.$$

Therefore, if Q at rest is 5 l/min, then R is $\sim$ 19 mmHg/min (95 mmHg/5 l/min) (Fig. 1B).

During exercise, blood pressure increases as a result of the accompanying increase in cardiac output or, more specifically, of increases in stroke volume and heart rate

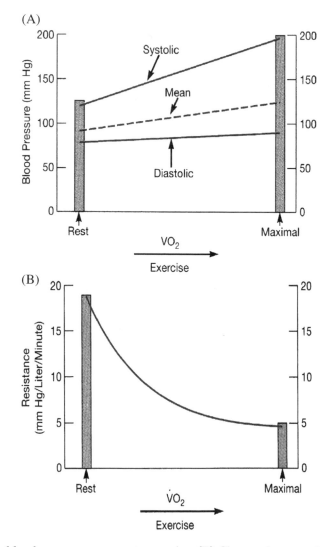

Fig. 1. (A) Acute blood pressure response to exercise. (B) Changes in systemic vascular resistance to flow during exercise.

brought about by changes in the autonomic nervous system and hormonal influences. Actually, as shown in Fig. 1A, this affects systolic pressure more than diastolic or mean pressure. The reason for this is that during exercise there is a simultaneous decrease in resistance due to vasodilation of the arterioles supplying blood to the more metabolically active skeletal muscles. This means that more blood will drain from the arteries through the arterioles and into the active muscle capillaries, thus minimizing changes in diastolic pressure. In turn, changes in mean arterial pressure will also be minimized. These changes in resistance during exercise are impressive. For example, at maximal exercise, with $P_{mean} = 126\,mmHg$ and $Q = 30\,l/min$, resistance would be $126/30 = 4.2\,mmHg/l/min$. This represents a 4.5-fold decrease from that at rest.

The blood pressure response to exercise differs between normotensive and hypertensive people. In normotensive individuals, acute bouts of dynamic exercise result in a higher SBP (usually $< 220\,mmHg$) and a reduction in peripheral vascular resistance as described above. However, because of an elevated baseline level, the absolute level of SBP attained during dynamic exercise is usually higher in persons with hypertension ($> 220\,mmHg$). In addition, DBP may not change, or may even slightly rise, during dynamic exercise, probably as a result of impaired endothelial function and increased sympathetic outflow. Patients with hypertension exhibit an increase in the total peripheral resistance and increases in myocardial oxygen consumption and impaired vasodilation *(5)*. The blood pressure response in normal and borderline hypertensive men is illustrated in Fig. 2.

Immediately following an acute bout of exercise, a postexercise hypotension phenomenon has been recognized in both normotensive and hypertensive individuals. This response may last up to 22 h after exercise and, due to the decrease in systemic vascular resistance, usually drops the arterial blood pressure by 5–7 mmHg. The reduction in blood pressure after exercise can be sustained for up to 1–2 weeks, after three or more separate bouts of exercise *(6)*. Over time, these changes chronically translate into eccentric left ventricular hypertrophy with a preserved cardiac function *(7)*. Stretching caused by the overload from exercise translates into cardiomyocyte expansion, hypertrophic remodeling, and an increase in the contractile force per cell *(8)*. This homogenous, physiologic remodeling is beneficial, as opposed to the pathologic concentric hypertrophy related to chronic hypertension, which involves apoptotic processes and the replacement of necrotic tissue by fibroblasts and collagen *(9)*.

A reduction in the cardiac output and/or a reduction in the peripheral vascular resistance are postulated as possible mechanisms for the antihypertensive effects of exercise training *(10–12)*. Aerobic exercise is also associated with a decrease in plasma noradrenaline, which correlates with the reductions in SBPs and DBPs that are common among hypertensive individuals with elevated resting catecholamine levels. This reduction in levels of sympathetic activity may correlate with the reduction in cardiac output as well as in peripheral resistance *(13)*. At the endothelial level, the elevated shear stress in the vessel walls, a product of the increased blood flow to muscles during exercise, likely serves as a stimulus for nitric oxide release, thus leading to smooth muscle-mediated vasodilation *(14)*. Reactive hyperemia, an index of the nitric oxide-related vasodilation, improved with long-term aerobic exercise in a study of Japanese patients with mild-to-moderate essential hypertension *(15)*.

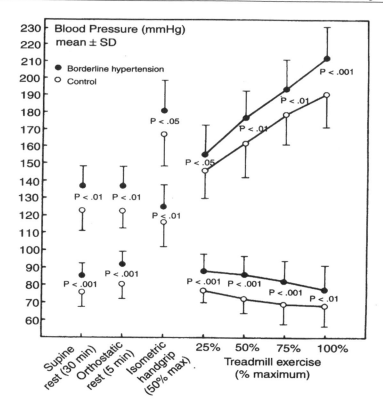

Fig. 2. Systolic blood pressure (SBP) and diastolic blood pressure (DBP) responses in normal and borderline hypertensive men.

There is also a depletion of whole blood and plasma volumes, as well as sodium depletion, noted by a significant correlation between the changes in the sodium/potassium ratio and SBP *(16)*. These changes were confirmed in a study where middle-aged men with essential hypertension subjected to regular exercise experienced a significant reduction in blood pressure, a higher serum Na:K ratio, a higher cardiac index, and lower total peripheral resistance *(17)*. These findings help explain the theory that exercise reduces blood pressure more effectively in volume-dependent hypertensives.

CLINICAL EVIDENCE

Data from the First National Health and Nutrition Examination Survey (NHANES I) with 9791 study subjects revealed a favorable association between exercise and outcomes (all-cause and cardiovascular mortality) in hypertensive individuals ($p < 0.001$ and $p = 0.002$, respectively), when compared to normotensive and prehypertensive subjects *(18)*. The chronic effects of regular exercise on individuals with hypertension are reflected by an average blood pressure reduction of 2.6–7.4 mmHg *(19)*. Thus, prescribing exercise should be a standard of practice, especially in patients with hypertension.

Data from multiple randomized controlled clinical trials support the use of exercise for blood pressure reduction *(20)*. Despite this overwhelming evidence, some aspects remain undefined; one example is whether the reduction in blood pressure is independent of weight reduction, body composition, and other modifiable risk factors. A meta-analysis of 44 randomized controlled clinical trials indicates that endurance exercise contributes to the control of blood pressure in overweight as well as in lean subjects, although a significant decrease in the BMI occurred in the obese population only *(21)*. Although exercise seems to exert its benefit independently from other modifiable factors, the PREMIER clinical trial established that blood pressure control was most successful among individuals undergoing multiple behavioral interventions including physical activity, weight loss, decreased sodium intake, decreased daily intake of alcohol, and a diet high in fruits and vegetables and low in saturated and total fat (DASH diet) *(22)*.

Another meta-analysis of 54 randomized controlled trials (2419 patients) evaluating the effect of aerobic exercise on blood pressure reported an overall significant reduction in mean SBP (-3.8 mmHg) and mean DBP (-2.6 mmHg) *(23)*. Aerobic exercise lowered BP in people who were normotensive or hypertensive, overweight or of normal weight, and Black, White, or Asian. These results are tabulated in Table 1. In addition, all frequencies, intensities, and types of aerobic exercise lowered BP. These results are summarized in Table 2. BP was significantly reduced even in trials whose participants did not lose weight.

Other factors such as daily emotional fluctuations, stress, and degree of physical activity have also been implicated in the severity of hypertension and its response to exercise. Regular aerobic exercise together with weight loss has particularly proven to be beneficial in the reduction of diastolic and mean arterial blood pressure during activities of daily living. In a study of 112 participants, the elevations of blood pressure

Table 1
Effect of Aerobic Exercise on Blood Pressure with Regard to Hypertensive Status, Ethnicity, and Baseline BMI

Parameters (# studies)	SBP (mmHg)	DBP (mmHg)
Hypertensive status		
Hypertensive (15)	-4.94	-3.73
Normotensive (27)	-4.04	-2.33
Ethnicity		
White (23)	-3.44	-2.61
Asian (6)	-6.22	-6.58
Black (4)	-10.96	-3.25
Baseline BMI		
< 24.5 (11)	-3.9	-2.4
24.5–26.4 (12)	-4.5	-3.6
> 26.4 (12)	-2.2	-1.8

BMI, body mass index; DBP, diastolic blood pressure; SBP, systolic blood pressure.

Table 2
Effect of Aerobic Exercise on Blood Pressure with Regard
to Exercise Type, Weekly Exercise, and Exercise Intensity

Parameters	SBP (mmHg)	DBP (mmHg)
Exercise type		
Bike (17)	−5.6	−4.0
Walk or Jog (23)	−2.6	1.7
Mixed or other (13)	−3.6	−2.3
Weekly exercise (min/week)		
< 120 (21)	−2.8	−2.2
120–150 (15)	−4.7	−2.1
> 150 (13)	−5.1	−2.8
Exercise intensity		
Low (7)	−4.1	−2.7
Moderate (28)	−4.3	−3.6
High (10)	−4.0	−1.5

DBP, diastolic blood pressure; SBP, systolic blood pressure.

associated with the emotional distress and physical activity variations during a typical day, notably improved with 55 min of daily exercise ($p < 0.005$); exercise alone only improved blood pressure during low degrees of activity and distress (24).

EXERCISE AND HYPERTENSION IN THE ELDERLY

The control of isolated systolic hypertension in the elderly is a topic of debate. Progressive degeneration of the arterial media and increased collagen and calcium deposition results in stiffening of the arteries in the elderly, hypertensive population (25). These changes seem to be hastened by the effect of prolonged high blood pressure levels. Clinically, this is manifested by an elevated SBP and has been implicated as a contributor to cardiovascular morbidity and mortality (26). However, moderate aerobic exercise training has failed to improve large-artery stiffness in patients with isolated systolic hypertension (27). Nonetheless, a study involving elderly individuals with essential hypertension that were randomized to a low- or moderate-intensity training program found that low-intensity exercise significantly reduces the systolic BP 7 mmHg after 9 months of regular training ($p < 0.05$). Both low- and moderate-intensity exercise, however, reduced the DBP and mean BP by 9 mmHg and 8 mmHg, respectively, when compared with the control group of patients not exercising (28). An increase in the total body fat, particularly abdominal fat that is more prominent with aging, is also directly related to the appearance of hypertension in this age group (29). Data obtained from the Senior Hypertension and Physical Exercise (SHAPE) study revealed that after a 6-month randomized controlled trial of aerobic and resistance training, exercisers failed to significantly reduce their SBP (change of −0.8 mmHg from baseline) (30). Aortic stiffening, as measured by aorto-femoral pulse-wave velocity, failed to improve with exercise as well; this would explain the resistance of systolic hypertension to improve with physical activity in the elderly.

However, a meta-analysis involving 802 normotensive and hypertensive patients older than 50 years demonstrated a significant reduction of 2 mmHg in SBP *(20)*. Younger adult populations exhibit a better response to exercise. For instance, a study involving postmenopausal women with an average age of 55 years revealed a significant reduction in the systolic (from 142 mmHg to 131 mmHg, 8%) and mean arterial blood pressure (from 103 mmHg to 98 mmHg, 5%) after 24 weeks of regular walking in prehypertensive and stage I hypertensive patients. Systolic BP and mean arterial BP remained constant in the control group throughout the 24 weeks. There was no significant change in resting DBP in either group across 24 weeks. The improvement was unrelated to body composition, diet, or fasting insulin levels *(31)*.

PRESCRIPTION OF EXERCISE FOR PATIENTS WITH HYPERTENSION

As a consensus, patients with hypertension should exercise most or all days of the week, for a minimum of 30 min of moderate aerobic exercise. Resistance training should serve as an adjunct to an aerobic-based program *(32)*. Moderate-intensity exercise should be defined as one producing an elevation to 50–60% of the maximum heart rate and associated with 40–60% of the heart rate reserve or VO_2 reserve. For endurance exercise training, it appears prudent to maintain exercise blood pressure values less than 220/105 mmHg. Moderate-intensity exercise has been proven to be as effective as vigorous activity in lowering blood pressure and is associated with fewer cardiovascular and musculoskeletal adverse effects *(33)*. Hypertensive patients seem to maximally benefit from aerobic exercise involving large muscle groups such as walking, running, cycling, or swimming.

The prescription of exercise will vary according to the stage of hypertension (Table 3), the cardiovascular status in general, and the patient's age. These factors will determine the frequency, intensity, duration, and type of exercise advised, and whether exercise testing and monitoring is required. For instance, patients who are older (> 50), with documented hypertension and suspected cardiovascular disease, will need evaluation and/or monitoring by a clinical exercise physiologist; in these cases only light-to-moderate physical activity is recommended (Table 4). Conversely, younger prehypertensive patients with no documented atherosclerotic disease may engage in more strenuous activities and likely do not require initial testing or monitoring *(36)*.

The evaluation of patients who will start to exercise depends on the intensity of the anticipated activity and on the patient's cardiovascular risk factors. Peak or symptom-limited exercise testing is warranted in patients with hypertension about to engage into hard physical activity or in those individuals with cardiovascular disease. Patients without cardiovascular disease, but with blood pressure > 180/110 mmHg, may benefit from exercise testing before moderate activity but not before light activity. Commonly used criteria for discontinuation of exercise testing include SBP and/or DBP values > 250 mmHg and 115 mmHg, respectively *(19)*. Conversely in asymptomatic individuals with BP < 180/110 mmHg who are about to engage in light-to-moderate physical activity, no further testing is advised (Table 4). All hypertensive patients, however, must be carefully screened with a history and physical examination for the presence of secondary causes of hypertension, the presence of risk factors, target-organ damage, and the presence of cardiovascular disease *(19)*.

Table 3

Classification and Management of Blood Pressure for Adults Aged 18 Years or Older

BP classification	SBP (mmHg*)		DBP (mmHg*)	Lifestyle modification	Management	
					Initial drug therapy	
					Without compelling indication	With compelling indications
Normal	< 120	and	< 80	Encourage		
Prehypertension	120–139	or	80–89	Yes	No antihypertensive drug indicated	Drug(s) for the compelling indications[†]
Stage 1 hypertension	140–159	or	90–99	Yes	Thiazide-type diuretics for most; may consider ACE inhibitor, ARB, BB, CCB, or combination	Drug(s) for the compelling indications Other antihypertensive drugs (diuretics, ACE inhibitor, ARB, BB, CCB) as needed
Stage 2 hypertension	≥ 160	or	≥ 100	Yes	Two-drug combination for most (usually thiazide-type diuretic and ACEI or ARB or BB or CCB)[‡]	Drug(s) for the compelling indications Other antihypertensive drugs (diuretics, ACE inhibitor, ARB, BB, CCB) as needed

ACE, angiotensin-converting enzyme inhibitor; ARB, angiotensin-receptor blocker; BB, beta-blocker; CCB, calcium channel blocker; DBP, diastolic blood pressure; SBP, systolic blood pressure.

* Treatment determined by highest BP category.

[†] Treat patients with chronic kidney disease or diabetes to BP goal of < 130/80 mmHg.

[‡] Initial combined therapy should be used cautiously in those at risk for orthostatic hypotension.

Reprinted from National Cholesterol Education Program (NCEP) (36).

Table 4
How to Prescribe Exercise to Hypertensive Patients Based on Health Status and Age

Patient category	Column A	Column B	Column C
	• Prehypertensives with no suspected CVD < 50 years • Stage 1 hypertensives < 50 years	• Prehypertensives with suspected CVD • Prehypertensives > 50 years with no suspected CVD • Stage 2 hypertensives with no suspected CVD < 50 years	• Stage 1 and Stage 2 hypertensives with no suspected CVD > 50 years • Stage 1 and Stage 2 hypertensives with suspected CVD
Exercise testing and monitoring	Not necessary	Recommended	Recommended
Exercise type	Aerobic activities: walking, jogging, cycling, swimming	Walking, cycling until medically evaluated	Low-impact activities such as walking, cycling, and swimming
	Resistance training for retaining muscle mass	Send to clinical exercise physiologist for conditioning and aerobic training advice	Resistance training for muscle maintenance
	Monitoring not necessary but suggest they seek advice from a clinical exercise physiologist for a conditioning and aerobic-based training program	Monitoring probably not necessary unless patient has been sedentary for a number of years and feels uncomfortable about exercise	Send to clinical exercise physiologist for monitored conditioning program
		Resistance training for muscle maintenance	Follow aerobic training program designed by a clinical exercise physiologist. Periodic monitoring may be necessary
Frequency	6–7 days/week	5–7 days/week	5–7 days/week
Intensity	Start with 20–30 min continuous aerobic activity at comfortable	Work at light-to-moderate intensity until	Light to moderate. Lower intensity can star with

(Continued)

Table 4 (Continued)

Patient category	Column A	Column B	Column C
	pace (50–65%) of maximum heart rate for 3–4 weeks for general conditioning	evaluated and conditioned	20–30 min/day of continuous activity then build to 45–60 min/day
	Then exercise at up to 85% of maximum heart rate	Then undertake a maintenance aerobic program at up to 85% of maximum heart rate	Maintain an endurance-based resistance training for muscle maintenance
	Maintain an endurance-based resistance training for muscle maintenance	Maintain an endurance-based resistance training for muscle maintenance	
Duration	Aim for 30–60 min/day (minimum 150 min/week of aerobic activity)	Start with 20–30 min/day of continuous activity. Build to 30–60 min/day (minimum 150 min/week)	Start with 20–30 min/day of continuous activity. Build to 30–60 min/day (minimum 150 min/week)
Weight problems	For patients who are overweight, emphasize weight reduction through diet modification. Goal is 60 min/day of aerobic exercise. Suggest alternating aerobic activity type to avoid injuries. Emphasize endurance resistance training of three sets of 12–15 repetitions. Do not make resistance training main exercise. It is important not to hold breath while lifting weights.		

CVD, cardiovascular disease. 2006 Australian Family Physician. Reproduced with permission from The Royal Australian College of General Practitioners *(35)*.

REFERENCES

1. Whelton PK, He J, Appel LJ. Primary Prevention of Hypertension: Clinical and Public Health Advisory from the National High Blood Pressure Education Program. *JAMA*. 2002;288:1882–1888.
2. Carnethon M, Gidding S, Nehgme R. Cardiorespiratory Fitness in Young Adulthood and the Development of Cardiovascular Disease Risk Factors. *JAMA* 2003;290(23):3092–3100.
3. Fagard R. The Role of Exercise in Blood Pressure Control: Supportive Evidence. *J Hypertens*. 1995;13:1223–1227.
4. Hagberg JM, Park JJ, Brown MD. The Role of Exercise Training in the Treatment of Hypertension: An Update. *Sports Med*. 2000;30(3):193–206.
5. Pickering T. Pathophysiology of Exercise Hypertension. *Herz*. 1987;12(2):119–124.
6. Thompson PD, Crouse SF, Goodpaster B. The Acute Versus the Chronic Response to Exercise. *Med Sci Sports Exerc*. 2001;33(6):S438–S445.
7. Shapiro L. Morphologic Consequences of Systemic Training. *Cardiol Clin*. 1992;10(2):219–226.
8. Wakatsuki T, Schlessinger J, Elson E. The Biochemical Response of the Heart to Hypertension and Exercise. *Trends Biochem Sci*. 2004;29(11):609–617.
9. Weber K. Fibrosis and Hypertensive Heart Disease. *Curr Opin Cardiol*. 2000;15:264–272.
10. De Plaen JF, Detry JM. Hemodynamic Effects of Physical Training in Established Arterial Hypertension. *Acta Cardiol*. 1980;35:179–188.
11. Hagberg JM, Goldring D, Ehsani A. Effect of Exercise Training on the Blood Pressure and Hemodynamic Features of Hypertensive Adolescents. *Am J Cardiol*. 1983;52:763–768.
12. Nelson L, Jennings G, Esler MD. Effect of Changing Levels of Physical Activity on Blood Pressure and Hemodynamics in Essential Hypertension. *Lancet*. 1986;2:473–476.
13. Duncan JJ, Farr JF, Upton SS. The Effects of Aerobic Exercise on Plasma Catecholamines and Blood Pressure in Patients with Mild Essential Hypertension. *JAMA*. 1985;254:2609–2613.
14. McAllister R, Hirai T, Musch T. Contribution of Endothelium-Derived Nitric Oxide (EDNO) to the Skeletal Muscle Blood Flow Response to Exercise. *Med Sci Sports Exerc*. 1995;27:1145–1151.
15. Higashi Y, Sasaki S, Sasaki N. Daily Aerobic Exercise Improves Reactive Hyperemia in Patients with Essential Hypertension. *Hypertension*. 1999;33:591–597.
16. Urata H, Tanabe Y, Kiyonaga A. Antihypertensive and Volume-Depleting Effects of Mild Exercise on Essential Hypertension. *Hypertension*. 1987;9:245–252.
17. Kinoshita A, Urata H, Tanabe Y. What Types of Hypertensives Respond Better to Mild Exercise Therapy? *J Hypertens*. 1998;6:S631–S633.
18. Fang J, Wylie-Rosett J, Alderman M. Exercise and Cardiovascular Outcomes by Hypertensive Status: NHANES I Epidemiologic Follow-up Study, 1971-1992. *Am J Hypertens*. 2005;18:751–758.
19. American College of Sports Medicine Position Stand. Exercise and Hypertension. *Med Sci Sports Exerc*. 2004;36:533–553.
20. Kelly G, Sharpe K. Aerobic Exercise and Resting Blood Pressure in Older Adults: A Meta-Analytic Review of Randomized Controlled Trials. *J Gerontol*. 2001;56:M298–M303.
21. Fagard R. Physical Activity in the Prevention and Treatment of Hypertension in the Obese. *Med Sci Sports Exerc*. 1999;31:S624–S630.
22. PREMIER Collaborative Research Group. Effects of Comprehensive Lifestyle Modification on Blood Pressure Control. *JAMA*. 2003;289(16):2083–2093.
23. Whelton S, Chin A, Xin X. Effect of Aerobic Exercise on Blood Pressure. *Ann Intern Med*. 2002;136(7):493–503.
24. Steffen P, Sherwood A, Gullette E. Effects of Exercise and Weight Loss on Blood Pressure During Daily Life. *Med Sci Sports Exerc*. 2001;33(10):1635–1640.
25. London G, Guerin A. Influence of Arterial Pulse and Reflective Waves on Systolic Blood Pressure and Cardiac Function. *J Hypertens Suppl*. 1999;17:S3–S6.

26. Antikainen R, Jousilahti P, Tuomilehto J. Systolic Blood Pressure, Isolated Systolic Hypertension and Risk of Coronary Heart Disease, Strokes, Cardiovascular Disease and All-Cause Mortality in the Middle-Aged Population. *J Hypertens*. 1998;16:577–583.

27. Ferrier K, Waddell T, Gatzka C. Aerobic Exercise Training Does Not Modify Large-Artery Compliance in Isolated Systolic Hypertension. *Hypertension*. 2001;38:222–226.

28. Hagberg J, Montain S, Martin W. Effect of Exercise Training in 60 to 69-Year-Old Persons with Essential Hypertension. *Am J Cardiol*. 1989;64:348–353.

29. Smith S, Lovejoy J, Greenway F. Contributions of Total Body Fat, Abdominal Subcutaneous Adipose Tissue Compartments, and Visceral Adipose Tissue to the Metabolic Complications of Obesity. *Metabolism*. 2001;50:425–435.

30. Stewart K, Bacher A, Turner K. Effect of Exercise on Blood Pressure in Older Persons. *Arch Intern Med*. 2005;165:756–762.

31. Moreau K, Degarmo R, Langley J. Increasing Daily Walking Lowers Blood Pressure in Postmenopausal Women. *Med Sci Sports Exerc*. 2001;33(11):1825–1831.

32. Pescatello L. Exercise and Hypertension: Recent Advances in Exercise Prescription. *Curr Hypertens Rep*. 2005;7(4):281–286.

33. Elley CR, Aroll B. Refining the Exercise Prescription for Hypertension. *Lancet*. 2005;366(9493):1248–1249.

34. National Cholesterol Education Program (NCEP). Executive Summary of the Third Report of the Expert Panel on Detection, Evaluation and Treatment of High Blood Cholesterol in Adults (Adult Treatment Panel III).*JAMA*. 2003;289(19):2560–2572.

35. Baster T, Baser-Brooks C. How to Prescribe Exercise to Hypertensive Patients Based on Health Status and Age. *Aust Fam Physician*. 2005;34:421.

36. American College of Sports Medicine. *Guidelines for Exercise Testing and Prescription*, 6th ed. Philadelphia, PA: Lippincott, Williams & Wilkins, 2000.

17 Diabetes Mellitus and Cardiac Rehabilitation in Clinical Practice

Jennifer B. Green, MD

OVERVIEW

The term diabetes mellitus refers to various conditions associated with disordered glucose metabolism and hyperglycemia. This group of conditions includes disease states caused by insulin deficiency, alteration in insulin activity, or both. Traditionally, diabetes has been broadly classified as either type 1 or type 2, primarily based on the presence or absence of endogenous insulin production. However, it is increasingly obvious that diabetes is a significantly heterogenous condition and that many individuals are not easily classified into one of these two groups. Aside from genetic and environmental effects, a large number of pancreatic conditions, drugs, infectious agents, and endocrine or metabolic conditions have been associated with the development of diabetes (1,2). Table 1 summarizes the wide variety of genetic defects, pancreatic disorders, endocrinopathies, infectious agents, and medications which may be associated with diabetes. For the purposes of this text, discussion will primarily focus on the commonly recognized features of type 1 and type 2 diabetes. Although these conditions may vary considerably with respect to pathophysiology, presentation, and management options, it is important to recognize that the complications of both types are the same and may be quite severe.

From: *Contemporary Cardiology: Cardiac Rehabilitation*
Edited by: W. E. Kraus and S. J. Keteyian © Humana Press Inc., Totowa, NJ

Table 1
Etiologic Classification of Diabetes Mellitus *(2)*

I. Type 1 diabetes (ß-cell destruction, usually leading to absolute insulin deficiency)
   A. Immune mediated
   B. Idiopathic
II. Type 2 diabetes (may range from predominantly insulin resistance with relative insulin deficiency to a predominantly secretory defect with insulin resistance)
III. Other specific types
   A. Genetic defects of ß-cell function
      1. Chromosome 12, HNF-1 (MODY3)
      2. Chromosome 7, glucokinase (MODY2)
      3. Chromosome 20, HNF-4 (MODY1)
      4. Chromosome 13, insulin promoter factor-1 (IPF-1; MODY4)
      5. Chromosome 17, HNF-1ß (MODY5)
      6. Chromosome 2, NeuroD1 (MODY6)
      7. Mitochondrial DNA
      8. Others
   B. Genetic defects in insulin action
      1. Type A insulin resistance
      2. Leprechaunism
      3. Rabson–Mendenhall syndrome
      4. Lipoatrophic diabetes
      5. Others
   C. Diseases of the exocrine pancreas
      1. Pancreatitis
      2. Trauma/pancreatectomy
      3. Neoplasia
      4. Cystic fibrosis
      5. Hemochromatosis
      6. Fibrocalculous pancreatopathy
      7. Others
   D. Endocrinopathies
      1. Acromegaly
      2. Cushing's syndrome
      3. Glucagonoma
      4. Pheochromocytoma
      5. Hyperthyroidism
      6. Somatostatinoma
      7. Aldosteronoma
      8. Others
   E. Drug- or chemical-induced
      1. Vacor
      2. Pentamidine
      3. Nicotinic acid
      4. Glucocorticoids
      5. Thyroid hormone
      6. Diazoxide
      7. ß-adrenergic agonists

        8. Thiazides
        9. Dilantin
     10. Alpha-interferon
     11. Others
  F. Infections
        1. Congenital rubella
        2. Cytomegalovirus
        3. Others
  G. Uncommon forms of immune-mediated diabetes
        1. "Stiff-man" syndrome
        2. Anti-insulin receptor antibodies
        3. Others
  H. Other genetic syndromes sometimes associated with diabetes
        1. Down's syndrome
        2. Klinefelter's syndrome
        3. Turner's syndrome
        4. Wolfram's syndrome
        5. Friedreich's ataxia
        6. Huntington's chorea
        7. Laurence–Moon–Biedl syndrome
        8. Myotonic dystrophy
        9. Porphyria
     10. Prader–Willi syndrome
     11. Others
IV. Gestational diabetes mellitus (GDM)

At present, diabetes is estimated to affect 170 million individuals worldwide, with the number of affected individuals estimated to rise to 300 million by the year 2025 *(3,4)*. Among the developed countries, the prevalence of diabetes is estimated to currently be 6–7%; however, certain ethnic groups such as African Americans, native Americans, and Hispanics are disproportionately affected *(1)*. Excess caloric consumption and decreased physical activity have contributed significantly to the increase in numbers of overweight and diabetic individuals.

TYPE 1 DIABETES MELLITUS

Type 1 diabetes is characterized by insulin deficiency secondary to autoimmune destruction of the pancreatic beta cells. Although this condition is usually diagnosed in childhood, it is known to occur at any age. At present, type 1 diabetes comprises only 10% of the U.S. population with diabetes. Clinical disease does not occur until at least 90% of the beta cells have been destroyed, at which point most individuals will develop the abrupt onset of symptoms including polydipsia, polyuria, polyphagia, and weight loss. Diabetic ketoacidosis is a severe complication of this condition, in which increased breakdown of adipose stores result in elevated levels of free fatty acids, which are metabolized in the liver to the ketone bodies acetoacetate and beta hydroxybutarate. Accumulation of these substances results in ketonemia, ketonuria, and a potentially life-threatening metabolic acidosis *(1)*.

A genetic predisposition to type 1 diabetes is clear, with a sibling's risk of developing disease being 100 times that of the general population *(5)*. The human leukocyte antigen (HLA) locus contributes the most significant genetic risk for type 1 diabetes, with the majority of affected individuals having HLA-DR3, HLA-DR4, or both. Susceptibility to or protection from disease is attributed to linked DQ alleles. However, the predictive ability of this testing is poor, as most persons with "susceptible" alleles will not develop clinical disease *(1)*. Environmental factors such as viruses may trigger the autoimmune response that causes type 1 diabetes *(6)*.

As would be expected, individuals with type 1 diabetes are dependent on exogenous insulin therapy. As is also seen in type 2 diabetes, tight glycemic control in type 1 diabetes has been associated with a reduction in the microvascular complications of retinopathy, nephropathy, and neuropathy *(7)*. However, strict glycemic management is generally associated with an increased incidence of hypoglycemic events. Intensive insulin management through insulin pump therapy or the administration of multiple daily injections has rapidly become the standard of care in management. Physiologic cure of diabetes, or a significant reduction in insulin requirements, may be achieved through transplantation of pancreatic islet cells or following transplantation of the organ itself. However, the disease may recur either due to rejection of the transplanted tissue or less likely due to recurrence of the primary autoimmune process *(6)*.

TYPE 2 DIABETES MELLITUS

Type 2 diabetes is a complex metabolic condition that is presently estimated to affect 5–7% of the U.S. population. The pathophysiology is less clear than in type 1 diabetes; however, the disease is generally characterized by resistance to insulin action as well as relative insulin deficiency. Conditions including overweight and obesity, inactivity, and aging all contribute significantly to the risk of type 2 diabetes, but genetic factors are also important *(1)*. This condition is most prevalent in overweight or obese individuals over the age of 40 years; however, an increasing number of children and adolescents are also affected by type 2 diabetes.

It is felt most likely that an increase in insulin resistance occurs with aging, weight gain, and decreased physical activity. Insulin resistance is manifest by a decrease in peripheral glucose uptake and utilization, as well as ineffective suppression of hepatic glucose production. The pancreas is able to compensate for the insulin resistance for some time by producing a compensatory hyperinsulinism. Eventually, however, the pancreas is unable to maintain enough insulin production to maintain blood sugars within the normal range, resulting in hyperglycemia. Type 2 diabetes is associated with a disfavorable metabolic profile including hypertension; a prothrombotic tendency with elevation in plasminogen activator inhibitor-1 (PAI-1) and platelet dysfunction; and a dyslipidemia characterized by low levels of high-density lipoprotein (HDL) cholesterol, elevated triglycerides, and an increased ratio of small, dense, atherogenic low-density lipoprotein (LDL) cholesterol particles *(1)*.

The American Diabetes Association suggests that screening for type 2 diabetes (through fasting blood sugar or oral glucose tolerance testing) be performed every 3 years starting at age 45 years. However, glucose-tolerance testing should be performed earlier for those at increased risk, including those persons with risk factors such as overweight or obesity, dyslipidemia, hypertension, a family history of diabetes, history of gestational diabetes, known previous hyperglycemia, polycystic ovary syndrome, or belonging to high-risk ethnic groups (2).

The U.K. Prospective Diabetes Study (UKPDS) trial has clearly demonstrated that intensive glycemic control of type 2 diabetes will reduce microvascular complications (8). A reduction in cardiovascular events was also seen but did not reach statistical significance: further studies to determine the relationship between glycemic lowering and cardiovascular disease are ongoing. As individuals with type 2 diabetes are generally insulin deficient in a relative rather than absolute sense, insulin therapy is not always necessary. However, most persons with type 2 diabetes will eventually require insulin therapy to manage glycemia adequately. Given some degree of intrinsic insulin production, diabetic ketoacidosis is not commonly seen in type 2 diabetes. It may occur, however, in conditions that cause a significant increase in insulin requirements – for example, during serious infections, or following surgery or myocardial infarction (1). Various classes of oral diabetes medications are currently available, which work through mechanisms including an increase in insulin production, improved insulin sensitivity, or slowed absorption of dietary carbohydrates. Newer injectable agents are available which mimic the effects of naturally occurring pancreatic or small intestinal hormones. In addition, all currently available insulins may be used in the management of type 2 diabetes. A complete review of these drugs and their uses is beyond the scope of this text.

Given the complexity of the condition that is type 2 diabetes, potentially curative interventions are presently limited. Meaningful weight loss achieved through lifestyle, medical, or surgical intervention has been associated with significant improvements in glycemia. Perhaps most important, the Diabetes Prevention Program trial found that lifestyle modification significantly reduced the development of diabetes in an at-risk group of individuals. A reduction in risk was also found with the use of the insulin-sensitizing agent metformin but to a lesser degree than was seen with dietary and exercise intervention (9). Additionally, troglitazone therapy significantly reduced the likelihood of diabetes in at-risk women who had been previously diagnosed with gestational diabetes (10). It is clear, however, that regular physical activity and maintenance of a normal body weight are probably the most effective prevention strategies.

COMPLICATIONS OF DIABETES

Although the manifestations of diabetes may vary considerably among affected individuals, the potential complications of longstanding diabetes are similar in both type 1 and type 2 diabetes. Years of hyperglycemia result in damage to large and small arteries. Damage to the vasculature is broadly classified as either macrovascular (characterized by accelerated atherosclerosis and an increased risk of myocardial infarction, stroke, and peripheral vascular disease) or microvascular (with associated damage to the retina, kidneys, and nerves). The development of these complications is quite complex but appears to involve multiple mechanisms including the formation of advanced glycation end products, pro-coagulant effects, and alterations in the polyol pathway which increase cellular susceptibility to oxidative stress *(1)*. The increased cardiovascular risk associated with diabetes cannot be over-emphasized; in fact, cardiovascular disease (and in particular, coronary artery disease) is the leading cause of mortality in persons with diabetes. Risk reduction through smoking cessation, antiplatelet therapy, blood pressure control, and management of dyslipidemia is essential. The role of glycemic control in reducing cardiovascular risk is unclear but is under further investigation.

Diabetic retinopathy is a progressive condition characterized by proliferation of the retinal vessels and increased vasopermeability *(11)*. Visual loss occurs subsequent to macular involvement, vitreal hemorrhage, and/or retinal detachment. Cataract formation is a significant late complication of diabetes *(12)*. Good glycemic and blood pressure control, as well as regular ophthalmologic evaluation, are essential to the preservation of vision. Ophthalmologic screening should begin at the time of diagnosis of type 2 diabetes or 5 years after the onset of type 1 diabetes *(2)*.

Diabetic nephropathy is the primary cause of kidney failure among many developed countries in North America, Europe, and Asia *(12)*. Extensive vascular and other changes occur within the kidney, including damage to the glomeruli, basement membrane, collecting tubules, and interstitium. Early and frequent screening for the presence of albuminuria is essential in monitoring the progression of disease. As in diabetic retinopathy, control of glycemia and hypertension are of proven benefit in both prevention and management of this complication. Individuals who have evidence of nephropathy or are hypertensive should be started preferentially on either an angiotensin-converting enzyme (ACE) inhibitor or an angiotensin-receptor blocker (ARB) *(2)*. Documentation of nephropathy should prompt an evaluation for cardiovascular disease and retinopathy, as these complications are closely linked.

Most cases of neuropathy in the developed world are secondary to diabetes. In fact, this complication is responsible for the majority of diabetes-related hospitalizations, as well as the majority of nontraumatic amputations. A distal symmetric sensorimotor polyneuropathy is the most common presentation *(13)*. Small fiber neuropathy may cause a pain syndrome of hypersensitivity and hyperalgesia, which may progress to complete sensory loss. Peripheral neuropathy – particularly in association with peripheral vascular disease – predisposes to foot injury, foot deformity, ulceration, and limb loss. Nerve conduction studies are the most sensitive diagnostic test *(11)*; however, a thorough physical examination will also often reveal abnormalities in deep tendon reflexes, proprioception, nociception, temperature sensation, or vibratory sensation. Autonomic nerve dysfunction is present in an estimated 50% of individuals with diabetes. This complication is commonly manifest as nausea or emesis due to gastroparesis; constipation due to altered colonic motility; erectile dysfunction; or orthostatic hypotension with resting tachycardia. Altered cardiac sympathetic innervation is associated with a significantly increased risk of sudden death and should be suspected in persons with unexplained dyspnea, cough, fatigue, syncope, tachycardia, or bradycardia. A prolonged QT interval – a risk factor for arrhythmia – is characteristic of this condition. Heart rate variability measurement may be used as a means of formal diagnosis *(12)*.

EXERCISE IN DIABETES MELLITUS

As previously noted, individuals with diabetes have a markedly increased risk of cardiovascular disease. In fact, many will have established vascular disease at the time they are diagnosed with type 2 diabetes *(14)*. The benefits of exercise in those affected by diabetes are clear, including improvements in glycemia and other dysmetabolic parameters. However, patients with diabetes may require a very carefully structured exercise regimen to minimize the risk of hypoglycemia or worsening of their established complications.

Clinical trials have demonstrated that exercise will improve glycemia in those with diabetes, independent of effects on weight loss *(15)*. Short-term exercise also results in improvement in measures of endothelial-mediated vascular dilatation and arterial compliance *(16)*. Longer-term benefits of exercise include improvements in left ventricular diastolic function, decreases in markers of systemic inflammation, increased mobilization of fat from adipose stores with increases in fat oxidation, reduction in numbers of apoB-containing particles, and improvement in body composition with reduction in total body and visceral adiposity *(14,15)*. Consistent exercise training is associated with improved insulin sensitivity and increases in peripheral uptake and utilization of non-esterified fatty acids *(15)*. In addition, patients with diabetes involved in a cardiac rehabilitation and exercise program demonstrated fewer symptoms of depression and anxiety and reported an improved quality of life *(17)*. Men with diabetes and a high level of physical fitness were also found to have decreased rates of cardiovascular disease, death, and mortality compared with diabetic men with lesser degrees of physical fitness *(14,15)*. Physical activity is also essential to diabetes prevention: lifestyle intervention, including at least 150 min per week of moderately intensive exercise divided to be performed most days of the week, was associated with a significant reduction in rates of type 2 diabetes in individuals at high risk for this condition *(9)*. On the basis of these benefits, a regular exercise regimen including both aerobic and resistance training is recommended for most individuals with diabetes. This should include either a minimum of 150 min per week of moderate intensity aerobic exercise (50–70% of maximum heart rate) or at least 90 min per week of high-intensity exercise (> 70% of maximum heart rate). This overall dose should be divided among multiple sessions per week, preferably daily. Resistance training should be performed three times weekly, with an ultimate goal of three sets of 8–10 repetitions of the major muscle groups. As indicated, for all types of exercise, the sessions should be divided among several days per week, as some metabolic benefits of exercise tend to wane after approximately 72 h *(15)*.

Given the increased risk of cardiovascular disease in those with diabetes, an assessment of cardiovascular risk should be made prior to initiation of a moderately or highly intensive exercise regimen. Although some authors have suggested exercise stress testing in all persons with diabetes, it seems reasonable to recommend that this procedure be performed in those felt to have a greater than 10% 10-year risk of a cardiovascular event *(15)*. In addition to identification of ischemia, stress testing may be useful in the evaluation of heart rate and blood pressure responses to exercise, assessment of anginal thresholds or functional capacity, and detection of arrhythmia *(14,15)*.

Glucose uptake in muscle increases during exercise, due to an increase in blood flow to exercised tissues and intracellular transport of glucose. This increase in glucose uptake occurs in an insulin-independent fashion and will occur in nondiabetic as well as insulin-resistant individuals. Muscle glycogen stores serve as the primary source of fuel during early exercise, whereas more prolonged activity will consume circulating glucose and promote hepatic glycogenolysis and gluconeogenesis. Increases in insulin sensitivity are also seen in both the liver and the peripheral tissues. In the normal state, a reduction in insulin secretion and counter-regulatory increases in the levels of glucagon, catecholamines, cortisol, and growth hormone will prevent hypoglycemia during physical activity. Immediately following exercise, a rise in insulin secretion is seen which prevents hyperglycemia due to the increased levels of counter-regulatory substances. Replenishment of muscle glycogen stores will follow cessation of physical activity and may persist for up to 24 h *(15)*; however, ingestion of carbohydrates after exercise will shorten the time needed to replete these stores. As will be discussed further, these compensatory mechanisms may be impaired in persons with diabetes and may result in dramatic reductions in blood sugar during or after physical activity.

The likelihood of exercise-related hypoglycemia is increased in those patients using medications such as sulfonylureas, insulin secretagogues, or insulin. Hypoglycemia should not occur if diabetes is managed with diet or with classes of medications other than those mentioned. Hypoglycemia is often seen in those who are insulin deficient (as in type 1 diabetes or longstanding type 2 diabetes) due in part to a concomitant glucagon deficiency. Other risk factors for hypoglycemia include very intensive glycemic management, recent episodes of hypoglycemia or hypoglycemic unawareness, and renal insufficiency *(18)*. A careful review of the patient's medical history – including the type, dose, and timing of glucose-lowering medications – can help predict those persons at increased risk. Persons with hypoglycemic unawareness have an impaired sympathoadrenal response to exercise and may have few or no warning signs of severe hypoglycemia. Fortunately for these individuals, avoidance of hypoglycemia for several weeks will often result in an improved ability to sense impending low blood sugars *(18)*. It may be most prudent to delay initiation of a vigorous exercise regimen until this is accomplished. For most patients, modification of medication doses, frequent blood glucose testing, and increases in carbohydrate ingestion will generally prevent the occurrence of severe hypoglycemic episodes. However, all rehabilitation facilities should have glucose tablets, glucose gel, and injectable glucagon available to manage hypoglycemia should it occur *(17)*. Symptoms of hypoglycemia commonly include diaphoresis, hunger, tremor, and palpitations. Behavioral changes such as confusion or disorientation may occur, and severe hypoglycemia may result in obtundation, seizure, or coma. Should symptoms occur during or after exercise, it is most prudent to cease physical activity, treat with oral glucose, and test the finger stick blood glucose level at that point and again in 15 min. Treatment with glucagon injection should be reserved for individuals who are unable to ingest glucose orally, generally due to an altered mental status.

To exercise most safely, patients using insulin or oral hypoglycemic agents should monitor their blood sugar prior to exercise. If the blood sugar is under 100 at that point, ingestion of 15 g of carbohydrates is recommended before initiating activity. If insulin is used, the injection prior to exercise should be administered in the abdomen rather than in an extremity: insulin is absorbed at an increased rate from an arm or leg that is being exercised (17,19). It is also advisable to avoid exercise for 60–90 min after mealtime insulin is administered (17). Hypoglycemia may occur during or after exercise unless extra carbohydrate is ingested or medication doses are adjusted for activity. Reduction in the dose of insulin or insulin secretagogue used with the meal prior to exercise may be most prudent. However, as the hypoglycemic effects of exercise may persist for many hours, reductions in insulin or other medication doses following exercise may also be necessary (15).

Blood sugars should be tested immediately following exercise, as well as several hours later. Those persons exercising in the evening must be aware of the possibility of nocturnal hypoglycemia: if this occurs and does not resolve with medication or dietary adjustment, a change to morning exercise is recommended (17). For patients with diabetes who are at risk for hypoglycemia, a standardized exercise regimen will help to predict the blood sugar response to physical activity (20). Initiation of an exercise regimen – or intensification of an existing exercise regimen – should prompt careful monitoring of blood glucose levels and reassessment of medication dosages.

There are additional concerns for the physically active person with type 1 diabetes. Fixed doses of insulin given prior to exercise may cause hypoglycemia, due to an increase in glucose uptake as well as suppression of hepatic gluconeogenesis (19). Reductions in insulin doses prior to and following exercise are often necessary. It is also recommended that persons with type 1 diabetes consume glucose prior to and every 20–30 min during vigorous exercise (20). Blood sugars of 250 mg/dl or higher prior to exercise should prompt measurement of ketones in the blood or urine. If hyperglycemia and ketones are both present, exercise is contraindicated as physical activity may worsen existing ketosis (15). Exercise may be permitted if insulin administration results in improved glycemia and clearance of ketones (19). Some patients with type 1 diabetes may experience hyperglycemia following exercise: this is due to an inability to increase insulin levels in response to elevated catecholamines and other counter-regulatory hormones (15). This is most commonly seen after brief periods of intense exercise (20) and may in fact require increased doses of post-exercise insulin. Tables 2 and 3 outline a safety checklist for patients, as well as strategies to prevent or manage exercise-related fluctuations in blood sugars.

EXERCISE COMPLICATIONS ASSOCIATED WITH NEUROPATHIES

Conditions such as peripheral neuropathy and peripheral vascular disease are common in persons with diabetes: these conditions predispose to foot injury, impaired wound healing, and are responsible for the majority of nontraumatic lower extremity amputations (21). These complications may impair stability, gait, and performance of daily activities. The initial evaluation of patients with diabetes should include a thorough inspection of the lower extremities, with assessment for foot deformity, foot injury, or neurovascular compromise. Patients should be counseled to inspect their feet prior to and following exercise, and to wear well-fitting, shock-absorbent shoes (17,22). Foot care can often be aided by a physical therapist, should one be involved with the program. Individuals with partial foot amputations will require orthotics to prevent excessive plantar forces and skin breakdown (21). Exercises such as swimming, using

Table 2
Checklist for Patients with Diabetes Prior to Starting Exercise *(19)*

1. *The exercise plan*
    (a) Will the exercise be regular or sporadic?
    (b) What is the anticipated intensity of the activity?
    (c) How does it relate to the level of physical training?
    (d) How long will it last?
    (e) Will it be continuous or intermittent?
    (f) How many calories will be expended?
2. *The plan for meals and supplemental feedings*
    (a) When was the last meal eaten?
    (b) Should a high-carbohydrate snack be eaten before starting?
    (c) Should supplemental carbohydrate feedings be taken during exercise? If so, how much and how often?
    (d) Will extra food be required after exercise to avoid post-exercise hypoglycemia?
3. *The insulin regimen*
    (a) What is the usual insulin mixture and dosage? Should it be decreased prior to or after exercise?
    (b) When was the last insulin injection?
    (c) Should the injection site be changed to avoid exercising areas?
4. *The pre-exercise blood glucose concentration*
    (a) Is the blood glucose concentration in a safe range to exercise (100–250 mg/dl)?
    (b) If the blood glucose is less than 100 mg/dl, a pre-exercise carbohydrate snack should be taken to decrease the risk of exercise-induced hypoglycemia
    (c) If the blood glucose is greater than 250 mg/dl, urine or serum ketones should be checked. If they are negative and the high glucose is due to recent food intake, it is generally safe to exercise. If ketones are positive, supplemental insulin should be taken and exercise delayed until ketones are negative and blood glucose is less than 250 mg/dl.

a stationary bike, or upper extremity exercises may be preferable to weight-bearing exercise in those with advanced neuropathy *(15)*.

Common manifestations of autonomic neuropathy include an elevated resting heart rate without appropriate response to exercise, orthostatic blood pressure changes, reduced gastrointestinal motility, and predisposition to dehydration due to altered thermoregulation and thirst. Delayed gastric emptying with slowed absorption of carbohydrates as well as impaired counter-regulatory mechanisms may increase the risk of hypoglycemia in affected individuals: frequent monitoring of blood sugars, medication adjustment, and periodic ingestion of glucose may be necessary to stabilize blood sugars adequately during exercise. Orthostatic changes may be alleviated by interventions such as the use of support hose, adequate hydration, and avoidance of exercise in the immediate postprandial state *(17)*. In addition, a less-intensive blood pressure goal may be appropriate for affected individuals. As the heart rate response to exercise may be limited, a lower heart rate goal or a perceived exertion scale may be most useful in monitoring the intensity of exercise in those affected by autonomic neuropathy *(14,15)*.

Table 3
Strategies for Prevention and Treatment of Adverse Effects of Exercise *(19)*

1. *Acute hypoglycemia*
   (a) Pre-exercise meal
   (b) Supplemental carbohydrate during exercise
   (c) At least 1–1.5 h between insulin administration and activity
   (d) Frequent blood glucose monitoring
   (e) Emergency therapy
       (i) Oral glucose or carbohydrate
       (ii) Glucagon i.m. or s.c.
       (iii) Paramedics and IV glucose
2. *Postexercise hypoglycemia*
   (a) Supplemental food/carbohydrate after exercise
   (b) Decrease insulin dose
   (c) Emergency therapy
       (i) Oral glucose or carbohydrate
       (ii) Glucagon i.m. or s.c.
       (iii) Paramedics and IV glucose
3. *Acute hyperglycemia*
   (a) Frequent blood glucose monitoring
   (b) Supplemental insulin after exercise if hyperglycemia is sustained
4. *Hyperglycemia and exercise-induced ketosis*
   (a) Pre-exercise blood glucose monitoring and urine/blood ketone check
   (b) If glucose greater than 250 mg/dl and ketones present
       (i) Delay exercise
       (ii) Supplemental insulin
       (iii) Recheck blood glucose in 1–2 h

NEPHROPATHY AND RETINOPATHY

Although no restriction in physical activity is necessary in the patient with mild diabetic retinopathy, exercise may be contraindicated in those with severe proliferative disease. In this circumstance, vigorous physical activity (including resistance training) may increase the risk of retinal detachment or vitreal hemorrhage. It is generally advised that such exercise be avoided for 3–6 months following laser photocoagulation therapy *(15,19)*. There are no specific contraindications to exercise in persons with nephropathy: although exercise may transiently increase urinary protein excretion, physical activity is not associated with progression of diabetic renal disease *(15)*.

CONCLUSIONS

It is apparent that a more sedentary lifestyle, coupled with excessive caloric intake, has contributed significantly to the recent dramatic increase in type 2 diabetes. Although an ever-increasing number of pharmaceutical agents are available to facilitate management, a considerable percentage of persons with diabetes remain very poorly controlled. The complications of this condition contribute significantly to disease-associated morbidity and mortality in the developed world. Future efforts should be directed toward disease prevention, earlier detection, and intensive management of hyperglycemia and associated dysmetabolic conditions from the time of diagnosis.

Regular physical activity is recommended for all persons with diabetes and may be one of the most effective interventions in diabetes prevention. Exercise programs in those with diabetes have demonstrated beneficial effects on glucose control, body composition, mood, and markers of cardiovascular health. Although certain medications used to manage diabetes may predispose to an increased risk of hypoglycemia, careful management of medication doses and carbohydrate ingestion will permit safe exercise in most. A thorough review of the individual's medical history, medication uses, and assessment for diabetic complications will minimize the risks associated with an exercise regimen *(2)*.

REFERENCES

1. Abbas AK, Fausto N, Kumar V. The Endocrine Pancreas. *Robbins and Cotran Pathologic Basis of Disease*, 7th ed. Saunders, Philadelphia; 2005;1189–1205.
2. American Diabetes Association. Clinical Practice Recommendations 2005. *Diabetes Care.* 2005;28(Suppl 1):S1–S79.
3. Stumvoll M, Goldstein BJ, van Haeften TW. Type 2 Diabetes: Principles of Pathogenesis and Therapy. *Lancet.* 2005;365:1333–1346.
4. Buse JB, Polonsky KS, Burant CF. Type 2 Diabetes Mellitus. In *Williams Textbook of Endocrinology*, 10th ed., PR Larsen (ed.). Philadelphia: Saunders; 2003:1427–1468.
5. Permutt MJ, Wasson J, Cox N. Genetic Epidemiology of Diabetes. *J Clin Invest.* 2005;115(6): 1431–1439.
6. Eisenbarth GS, Polonsky KS, Buse JB. Type 1 Diabetes Mellitus. *Williams Textbook of Endocrinology*, 10th ed., PR Larsen (ed.). Philadelphia: Saunders; 2003:1485–1504.
7. The Diabetes Control and Complications Trial Research Group. The Effect of Intensive Treatment of Diabetes on the Development and Progression of Long-Term Complications in Insulin-Dependent Diabetes Mellitus. *N Engl J Med.* 1993;329:977–986.
8. UK Prospective Diabetes Study (UKPDS) Group. Intensive Blood-Glucose Control with Sulphony-lureas or Insulin Compared with Conventional Treatment and Risk of Complications in Patients with Type 2 Diabetes (UKPDS 33). *Lancet.* 1998;352:837–853.
9. Knowler WC, Barrett-Connor E, Fowler SE, Hamman RF, Lachin JM, Walker EA, Nathan DM. Reduction in the Incidence of Type 2 Diabetes with Lifestyle Intervention or Metformin. *N Engl J Med.* 2002;346:393–403.
10. Buchanan TA, Xiang AH, Peters RK, Kjos SL, Marroquin A, Goico J, Ochoa C, Tan S, Berkowitz K, Hodis HN, Azen SP. Preservation of Pancreatic Beta-Cell Function and Prevention of Type 2 Diabetes by Pharmacological Treatment of Insulin Resistance in High-Risk Hispanic Women. *Diabetes.* 2002;51:2796–2803.
11. Bloomgarden ZT. Diabetic retinopathy and neuropathy. *Diabetes Care.* 2005;28(4):963–970.
12. Brownlee M, Aiello LP, Friedman E, Vinik AI, Nesto RW, Boulton AJM. Complications of Diabetes Mellitus. In *Williams Textbook of Endocrinology*, 10th ed., PR Larsen (ed.). Philadelphia: Saunders; 2003:1509–1565.
13. Boulton AJM, Vinik AI, Arezzo JC, Bril V, Feldman EL, Freeman R, Malik RA, Maser RE, Sosenko JM, Ziegler D. Diabetic Neuropathies. *Diabetes Care.* 2005;28(4):956–962.
14. Stewart KJ. Exercise Training: Can It Improve Cardiovascular Health in Patients with Type 2 Diabetes? *Br J Sports Med.* 2004;38:250–252.

15. Sigal RJ, Kenny GP, Wasserman DH, Castaneda-Sceppa C. Physical Activity/Exercise and Type 2 Diabetes. *Diabetes Care*. 2004;27(10):2518–2539.
16. McGavock JM, Eves ND, Mandic S, Glenn NM, Quinney HA, Haykowsky MJ. The Role of Exercise in the Treatment of Cardiovascular Disease Associated with Type 2 Diabetes Mellitus. *Sports Med*. 2004;34(1):27–48.
17. Lavie CJ, Milani RV. Cardiac Rehabilitation and Exercise Training Programs in Metabolic Syndrome and Diabetes. *J Cardiopulm Rehabil*. 2005;25:59–66.
18. American Diabetes Association Workgroup on Hypoglycemia. Defining and Reporting Hypoglycemia in Diabetes. *Diabetes Care*. 2005;28(5):1245–1249.
19. Steppel JH, Horton ES. Exercise in the Management of Type 1 Diabetes Mellitus. *Rev Endocr Metab Disord*. 2003;4:355–360.
20. Ertl AC, Davis SN. Evidence for a Vicious Cycle of Exercise and Hypoglycemia in Type 1 Diabetes Mellitus. *Diabetes Metab Res Rev*. 2004;20:124–130.
21. Witzke KA, Vinik AI. Diabetic Neuropathy in Older Adults. *Rev Endocr Metab Disord*. 2005;6: 117–127.
22. Ades PA, Balady GJ, Berra K. Transforming Exercise-Based Cardiac Rehabilitation Programs into Secondary Prevention Centers: A National Imperative. *J Cardiopulm Rehabil*. 2001;21:263–272.

18 Pulmonary Issues Related to Cardiac Rehabilitation

Neil MacIntyre, MD

CONTENTS

INTRODUCTION

Chronic cardiac diseases and chronic pulmonary diseases coexist in many patients. In a review of the National Hospital Discharge Survey (1979–2001), 16% of chronic obstructive pulmonary disease (COPD) patients had coexistent hypertension, 15% had coexistent ischemic heart disease, and 10% had coexistent congestive heart failure (1). In the outpatient setting, the majority of the patients entering a pulmonary rehabilitation program were identified as having important cardiovascular issues such as hypertension (34%) and arrhythmias or coronary artery disease (27%) (2). The fact that these two categories of disease have so much overlap is important when considering these patients for rehabilitation programs. Indeed, although the principles of rehabilitation are similar for both types of patients, there are important differences in focus, assessment, monitoring, and rehabilitation methods that need to be understood. The remainder of this chapter will draw from the pulmonary rehabilitation evidence base to illustrate the mechanisms by which pulmonary disease can impact cardiac patients and to provide approaches to cardiac patients with pulmonary disease in terms of pulmonary assessment, rehabilitation strategies, and expected outcomes.

From: *Contemporary Cardiology: Cardiac Rehabilitation*
Edited by: W. E. Kraus and S. J. Keteyian © Humana Press Inc., Totowa, NJ

MECHANISMS OF FUNCTIONAL DETERIORATION IN CHRONIC LUNG DISEASE

The tempo of progressive disability is different if it comes from pulmonary, as opposed to cardiac, causes. Chronic lung disease progressively damages lung tissue and airways and, over a period of years, ultimately results in a depletion of ventilatory reserves and a resulting slow downhill course. Complicating this physiologically are abnormalities in gas exchange (hypoxemia) and elevations in pulmonary vascular pressures that lead to right ventricular dysfunction (3). All these factors contribute to the sensation of dyspnea and the resultant limitation on physical activity.

As dyspnea and exercise capacity worsen, the need for medical care increases, and the patient's ability for self-care decreases; a confusing combination of functional limitations and dependence on others is thrust on the patient. The net effect is a profound sense of "loss of control," with consequent depression and anxiety (4).

These factors are further worsened by the vicious cycle of inactivity. Exertional dyspnea promotes fear of exertion which then leads to an "exertion phobia" and a reduction in physical activity. The lack of exercise, in turn, leads to both central and peripheral deconditioning and, ultimately, to decreased endurance and weakness (5), and often to muscular atrophy (6). As a result of this, the patient experiences greater dyspnea, an even greater intolerance to exertion, and further loss of functional capacity. The progressive loss of exercise capacity resulting from this vicious cycle of inactivity is super-imposed on the underlying functional reduction caused by the lung disease and is further magnified by the presence of coexisting cardiac dysfunction.

Concern that exercise might precipitate respiratory failure by overloading weakened respiratory muscles leads to speculation that exercise training might be contraindicated in hypercapnic COPD patients. It has been shown, however, that hypercapnic COPD patients with severe ventilatory impairment and respiratory muscle weakness tolerate exercise and benefit significantly from intensive pulmonary rehabilitation (7,8). Similarly, exercise hypoxemia has been considered by some to be a contraindication to an exercise program, and this may be a particular concern in patients with ischemic cardiac disease. Our experience, however, has been that appropriate supplemental oxygen and proper monitoring (e.g., oximetry) in patients with stable and well-controlled cardiac symptoms allow such patients to participate fully in all aspects of the exercise program (9–11).

PATIENT ASSESSMENT

In the patient with combined cardiac and pulmonary disability, stable and well-controlled disease processes should not exclude the patient from participation in rehabilitation programs. The only real requirements are that the patient be free of acute illness, be on proper maintenance medications (see Figure 1) and be motivated to lead a more active life (12,13).

A comprehensive patient evaluation is essential to attaining the goals of rehabilitation and is the foundation on which the individually tailored program is constructed. From the pulmonary perspective, the first step in this assessment is to make an accurate diagnosis substantiated by history, physical examination, pulmonary function testing, and, as needed, chest radiography and other laboratory tests. The importance of this initial step is evidenced by the inability of many patients to report a correct diagnosis. In our experience, up to half of the patients entering our pulmonary rehabilitation program reported an incorrect diagnosis of their pulmonary problem.

Once proper diagnoses are made, an appropriate medication regimen can be established. For the patient with the most common pulmonary disorder, COPD, it is particularly important to assure proper medication regimens according to recent guidelines (Fig. 1) *(14,15)*.

Exercise assessment is a critical component of participants prior to entering a rehabilitation program *(12,13,16,17)*. In the patient with pulmonary disease, these assessments should stress the patient maximally and measure the maximum workload (and O_2 consumption, CO_2 production in selected patients), ventilatory response [minute ventilation and post exercise spirometry in all; dead space development, ventilatory equivalent for CO_2 production (VE/VCO_2), and arterial PCO_2 in selected patients], and gas exchange (pulse oximetry in all and arterial PO_2 in selected patients). These should be done in conjunction with the cardiovascular assessments required for cardiac rehabilitation.

These pulmonary exercise assessments perform two functions:

- They provide insight into the various respiratory factors that are involved in the functional disabilities (Table 1). This permits focused therapies to be done. For instance, detecting exercise hemoglobin desaturation (e.g., $SpO_2 < 88\%$) will lead to appropriate oxygen therapy, and detecting ventilatory limitations from air trapping or exercise bronchospasm (> 20% drop in FEV1) will lead to better bronchodilator therapy.
- They quantify the level of disability. This provides information for setting initial exercise loads (see Exercise Training Prescription section below) and program expectations [e.g., pulmonary patients who do not reach ventilatory or gas exchange limits during the exercise test have a greater exercise response to rehabilitation *(17)*].

New	0: At Risk	I: Mild	II: Moderate	III: Severe	IV: Very Severe
Characteristics	• Chronic symptoms • Exposure to risk factors • Normal spirometry	• $FEV_1/FVC < 70\%$ • $FEV_1 \geq 80\%$ • With or without symptoms	• $FEV_1/FVC < 70\%$ • $50\% \leq FEV_1 < 80\%$ • With or without symptoms	• $FEV_1/FVC < 70\%$ • $30\% \leq FEV_1 < 50\%$ • With or without symptoms	• $FEV_1/FVC < 70\%$ • $FEV_1 < 30\%$ or presence of chronic respiratory failure or right heart failure
	Avoidance of risk factor(s); influenza vaccination				
		Add short-acting bronchodilator when needed			
			Add regular treatment with one or more long-acting bronchodilators Add rehabilitation		
				Add inhaled glucocorticosteroids if repeated exacerbations	
					Add long-term oxygen if chronic respiratory failure Consider surgical treatments

Fig. 1. Recommended therapies for COPD patients based upon severity of disease by the Global Obstructive Lung Disease (GOLD) group. Reprinted with permission *(14)*.

Table 1
Patterns of Exercise Limitation in Patients with Chronic Lung Disease During Maximal
Exercise Testing

Primary exercise limitation	Maximum Ve/MVV	Peak HR	SpO_2 (%)
Ventilatory	> 0.8	< 0.8	> 90
Gas exchange	< 0.8	< 0.8	< 90
Cardiovascular	< 0.8	> 0.8	> 90
Ventilatory + cardiovascular	> 0.8	> 0.8	> 90
Ventilatory + gas exchange	> 0.8	< 0.8	< 90
Gas exchange + cardiovascular	< 0.8	> 0.8	< 90
Ventilatory + gas exchange + cardiovascular	> 0.8	> 0.8	< 90

Maximum Ve/MVV, maximal exercise ventilation as a fraction of the maximum voluntary ventilation;
Peak HR, peak exercise heart rate as a fraction of the predicted maximum heart rate. Adapted from *(17)*.

Because psychological disturbances are common in patients with chronic lung disease, psychosocial assessment is important prior to participation in a rehabilitation program *(4)*. The most common emotional consequences of COPD are depression and anxiety, which can further reinforce social isolation and inactivity. Cognitive function has also been shown to be impaired in these patients, perhaps as a consequence of chronic hypoxemia. Medications and psychotherapy can be provided as necessary.

Other assessments necessary in patients with pulmonary disease prior to beginning rehabilitation include physical therapy evaluations, nutritional evaluations, occupational therapy [especially activities of daily living (ADL)] evaluations, and an education assessment for the patient's knowledge and understanding of the disease process and its management *(12,13)*. A particularly important assessment is tobacco usage. Although it is reasonable to allow current smokers to participate in a rehabilitation program, formal efforts should be made to discontinue smoking.

PULMONARY-SPECIFIC COMPONENTS TO REHABILITATION

Education

A primary purpose of the educational component of any rehabilitation program (both cardiac and pulmonary) is to provide the framework for self-care. Through an educational process of instruction, supervision, and practice, patients can acquire an awareness of their disease and its management that allows them to take responsibility for their own care. A spouse, family member, or close friend who participates in the educational activities can provide familial understanding of the disease process and can reinforce the recommended self-care techniques in the home setting.

The educational process usually consists of a combination of lectures, discussions, demonstrations, and practice sessions. During all program activities, the patient's knowledge and ability to perform self-management techniques are continually reinforced. Topics typically covered in formal lectures and discussion sessions include the anatomy and physiology of the lung, the pathophysiology of chronic lung disease, pulmonary medications, nutrition, physiologic responses to exercise, sexual concerns, travel concerns, coping with chronic lung disease, and psychosocial issues. A growing educational need in the COPD patient is inhaler operations *(18)*. Newer medications are becoming available in an array of metered-dose inhalers and dry powder inhalers that can be bewildering to these patients. Chronic lung disease patients should also be instructed on an action plan in the event of an acute exacerbation. Undo delay in starting antibiotics and steroids (in appropriate patients) can be costly in terms of subsequent needs for health care utilization.

Respiratory therapy and physical therapy techniques for the pulmonary patient are more appropriately presented in either individual or group demonstrations and in practice sessions. These topics include cleaning and care of equipment, proper use of metered-dose inhalers and spacers, relaxation techniques, clearing of secretions using techniques of controlled coughing, postural drainage, percussion and vibration, and supplemental oxygen therapy. Educational material in the form of pamphlets, booklets, and books is available from a multitude of sources, including the American Lung Association. This additional information should be used to support and reinforce the information the patient receives in the lectures, discussions, and demonstrations.

Breathing retraining traditionally has been a key aspect of the educational component of a pulmonary rehabilitation program. Pursed-lip breathing and diaphragmatic breathing are commonly used concomitantly to reduce shortness of breath and improve gas exchange. By using pursed-lip breathing, patients may be able to maintain adequate oxygenation without supplemental oxygen.

Exercise Training Prescription

In general, exercise training for patients with pulmonary disease should be a balance of three types of exercise: stretching and flexibility exercises, strengthening exercises, and endurance exercises *(12,13)*. Stretching and flexibility exercises are usually part of a floor exercise routine that develops suppleness, improves range of motion, and helps provide a general warm-up. Strength training may be obtained as part of the floor exercise routine by performing exercises with dumbbells, cuff weights, or a stretch band. Pulmonary patients also do well with free weights and weight machines for strength training. Strength exercises require a stimulus of high intensity and low frequency. General endurance training involves exercises that produce a cardiopulmonary stress that results in elevated heart rate and ventilation. Such exercises include walking, rowing, swimming, water aerobics, cycling (arm or leg), stair climbing, and so on, provided that the exercise intensity produces sufficient cardiopulmonary stress. Compared with strength training, endurance training is of lower intensity and higher frequency.

The initial load prescription from the pulmonary perspective should be of sufficiently low intensity that it can be accomplished by the patient without discomfort. Nothing destroys the patient's motivation faster than failure to complete the initial exercise or experiencing significant discomfort during or after the first exercise session. The initial loads used by our program for the stationary bicycle and arm ergometer are based on the maximum workload reached during the exercise stress test (W_{max}). The initial bicycle workload (W_{bike}) is set at 50% of the maximum workload ($0.5 \times W_{max}$). This value is based on data suggesting that an individual can be expected to work for 8 h at 50% of maximum work capacity without undue fatigue. The initial load prescription for arm exercise is 30% of W_{max} (or 60% of W_{bike}) and is based on studies showing that the aerobic power of the arms ranges from 50 to 70% of the maximum power output of the legs.

Workloads must be reassessed at each exercise session and adjusted according to the patient's progress. Following the initial settings, the appropriate intensity for subsequent target workload (the desired training load) has been an area of controversy. Work from Casaburi (19) suggests that training intensity in COPD patients should be pushed to a training effect (e.g., up to 70–80% predicted maximal HR) if at all possible. Even patients with ventilatory or gas exchange limitations who cannot reach these target heart rates also appear to benefit from higher rather than lower levels of exercise. Thus, strategies using target intensities reaching the highest level attained on the initial exercise stress test should be the ultimate goal.

To accomplish the transition from the relatively low initial loads to the higher target loads, our pulmonary program relies on the Borg Scale of Perceived Exertion as a measure of perceived stress and the exercise heart rate as a measure of cardiopulmonary stress (20). If the Borg rating of the previous exercise session is less than 15 and the HR during exercise is less than the HR achieved during the assessment exercise test, consideration is given to increase the intensity. Whenever the patient is capable of performing a given load for the duration of the exercise session, the load is increased by about 12.5W for the bicycle ergometer and about 9W for the arm ergometer. After approximately six exercise sessions, most patients will have attained an exercise level representing a high percentage of the target workload.

Whenever the pulmonary patient experiences significant symptoms of fatigue or dyspnea, instead of stopping exercise, the load is reduced while the patient is encouraged to complete the exercise if possible. When the initial load is already the lowest possible, the patient stops until the symptoms subside and then continues the exercise to completion. The duration of the rest period is considered part of the exercise period. The short-term goal then becomes reducing the number of rests during the exercise period.

The recommended minimum duration and frequency of endurance exercise in pulmonary patients is no less than 20 min, three times per week (12,13). Increasing the duration and frequency beyond this minimum must take into consideration the motivation and goals of the patient and balance the time spent in training against the benefits derived from a more intense training regimen. The primary benefits of spending additional time on training are faster and greater improvement in physical capacity.

All exercise training should be performed under conditions of adequate arterial oxygenation ($PaO_2 > 55$ mm Hg, O_2 saturation $> 88\%$ in pulmonary patients and probably higher in patients with ischemic cardiac disease) (9,11,21). If the initial patient assessment has determined that the resting oxygenation is low or that significant desaturation occurs with exertion, supplemental oxygen must be provided to the patient to maintain adequate oxygen saturation. Usually, oxygen delivered at 2l/min through nasal cannula is sufficient. In some cases, however, it may be difficult to provide adequate oxygenation during exertion with even a partial rebreathing system. When adequate oxygenation cannot be maintained, either the intensity of the exercise must be reduced or the patient must be instructed to stop exercising until oxygenation is again adequate. Besides reducing the medical risk associated with low oxygenation, supplemental oxygen often allows the patient who needs oxygen to exercise for a longer duration at a higher intensity, thereby enhancing the beneficial effects of the exercise.

In patients on chronic bronchodilators or those who have been shown to have exercise bronchospasm, aerosolized bronchodilators (e.g., albuterol, ipratropium, or both) should be given prior to the exercise program. This can be administered as the patients regular dose with a time adjustment to coincide with exercise or as an additional treatment provided there is no tachycardia or tremor present.

Psychosocial and Other Focused Therapies

Other focused interventions are often dependent upon the individual patient. Pulmonary patients with clinically important depression/anxiety may need focused psychological therapies *(4,22)*. This is particularly important in patients with chronic lung disease where depression and anxiety are common and can significantly impair function as well as rehabilitation potential. Therapies can range from antidepressant or anxiolytic medications to group therapy sessions to formal psychiatric care.

OUTCOMES ASSOCIATED WITH REHABILITATION IN PULMONARY DISEASE PATIENTS

Evidence supporting the benefits of exercise training in chronic lung disease is compelling and has been reviewed in several publications *(2,12,13,23–29)*. Lower extremity exercise programs consistently improved walk distance (6–33%) and maximal work load (10–102%) in all studies reviewed. Proposed mechanisms of improvement include improved aerobic capacity (in those who can reach cardiovascular training levels), increased motivation, desensitization to dyspnea, improved ventilatory muscle function, and improved techniques of performance. Data from upper extremity exercise programs were less extensive but do support the concept that upper extremity exercise might improve the thoracic cage muscles of ventilation and improve activities of daily living.

Evidence supporting the effectiveness of pulmonary rehabilitation in reducing dyspnea is also strong *(12,26)*. This is a consistent finding using any number of dyspnea grading scales (e.g., visual analogue scales, baseline dyspnea index, transitional dyspnea index, and other respiratory questionnaires). The mechanisms of reduced dyspnea are no doubt multifactorial but would include better exercise tolerance (and reduced ventilation for a given load), better breathing patterns, better medications, and a better comprehension by the patient of his/her disease and how it can be effectively managed.

Many studies have demonstrated that improved psychosocial function occurs as a result of pulmonary rehabilitation *(12,22,30)*. Much of this benefit seems to come from improved exercise tolerance, reduced dyspnea, and a better understanding of the disease process and management by the patient, as routine psychological or psychiatric services have not been shown to impact outcomes.

Quality-of-life indicators have consistently shown benefit from pulmonary rehabilitation *(12)*. Like improvements in dyspnea and psychosocial function, the mechanisms for improved quality of life following pulmonary rehabilitation are probably multifactorial. An important outcome benefit to pulmonary rehabilitation has been a reduction in health care utilizations and costs *(12)*.

Evidence supporting a survival benefit for pulmonary rehabilitation does not exist. This should not be surprising as the goals of pulmonary rehabilitation are not to reverse the disease process but rather to improve the patient's functional capabilities within the constraints of the reduced lung function.

CONCLUSIONS

Patients with disabilities from both cardiac and pulmonary diseases clearly benefit from rehabilitation programs. Because these disease states often coexist, rehabilitation programs need to be aware of the specific assessments, rehabilitation methods, and outcomes associated with each. Successful rehabilitation can be provided for patients with both disease processes as long as the rehabilitation team is aware of these principles.

REFERENCES

1. Holguin F, Foch E, Redd C, Mannino DM. Comorbidity and Comortality in COPD Related Hospitalizations in the United States. *Chest.* 2005;128:2005–2011.
2. Bickford LS, Hodgkin JE, McInturff SL. National Pulmonary Rehabilitation Survey. Update. *J Cardiopulm Rehabil.* 1995;15:406–411.
3. MacNee W. Pathophysiology of Cor Pulmonale in Chronic Obstructive Pulmonary Disease. Part One. *Am J Respir Crit Care Med.* 1994;150:833–852.
4. Singer HK, Ruchinskas RA, Riley KC. The Psychological Impact of End-Stage Lung Disease. *Chest.* 2001;120:1246–1252.
5. Killian KJ, LeBlanc P, Martin DH, et al. Exercise Capacity and Ventilatory Circulatory, and Symptom Limitation in Patients with Chronic Airflow Limitation. *Am Rev Respir Dis.* 1992;146:935–940.
6. Skeletal Muscle Dysfunction in Chronic Obstructive Pulmonary Disease. A Statement of the American Thoracic Society and European Respiratory Society. *Am J Respir Crit Care Med.* 1999;159:S1–S40.
7. Lacasse Y, Wong E, Guyatt GH, et al. Meta-Analysis of Respiratory Rehabilitation in COPD. *Lancet.* 1996;348:1115–1119.
8. Lacasse Y, Brosseau L, Milne S, et al. Pulmonary Rehabilitation for Chronic Obstructive Pulmonary Disease. *Cochrane Database Syst Rev.* 2002;(3):CD003793.
9. Fujimoto K, Matsuzawa Y, Yamaguchi S, et al. Benefits of Oxygen on Exercise Performance and Pulmonary Hemodynamics in Patients with COPD with Mild Hypoxemia. *Chest.* 2002;122:457–463.
10. Emtner M, Porszasz J, Burns M, et al. Benefits of Supplemental Oxygen in Exercise Training in Nonhypoxemic COPD Patients. *Am J Resp Crit Care Med.* 2003;168:1034–1042.
11. Garrod R, Paul EA, Wedzicha JA. Supplemental Oxygen During Pulmonary Rehabilitation in Patients with COPD with Exercise Hypoxaemia. *Thorax,* 2000;55:539–543.
12. Pulmonary Rehabilitation: Joint ACCP/AACVPR Evidence-Based Guidelines. ACCP/AACVPR Pulmonary Rehabilitation Guidelines Panel. American College of Chest Physicians. American Association of Cardiovascular and Pulmonary Rehabilitation. *Chest.* 1997;112:1363–1396.
13. American Association of Cardiovascular and Pulmonary Rehabilitation. *Guidelines for Pulmonary Rehabilitation Programs*, 3rd ed., RZ ZuWallack and R Crouch (eds.). Human Kinetics; Champaign, IL 2004.

14. Global Initiative for Chronic Obstructive Pulmonary Disease Workshop Report: Updated 2003. Available at http://www.goldcopd.com, accessed July 2003.
15. American Thoracic Society/European Respiratory Society. Standards for the Diagnosis and Management of Patients with COPD; 2004. Available at http://www.throacic.org/copd
16. Weisman IM, Zeballos RJ. Clinical Exercise Testing. *Clin Chest Med.* 2001;22:679–701.
17. Plankeel JF, McMullen B, MacIntyre NR. Exercise Outcomes After Pulmonary Rehabilitation Depend on the Initial Mechanisms of Exercise Limitation Among Non-Oxygen-Dependent COPD Patients. *Chest.* 2005;127(1):110–116.
18. Geller DE. Comparing Clinical Features of the Nebulizer, Metered-Dose Inhaler, and Dry Powder Inhaler. *Respir Care.* 2005;50:1313–1322.
19. Casaburi R, Petessio A, Ioli F, et al. Reductions in Exercise Lactic Acidosis and Ventilation as a Result of Training in Patients with Obstructive Lung Disease. *Am Rev Resp Dis.* 1991;143:9–18.
20. Borg GA. Psychophysical Bases for Perceived Exertion. *Med Sci Sports Exer.* 1982;14:377–381.
21. MacIntyre, NR. Oxygen Therapy and Exercise Response in Lung Disease. *Resp Care.* 2000;45: 194–203.
22. Emery CF, Schein RL, Hauck ER, et al. Psychological and Cognitive Outcomes of a Randomized Trial of Exercise Among Patients with Chronic Obstructive Pulmonary Disease. *Health Psychol.* 1998;15:232–240.
23. Casaburi R, Porszasz J, Burns MR, et al. Physiologic Benefits of Exercise Training in Rehabilitation of Patients with Severe Chronic Obstructive Pulmonary Disease. *Am J Respir Crit Care Med.* 1997;155:1541–1551.
24. Maltais F, LeBlanc P, Jobin J. Intensity of Training and Physiological Adaptation in Patients with Chronic Obstructive Pulmonary Disease. *Am J Respir Crit Care Med.* 1997;155:555–561.
25. Bernard S, Whittom F, LeBlanc P, et al. Aerobic and Strength Training in Patients with Chronic Obstructive Pulmonary Disease. *Am J Respir Crit Care Med.* 1999;159:896–900.
26. O'Donnell DE, McGuire M, Samis L, et al. The Impact of Exercise Reconditioning on Breathlessness in Severe Chronic Airflow Limitation. *Am J Respir Crit Care Med.* 1995;152:2005–2013.
27. Puente-Maestu L, Sanz ML, Sanz P, et al. Comparison of Effects of Supervised Versus Self-Monitored Training Programs in Patients with Chronic Obstructive Pulmonary Disease. Eur Respir J. 2000;15:517–525.
28. O'Donnell DE, McGuire M, Samis L, et al. General exercise Training Improves Ventilatory and Peripheral Muscle Strength and Endurance in Chronic Airflow Limitation. Am J Respir Crit Care Med. 1998;157:1489–1497.
29. Ries AL, Kaplan RM, Linberg TM, et al. Effects of Pulmonary Rehabiltation on Physiological and Psychological Outcomes in Patients with COPD. *Ann Intern Med.* 1995;122:823–832.
30. Emery CF, Leatherman NE, Burker EJ, et al. Psychological Outcomes of a Pulmonary Rehabilitation Program. *Chest.* 1991;100:613–617.

19 Exercise Rehabilitation for Patients with Peripheral Arterial Disease

Christopher J. Womack, PhD, FACSM

CONTENTS

DEFINITION AND EPIDEMIOLOGY OF PERIPHERAL ARTERIAL DISEASE

Peripheral arterial disease (PAD) is characterized by atherosclerosis in peripheral arteries supplying blood to the legs. This form of atherosclerosis has a significant impact on peripheral circulation and ultimately on functional independence in older adults, as the leg pain (claudication) associated with PAD severely limits functional capacity and activities of daily living. Furthermore, patients with PAD are at much greater risk for other manifestations of cardiovascular disease (CVD) such as myocardial infarction or stroke. Specifically, there is an 11-fold increase in CVD-related mortality in patients symptomatic for PAD *(1)*.

PAD occurs in 16% of individuals > 55 years of age *(2)*. Interestingly, the majority (63%) of these individuals are asymptomatic for the disease in that they do not suffer claudication during ambulation *(2)*. This underscores the need for screening of older individuals for PAD as part of routine examination, especially among those patients with known CVD. Risk factors for PAD are similar to the traditional risk factors for CVD *(3)*, and cigarette smoking appears to be a particularly important risk factor, as heavy smoking results in a fourfold increase in risk for PAD *(4)*. Murabito et al. *(3)* have published a method that represents an easy way to estimate 4-year probability for the development of intermittent claudication based on traditional risk factors.

From: *Contemporary Cardiology: Cardiac Rehabilitation*
Edited by: W. E. Kraus and S. J. Keteyian © Humana Press Inc., Totowa, NJ

PATHOPHYSIOLOGY

The development of atherosclerosis in patients with PAD is similar to atherosclerotic plaque development in other arteries. As plaque progression develops, peripheral blood flow and resultant symptoms associated with PAD change across the Fontaine stages that are summarized in Table 1.

The presence of claudication can be easily assessed using the Rose questionnaire *(7)* or other appropriate device. The asymptomatic stage (Stage I) is characterized by an ankle to brachial systolic pressure ratio (ABI) of less than 0.94 or less than 0.73 after exercise *(5)*. Therefore, it is important to screen individuals at risk for PAD by obtaining ankle and brachial pressure measurements. The addition of an ankle pressure measurement is easily obtained in any clinical setting as the extra equipment required typically only consists of an ankle blood pressure cuff and a Doppler machine. This enables the clinician to intervene prior to symptomatic stages and minimize the impact of this disease on activities of daily living.

Complications

Although the disease process and associated risk factors are identical to those for coronary artery disease (CAD), there are unique clinical complications for PAD. Specifically, there is no acute event similar to a myocardial infarction in the lower limbs. Instead, prolonged ischemia due to the reduction in peripheral vasculature can ultimately result in ulcerations, gangrene, and even limb loss. In patients without these severe manifestations, there are still pronounced changes in muscle metabolism *(8,9)*.

Paradoxically, the reduction in blood flow appears to increase mitochondrial density in the affected limb *(9)*. However, despite the increased mitochondrial density, electron transport chain function is compromised in these patients *(10)*. Therefore, the increased mitochondrial density is likely an adaptation to offset the reduction in oxidative phosphorylation. Furthermore, the decreased electron transport chain function inhibits Krebs cycle activity, as there is an increase in acylcarnitine in gastrocnemius muscle of patients with PAD *(8)*. Hiatt et al. *(8)* found that muscle acylcarnitine was highly correlated with peak VO_2 ($r = -0.75$) in patients with unilateral PAD, suggesting that the ischemic state may result in metabolic changes that ultimately control the level of functional capacity in these patients.

Table 1
Fontaine Stages of Peripheral Arterial Disease

Stage	Symptoms	Diagnostic hemodynamic measures (5,6)
I	Asymptomatic	ABI < 0.94
II	Intermittent claudication	ABI < 0.90
III	Rest pain	Ankle pressure ≤ 50 mmHg
IV	Tissue necrosis	Ankle pressure ≤ 50 mmHg

TREATMENT STRATEGIES

Medications

Because patients with PAD have identical risk factors as patients with CAD, the medication regimen will be relatively similar. In general, several of these patients will take beta-blockers, angiotensin-converting enzyme inhibitors, statins, aspirin, and/or other antiplatelet drugs. Furthermore, an estimated 26% of patients will have type 2 diabetes *(11)* and may be on a medication for such. In addition to these medications designed to improve risk factors and prevent cardiovascular events, some medications may be prescribed to diminish peripheral ischemia and resultant claudication. Pentoxifylline was originally the most commonly prescribed medication to serve this purpose. However, more recent data suggest that the improvement in claudication due to this medication may be relatively small *(12)*. To date, the most efficacious drug for diminishing claudication is cilostazol, a phosphodiesterase inhibitor. In a 24-week clinical trial, cilostazol increased average maximal treadmill walking distance by approximately 44% (from 241–350 m) as compared with a 27% improvement with Pentoxifylline *(12)*.

One potential promising supplement to decrease claudication is carnitine. Early research suggested that supplemental carnitine improves treadmill performance in patients with PAD *(13)*. The purported effect of carnitine is that it binds to Acetyl CoA, which leads to a subsequent activation of pyruvate dehydrogenase and decrease in lactate accumulation *(13)*. Further research is needed to quantify the efficacy of carnitine supplementation against medications such as cilostazol. However, this does represent a promising area of treatment, as carnitine supplementation may result in fewer side effects than pharmacological interventions.

Surgical Interventions

The most common interventions designed to treat patients with PAD are femoral bypass graft and peripheral angioplasty, the latter performed either with or without the insertion of a stent. These interventions are typically not considered unless that patient is experiencing claudication at rest (Fontaine stage III) or similar severe manifestations of the disease *(14)*. Unlike exercise and pharmacological intervention, surgery does not specifically address the reduction of associated risk factors. Furthermore, recent research suggests that 6 months of exercise therapy is more effective and costs less than angioplasty *(15)*. Specifically, exercise therapy improved maximal walking distance by an average of 250 m at a total cost of $4968 dollars per patient versus an increase in 113 m at a total cost of $9303 dollars for angioplasty *(15)*. Thus, relevant lifestyle interventions (exercise rehabilitation, smoking cessation, and behavioral therapy) should be considered whenever possible in place of, or in addition to, surgical procedures.

IMPLICATIONS FOR REHABILITATION AND EXERCISE MANAGEMENT

Unique/Disease-Specific Adjustments to Acute Exercise

Because of the peripheral limitations, unique factors must be considered related to exercise responses in patients with PAD. Because of the decreased blood flow and altered skeletal muscle metabolism, oxygen uptake kinetics are notably altered. First, there is a delayed attainment of steady-state oxygen consumption *(16)*. Furthermore, instead of steady-state oxygen uptake kinetics during constant-intensity exercise, patients with PAD will typically exhibit a progressive increase in oxygen uptake with increasing exercise duration *(17)*. This can cause a progressive increase in the relative intensity of exercise during a submaximal bout of exercise. Perhaps the most important consideration, however, is that functional capacity in these patients is limited, not by the heart's ability to distribute blood but by pain specific to the periphery as a result of decreased local peripheral flow to the ischemic muscle. Thus, the target of rehabilitation is to decrease claudication during ambulation.

Unique Adjustments to the Exercise Prescription

Because of the unique considerations for exercise in patients with PAD, several considerations must be given to the exercise prescription. First, because claudication will often severely limit the duration of exercise, intermittent exercise should be prescribed, so that the patient accumulates an appropriate duration. The initial phase of training can include approximately 15 min of exercise per session with steady progression to 60 min per session. Patients should begin each interval at the prescribed intensity and continue until they perceive the claudication at a level of "3" on the pain scale, as shown in Table 2. After reaching a "3" on the claudication scale, the patient should then rest until the pain subsides, at which point they will begin exercising again. The rest periods should be monitored and recorded, as both the number and duration of the rest periods should decrease over the course of the rehabilitation program.

Exercise intensity should correspond to approximately 40–70% of Heart Rate Reserve *(18)*. However, it appears that the total volume of training is the primary determinant of the efficacy of rehabilitation, as low intensity (40% functional capacity) is as effective as high intensity (80% functional capacity) for eliciting functional improvements, provided the duration of the low-intensity program is increased *(19)*. A recently published meta-analysis suggests that the optimal training frequency in patients with PAD is 3 days per week, based on the observation that improvements in walking ability appear to be no better with 4 or 5 days per week than for 3 days per week *(20)*. However, because exercise therapy is often also prescribed for weight control and CVD risk factor modification, prescribing exercise for more than 3 days per week may be necessary.

Because PAD specifically limits the ability to ambulate, a significant portion, if not all, of the training should be done using walking as the mode of choice. This should facilitate program compliance as walking can be accomplished in various settings.

Table 2
Scale for the Ration of Perceived
Claudication

0	No pain
1	Onset of pain
2	Moderate pain
3	Intense pain
4	Maximal pain

There is also some recent evidence that pole-striding exercise is at least as beneficial as walking for improving functional capacity *(21)*; however, no direct comparison between pole striding and walking has been made in a single study. Other modes that utilize similar muscle groups as walking, such as stair climbing, may be considered for variety purposes, but should not comprise the bulk of the program, as walking has been shown to be superior to stair climbing in improving time to claudication during constant-intensity and incremental exercise tests *(22)*. Arm and leg ergometry both significantly improve time to claudication and functional capacity in patients with PAD *(23)*, but the efficacy of these modes in comparison with walking has yet to be determined.

Hiatt et al. *(24)* observed that treadmill training is superior to strength training, as strength training did not increase walking time to claudication onset and resulted in a lower improvement in peak walking time (36 versus 74%, respectively). Furthermore, previous research has shown that combining treadmill and strength training does not result in larger improvements than treadmill training alone *(25)*. However, the full impact and potential benefit of strength training is not known in this population and promises to be a compelling area for future research.

Supplemental strength training may be of benefit in patients with PAD. Specifically, strength training increases bone density, improves muscular strength and endurance, and can improve activities of daily living in older individuals *(26)*. Furthermore, strength training was shown to increase capillary density and decrease the proportion of skeletal muscle IIB/IIA fibers in patients with PAD *(27)*. This may be clinically significant, as recent data suggest that muscle capillarization and type I fiber area are correlated with exercise tolerance in patients with PAD *(28)*. Therefore, this intervention could improve the metabolic characteristics of skeletal muscle. Further research is needed to quantify the adaptations that patients with PAD make to strength training and the specific prescription considerations necessary to elicit these adaptations.

Chronic Adaptations to Exercise Training

Obviously, the most important adaptations that occur with exercise rehabilitation are an increased time to claudication during ambulation and an increased functional capacity. These adaptations directly translate into increased voluntary physical activity in this population. Additionally, economy of movement increases along with functional capacity *(17)*. The result of these two changes is that the relative intensity (% of functional capacity) of a given submaximal walking velocity can decrease by as much as 21% *(17)*. The cause of the improvement in exercise economy is unknown. It is possible that diminished claudication minimizes the altered gait mechanics in these patients. Furthermore, metabolic adaptations favoring better oxidative metabolism could contribute to the decrease in oxygen consumption at a given walking velocity. Future research is necessary to fully evaluate the mechanisms responsible for these adaptations.

One of the persistent misunderstandings regarding exercise rehabilitation in patients with PAD is that the major outcome is an improved peripheral blood flow. In fact,

although there is some evidence for improved peripheral flow in patients with PAD
(29,30), these adaptations are relatively minor and not highly correlated with improvements in functional status *(31)*. Resting ABI shows little to no change as an adaptation
to exercise training *(17,29)*, suggesting that exercise does not effectively cure the
patient of PAD. It appears that exercise adaptations related to blood flow in this
population occur primarily in relation to exercise and postexercise flow. As evidence
of this, increases in ABI during the postexercise period are evident within as few as 2
months of exercise rehabilitation *(17)*.

The mechanisms responsible for the improvements in blood flow have not been
clearly established. It is possible that exercise rehabilitation contributes to a regression
of atherosclerosis and subsequent improvements in blood flow. However, because the
adaptations appear confined to exercise and postexercise blood flow, this is not likely
to be the overriding factor. It is also possible that a large-enough volume of training
could effectively lead to the development of collateral vessels that could compensate
for the occluded vessels. However, it is not definitively known at this time whether
these adaptations occur in patients with PAD.

Some of the most important adaptations that occur as a result of exercise
rehabilitation in patients with PAD are metabolic adaptations in the affected skeletal
muscle. As mentioned previously, the affected muscles typically have a low carnitine :
acylcarnitine ratio *(8)*, indicative of impaired Krebs cycle activity. However, exercise
increases this ratio *(31)*, suggesting that the impaired metabolic state is at least partially
offset with exercise training. Furthermore, there is evident hypertrophy of both type
I and II fibers and an increase in muscle capillarization with strength training in this
population *(27)*. Thus, the peripheral skeletal muscle adaptations that occur may be
the most important changes that result in enhanced functional capacity in patients
with PAD.

Much like exercise rehabilitation programs in other patients with CVD, patients
with PAD exhibit an improvement in their risk factor profile. Specifically, previous
research has documented that exercise rehabilitation can (i) increase tissue plasminogen
activator activity (a marker of fibrinolytic potential) by 28% *(32)*, (ii) decrease total
cholesterol and LDL by 8 and 5%, respectively *(33)*, (iii) decrease systolic blood
pressure by 6% *(33)*, and (iv) increase voluntary physical activity by 38% *(29)*. For
patients who are smokers, smoking cessation should be included in the intervention
strategy to effectively address this risk factor as well. By incorporating the use of
exercise and smoking cessation, exercise not only improves quality of life in patients
with PAD, but it is also part of an effective strategy for decreasing the increased risk
of CVD mortality in these patients.

Testing and Assessment

As mentioned previously, the major goal of exercise therapy is to decrease the
degree of claudication during ambulation. Fortunately, this can be easily assessed and
quantified in almost any clinical setting. For facilities without treadmill exercise testing
equipment, the 6-min walk represents an excellent assessment tool. By having the
patient self-pace to achieve the maximum distance possible in 6 min, time and distance
to the onset of claudication pain can be measured. This evaluation can be an excellent
way to monitor patient progress in an inexpensive manner (see chapter 12).

If a more specific assessment is required, exercise protocols can be implemented, with and without oxygen consumption being measured. The advantage of these protocols is that they allow the clinician to standardize the intensity for comparison across patients and to compare particular patients to pre-rehabilitation data. These data can also be used to accurately provide an exercise prescription. If a facility is equipped with a metabolic measurement system, walking economy can be quantified and evaluated as an outcome of rehabilitation. In addition, direct, rather than estimated, measurements of functional capacity can be made. However, it should be noted that follow-up testing should be consistent with baseline testing with respect to the collection of metabolic data such as oxygen consumption.

Previous research has shown that treadmill walking protocols, with and without an inclined treadmill, and stair climbing protocols yield very similar values for onset of claudication, time to maximal claudication pain, and hemodynamic measures (34). Both constant-intensity protocols and graded exercise tests, where the intensity is progressively increased through increases in treadmill speed and/or grade, have been utilized for this population. However, prior research suggests that graded protocols are superior due to more reliable measurements for both onset of claudication pain and time to maximal claudication pain (35). One highly reliable treadmill protocol utilizes a constant speed of 2.0 mph with grade increases of 2% every 2 min (18). Blood pressure (ankle and brachial) and heart rate measurements can be made both during and after the exercise tests. These measurements are important in that they can (i) provide information that can be used to prescribe an exercise heart rate range, (ii) be used to screen for abnormal blood pressure and heart rate responses, and (iii) provide valuable feedback in terms of cardiovascular adaptations to training.

One clinical consideration with respect to exercise testing in patients with PAD is the use of treadmill tests to screen for CAD. It is possible that claudication limits exercise tolerance to the point where intensity is not sufficient to detect myocardial ischemia during the exercise test. Thus, occult CAD may become evident during follow-up testing, because the patient is able to achieve a higher workload, one that is sufficient to reveal ischemia. Therefore, EKG monitoring during follow-up stress tests is highly important, perhaps even more important than during the baseline evaluation.

SUMMARY

PAD is a disease that drastically affects mortality risk and quality of life. The majority of individuals with PAD are in the asymptomatic stage, reflecting the need for regular screening for this disease by clinicians. Ultimately, PAD can result in tissue necrosis, gangrene, and limb loss; yet profound metabolic changes occur in ischemic muscle of patients who do not experience these disease manifestations. Risk factors for this disease are similar to those for CAD; however, smoking is a particularly important risk factor for the development of PAD. Therapeutic treatment for patients with PAD includes various pharmacological interventions, smoking cessation, and exercise. Because exercise is limited by peripheral claudication pain, the major goal of this therapy is to diminish claudication symptoms during ambulation. This is best accomplished with 3 or more days per week of intermittent walking exercise. During each exercise session, patients should exercise to a perceived "moderate" claudication rating and then rest until the pain subsides. Strength training can be implemented as an adjunct, but it does not appear to supplement the improvements in functional capacity beyond those observed for walking. Clinical assessment of functional capacity and follow-up testing can be done using the 6-min walk and/or treadmill protocols.

REFERENCES

1. Criqui MH, Langer RD, Fronek A, Feigelson HS, Klauber MR, McCann TJ, Browner D. Mortality Over a Period of 10 Years in Patients with Peripheral Arterial Disease. *N Engl J Med.* 1992;326: 381–386.

2. Weitz JI, Byrne J, Clagett GP, Farkouh ME, Porter JM, Sackett DL, Strandness DE Jr, Taylor LM. Diagnosis and Treatment of Chronic Arterial Insufficiency of the Lower Extremities: A Critical Review. *Circulation.* 1996;94:3026–3049.

3. Murabito JM, D'Agostino RB, Silbershatz H, Wilson WF. Intermittent Claudication. A Risk Profile from The Framingham Heart Study. *Circulation.* 1997;96:44–49.

4. Kannel WB, McGee DL. Update on some Epidemiologic Features of Intermittent Claudication: the Framingham Study. *J Am Geriatr Soc.* 1985;33:13–18.

5. Hiatt WR, Marshall JA, Baxter J, Sandoval R, Hildebrandt W, Kahn LR, Hamman RF. Diagnostic Methods for Peripheral Arterial Disease in the San Luis Valley Diabetes Study. *J Clin Epidemiol.* 1990;43:597–606.

6. Labs KH, Dormandy JA, Jaeger KA, Stuerzebecher CS, Hiatt WR. Transatlantic Conference on Clinical Trial Guidelines in Peripheral Arterial Disease: Clinical Trial Methodology. Basel PAD Clinical Trial Methodology Group. *Circulation.* 1999;100:e75–e81.

7. Rose G, McCartney P, Reid DD. Self-Administration of a Questionnaire on Chest Pain and Inter-mittent Claudication. *Br J Prev Soc Med.* 1977;31:42–48.

8. Hiatt WR, Wolfel EE, Regensteiner JG, Brass EP. Skeletal Muscle Carnitine Metabolism in Patients with Unilateral Peripheral Arterial Disease. *J Appl Physiol.* 1992;73:346–353.

9. Jansson E, Johansson J, Sylven C, Kaijser L. Calf Muscle Adaptation in Intermittent Claudication. Side-Differences in Muscle Metabolic Characteristics in Patients with Unilateral Arterial Disease. *Clin Physiol.* 1988;8:17–29.

10. Brass EP, Hiatt WR, Gardner AW, Hoppel CL. Decreased NADH Dehydrogenase and Ubiquinol-Cytochrome c Oxidoreductase in Peripheral Arterial Disease. *Am J Physiol Heart Circ Physiol.* 2001;280:H603–H609.

11. Novo S, Avellone G, Di Garbo V, Abrignani MG, Liquori M, Panno AV, Strano A. Prevalence of Risk Factors in Patients with Peripheral Arterial Disease. A Clinical and Epidemiological Evaluation. *Int Angiol.* 1992;11:218–229.

12. Dawson DL, Cutler BS, Hiatt WR, Hobson RW 2nd, Martin JD, Bortey EB, Forbes WP, Strandness DE Jr. A Comparison of Cilostazol and Pentoxifylline for Treating Intermittent Claudi-cation. *Am J Med.* 2000;109:523–530.

13. Brevetti G, Chiariello M, Ferulano G, Policicchio A, Nevola E, Rossini A, Attisano T, Ambrosio G, Siliprandi N, Angelini C. Increases in Walking Distance in Patients with Peripheral Vascular Disease Treated with L-Carnitine: A Double-Blind, Cross-Over Study. *Circulation.* 1988;77:767–773.

14. Aronow WS. Management of Peripheral Arterial Disease. *Cardiol Rev.* 2005;13:61–68.

15. Treesak C, Kasemsup V, Treat-Jacobson D, Nyman JA, Hirsch AT. Cost-Effectiveness of Exercise Training to Improve Claudication Symptoms in Patients with Peripheral Arterial Disease. *Vasc Med.* 2004;9:279–285.

16. Barker GA, Green S, Green AA, Walker PJ. Walking Performance, Oxygen Uptake Kinetics and Resting Muscle Pyruvate Dehydrogenase Complex Activity in Peripheral Arterial Disease. *Clin Sci (Lond).* 2004;106:241–249.

17. Womack CJ, Sieminski DJ, Katzel LI, Yataco A, Gardner AW. Improved Walking Economy in Patients with Peripheral Arterial Occlusive Disease. *Med Sci Sports Exerc.* 1997;29: 1286–1290.

18. Womack CJ, Gardner AW. Peripheral Arterial Disease. In *ACSM's Exercise Management for Persons with Chronic Diseases and Disabilities*, JL Durstine and GE Moore (eds.). Champaign, IL: Human Kinetics; 2003:81–90.

19. Gardner AW, Montgomery PS, Flinn WR, Katzel LI. The Effect of Exercise Intensity on the Response to Exercise Rehabilitation in Patients with Intermittent Claudication. *J Vasc Surg.* 2005;42:702–709.

20. Bulmer AC, Coombes JS. Optimising Exercise Training in Peripheral Arterial Disease. *Sports Med.* 2004;34:983–1003.

21. Collins EG, Langbein WE, Orebaugh C, Bammert C, Hanson K, Reda D, Edwards LC, Littooy FN. Cardiovascular Training Effect Associated with Polestriding Exercise in Patients with Peripheral Arterial Disease. *J Cardiovasc Nurs.* 2005;20:177–185.

22. Jones PP, Skinner JS, Smith LK, John FM, Bryant CX. Functional Improvements Following Stair-Master Vs. Treadmill Exercise Training for Patients with Intermittent Claudication. *J Cardiopulm Rehabil.* 1996;16:47–55.

23. Walker RD, Nawaz S, Wilkinson CH, Saxton JM, Pockley AG, Wood RF. Influence of Upper- and Lower-Limb Exercise Training on Cardiovascular Function and Walking Distances in Patients with Intermittent Claudication. *J Vasc Surg.* 2000;31:662–669.

24. Hiatt WR, Wolfel EE, Meier RH, Regensteiner JG. Superiority of Treadmill Walking Exercise Versus Strength Training for Patients with Peripheral Arterial Disease. Implications for the Mechanism of the Training Response. *Circulation.* 1994;90:1866–1874.

25. Regensteiner JG, Steiner JF, Hiatt WR. Exercise Training Improves Functional Status in Patients with Peripheral Arterial Disease. *J Vasc Surg.* 1996;23:104–115.

26. Pollock ML, Franklin BA, Balady GJ, Chaitman BL, Fleg JL, Fletcher B, Limacher M, Pina IL, Stein RA, Williams M, Bazzarre T. AHA Science Advisory. Resistance Exercise in Individuals With and Without Cardiovascular Disease: Benefits, Rationale, Safety, and Prescription: An Advisory from the Committee on Exercise, Rehabilitation, and Prevention, Council on Clinical Cardiology, American Heart Association; Position paper endorsed by the American College of Sports Medicine. *Circulation.* 2000;101:828–833.

27. McGuigan MR, Bronks R, Newton RU, Sharman MJ, Graham JC, Cody DV, Kraemer WJ. Resistance Training in Patients with Peripheral Arterial Disease: Effects on Myosin Isoforms, Fiber Type Distribution, and Capillary Supply to Skeletal Muscle. *J Gerontol A Biol Sci Med Sci.* 2001; 56:B302–B310.

28. Askew CD, Green S, Walker PJ, Kerr GK, Green AA, Williams AD, Febbraio MA. Skeletal Muscle Phenotype is Associated with Exercise Tolerance in Patients with Peripheral Arterial Disease. *J Vasc Surg.* 2005;41:802–807.

29. Gardner AW, Katzel LI, Sorkin JD, Bradham DD, Hochberg MC, Flinn WR, Goldberg AP. Exercise Rehabilitation Improves Functional Outcomes and Peripheral Circulation in Patients with Intermittent Claudication: A Randomized Controlled Trial. *J Am Geriatr Soc.* 2001;49:755–762.

30. Hiatt WR, Regensteiner JG, Hargarten ME, Wolfel EE, Brass EP. Benefit of Exercise Conditioning for Patients with Peripheral Arterial Disease. *Circulation.* 1990;81:602–609.

31. Hiatt WR, Regensteiner JG, Wolfel EE, Carry MR, Brass EP. Effect of Exercise Training on Skeletal Muscle Histology and Metabolism in Peripheral Arterial Disease. *J Appl Physiol.* 1996;81:780–788.

32. Killewich LA, Macko RF, Montgomery PS, Wiley LA, Gardner AW. Exercise Training Enhances Endogenous Fibrinolysis in Peripheral Arterial Disease. *J Vasc Surg.* 2004;40:741–745.

33. Izquierdo-Porrera AM, Gardner AW, Powell CC, Katzel LI. Effects of Exercise Rehabilitation on Cardiovascular Risk Factors in Older Patients with Peripheral Arterial Occlusive Disease. *J Vasc Surg.* 2000;31:670–677.

34. Gardner AW, Skinner JS, Vaughan NR, Bryant CX, Smith LK. Comparison of Treadmill Walking
    and Stair Climbing over a Range of Exercise Intensities in Peripheral Vascular Occlusive Disease.
    Angiology. 1993;44:353–360.
35. Gardner AW, Skinner JS, Cantwell BW, Smith LK. Progressive Vs Single-Stage Treadmill Tests for
    Evaluation of Claudication. *Med Sci Sports Exerc*. 1991;23:402–408.

20

Dealing with Arthritis as a Comorbidity in Cardiac Rehabilitation Programs

Kim M. Huffman, MD, PhD

CONTENTS

BACKGROUND

"Arthritis" literally means inflammation within a joint, but this term is often used to encompass a wide range of conditions affecting bones, joints, and connective tissues with unique pathogeneses, epidemiologies, and disease manifestations. As many as 20% of adults in the US and approximately 49% of those over age 65 years report that they have arthritis *(1,2)*. Given the aging of our population, projected estimates suggest that close to 25% of the US adult population will be impacted by arthritis by 2030 *(2)*. Not surprisingly, arthritis is the leading reported cause of disability in the US *(3)*. Although many individuals presenting for cardiac rehabilitation (CR) will describe a history of "arthritis," the rehabilitative health professional should attempt to understand what particular form of arthritis afflicts the patient to optimize their rehabilitation (Table 1). Rheumatoid arthritis (RA) and osteoarthritis (OA) are particularly pervasive and have specific implications for CR.

From: *Contemporary Cardiology: Cardiac Rehabilitation*
Edited by: W. E. Kraus and S. J. Keteyian © Humana Press Inc., Totowa, NJ

Table 1
Distinguishing Features for Rheumatoid Arthritis and Osteoarthritis

	Rheumatoid arthritis	*Osteoarthritis*
Morning stiffness in active disease	One hour or more	Less than 30 min
Symmetric joint involvement	+++	+
DIP and CMC involvement	−	+++
Wrist and MCP involvement	+++	−
Cervical spine involvement	++	++
Lumbar and thoracic spine involvement	+	+++
Hip and knee involvement	++	+++
Metatarsal involvement	+++	+/−*
Rheumatoid factor and anti-CCP detected	++	−
Erosions on X-rays	++	−
Osteophytes on X-rays	−	+++
Treatment with immunosuppressive and biologic agents	+++	−

+++, typical; ++, often; +, occasional; −, rare to none.

CCP, cyclic citrullinated peptide; CMC, carpal–metacarpal joint; DIP, distal interphalangeal joint; MCP, metacarpal–phalangeal joint.

* Typically only first metatarsal–phalangeal joint involved.

RHEUMATOID ARTHRITIS

RA is a chronic, inflammatory arthritis and affects close to 1% of individuals *(4)*. Women are affected more often than men in a 3:1 ratio, and age of onset is typically after age 40 years in women and slightly older in men, although individuals can present with RA at any age. RA is associated with considerable morbidity and mortality such that more than 50% of individuals with RA are estimated to have severe disability *(4)*.

RA results from a combination of genetic and environmental predispositions. Some of the genetic associations of RA have been identified, such as an association between RA and human leukocyte antigen (HLA) DRB1 alleles, DR4, DR1, and DR14 *(5)*. Additionally, there appear to be associations between RA and cigarette smoking *(6)* and viral infections *(7)*, but precise genetic and environmental triggers have not yet been elucidated. The histopathology of RA demonstrates an accumulation of synovial fibroblasts, T cells, and macrophages within the joint synovium. While the inciting pathogenic events remain debated, the activated inflammatory cells produce pro-inflammatory mediators including cytokines, adhesion molecules, and matrix metallo-proteinases. These small molecules promote many characteristic manifestations, such as bony erosions and deformities, and symptoms, including joint swelling, stiffness, joint pain, and fatigue. Additionally, these molecules as well as the cells producing them are the targets for many of the current and developing treatments for RA *(8)*.

Typically, RA has an insidious onset followed by a steady course punctuated with periodic "flares" of activity. The pattern of joint involvement is characteristically symmetric. Initially, RA involves smaller joints such as the hands, feet, wrists, and ankles, although knees can also be commonly inflamed and damaged. Most remarkable in persons with established RA, disease activity in the cervical spine can produce devastating consequences; however, involvement of the thoracic and lumbar spine is much less common. Also, in contrast to OA, the distal interphalangeal (DIP) joints are rarely affected by RA. Over time, joint inflammation often results in fixed, characteristic deformities such as swan-neck and boutonniere deformities. These joint deformities may become a rare manifestation as disease-remitting treatments are being increasingly utilized in early disease but presently account for much of the disability associated with RA. Also, as a systemic inflammatory disease, RA can impact virtually any organ system in the body. Systemic manifestations are typically associated with severe active disease.

Diagnosis of RA is made based on the history, characteristic symmetric physical examination findings, laboratory tests such as rheumatoid factor and antibodies to cyclic citrullinated peptide, and radiographic changes such as erosions and periarticular osteopenia. Medical treatment of RA is complex, often managed by a rheumatologist or other specialist in RA, but typically includes a combination of medications ranging from nonsteroidal anti-inflammatory agents for very mild cases to disease modifying agents (methotrexate, leflunomide, azathioprine, sulfasalazine, hydroxychloroquine, and cyclosporine) and biologic agents (etanercept, infliximab, adalimumab, anakinra, rituximab, and abatacept) for more typical aggressive disease. Also, many individuals with RA are maintained on low doses of glucocorticoids (< 10 mg a day of prednisone), and steroids are commonly used in higher doses to treat joint "flares" and other systemic manifestations of this disease.

Individuals with RA are at increased risk of cardiovascular morbidity and mortality *(9,10)*. Women with RA appear particularly susceptible to cardiovascular disease *(11,12)* with evidence of twofold increases in risk of myocardial infarction *(13)*. Likely a complex interplay of genetic predisposition, inflammation, endothelial dysfunction, glucocorticoid use, and insulin resistance results in an increased prevalence of cardiovascular disease in individuals with RA.

OSTEOARTHRITIS

OA is an especially prevalent form of arthritis, often referred to as degenerative arthritis. As many persons have radiographic evidence of OA without symptoms, estimates for the prevalence of OA vary depending on whether radiographic evidence alone is used to define the disease. When requiring both radiographic changes and symptoms as a definition of OA, conservative estimates suggest that 2% of the US population and 10–15% of those over 65 years appear affected *(1,14)*. Regardless of the definition, the prevalence increases with age such that some estimates report over 75% of individuals over age 65 years have radiographic evidence of OA in at least one joint *(1,14)*. At all ages, women are commonly affected more than men.

Similar to RA, the pathogenesis of OA has not yet been completely elucidated, but OA is commonly understood to be a disease of articular cartilage and subchondral bone. Cartilage damage can result from abnormal or extreme forces, such as that which occurs with morbid obesity, distributed over normal joint tissues. Alternatively, normal forces can injure cartilage in the setting of abnormal joint tissues, for example, cartilage found in individuals with metabolic deposition diseases such as hemochromatosis. During and after cartilage injury, chondrocytes (the main cellular constituent of cartilage) release degradative enzymes, which result in a net loss of cartilage proteoglycan (an important molecule involved in the shock-absorbing capacity of the joint). Defects within cartilage occur, and, as a result, bone is exposed to synovial fluid and the degradative enzymes that initiate damage within underlying, subchondral bone. These effects result in the joint space narrowing found in radiographs of individuals with OA. Remodeling within subchondral bone results in many of the remaining radiographic findings (subchondral sclerosis, osteophytes, and subchondral cysts) associated with OA *(15)*.

Clinically, OA affects the hands and weight-bearing joints, such as knees and hips. When affecting the hands, OA commonly occurs in the first carpal–metacarpal joints and proximal interphalangeal and DIP joints. Deformities in the DIPs (referred to as Heberden's nodes) are often helpful in distinguishing OA from other types of arthritis, but DIP joints can also be deformed as a peripheral manifestation of psoriatic arthritis. Individuals with OA often describe joint pain, swelling (especially in the knees), and stiffness. Likely a manifestation of the degree of inflammation involved, the stiffness component of OA is typically limited to less than 30 min after prolonged inactivity. Also, with severe disease and joint damage, alterations in range of motion and deformities become prevalent. Diagnosis is made using characteristic findings in the history, physical examination, and radiographic evaluation of the patient. Laboratory studies may be helpful to evaluate causes of secondary OA but are not diagnostic for OA itself.

Treatment of OA includes treatment with pharmacologic and nonpharmacologic modalities. Pharmacotherapy is directed at reducing pain with nonsteroidal anti-inflammatory agents, acetaminophen, and occasionally narcotics. Although findings have been mixed, the "nutraceutical" glucosamine appears to improve pain and function in OA *(16)*. Additionally, topical medications, such as capsaicin cream, and intra-articular injections of steroids and hyaluronic acid derivatives are also routinely used, although the clinical effectiveness of the latter has not been unequivocally proven *(17)*. Currently, no disease modifying pharmacologic agents exist for OA, but clinical trials are ongoing. Nonpharmacologic treatment recommendations include patient education, weight loss for the obese, quadriceps strengthening for those with knee OA, braces designed to unload forces from affected weight-bearing joints, assistive walking devices when necessary, and paraffin baths for painful hand OA. Severe OA of the hip or knee causing pain that interrupts sleep or significantly impacts daily activities is often treated surgically with osteotomy or replacement of the joint.

IMPLICATIONS FOR REHABILITATION AND EXERCISE MANAGEMENT

As with any other patient enrolling in a CR program, for the patient with arthritis, it is imperative to devote attention to secondary prevention items, such as optimizing nutrition, risk factor management, and performing a psychosocial assessment. Nutritional recommendations should not differ for individuals with arthritis as a direct consequence of the presence of disease. However, persons with RA are at increased risk of osteoporosis; therefore, calcium and vitamin D intake, which are usually less than recommended levels in the American population, should be paid particular attention. Also, patients prescribed methotrexate for RA should be simultaneously prescribed a supplemental folic acid (typically 1 mg a day) to help minimize hyper-homocystinemia and side effects associated with this medication. In the obese patient with OA and cardiovascular disease, nutritional assessments and recommendations should follow those outlined for obese patients such that a comprehensive program should be designed to promote improved nutritional quality and weight loss.

In patients with known coronary disease, cardiovascular risk factor assessment should proceed similarly for those with arthritis as for those without. It is worth noting that many physicians believe that prior to a cardiovascular event or evidence of overt cardiovascular disease, individuals with RA should be managed with lipid and blood pressure guidelines similar to those for patients with diabetes. Similarly, given increasing evidence of metabolic derangements likely related to arthritis-associated reductions in physical activity levels, evaluation for possible diabetes should be undertaken in individuals with both arthritis and cardiovascular disease.

Psychosocial assessment is especially important in those with arthritis and cardiovascular disease. Depression commonly occurs in individuals with chronic illnesses and should be addressed in a comprehensive assessment (18). Additionally, in individuals with chronic diseases, higher levels of self-efficacy (confidence in one's ability to perform a specific task) predict better health outcomes [reviewed in (19)]. Assessing self-efficacy for each component of the rehabilitation program can be achieved simply by asking the patient whether he/she believes they will be able to accomplish a specific task, such as weight loss or smoking cessation.

Recommendations for Promoting Self-Efficacy in the Patient With Arthritis

- Have the patient practice the activity to improve necessary skills: utilize a physical and/or occupational therapist's guidance for those with severe deformities.
- Demonstrate other patients with arthritis who have succeeded in attaining arthritis-specific goals, such as weight loss and maintaining successful exercise programs.
- Involve persons who will provide positive reinforcement and encouragement: incorporate family members in the exercise program or suggest a group program such as aquatics therapy.
- Assess and discuss anxiety levels about particular exercise activities before and after the task: address whether the patient feels that his/her arthritis may impact their ability to perform the activity.

ARTHRITIS-SPECIFIC ADJUSTMENTS TO ACUTE EXERCISE AND EXERCISE TESTING

The most notable adjustment for acute exercise in individuals with arthritis is to recognize disease exacerbations, joint infections, and acute regional musculoskeletal problems. Although exercise has not been shown to promote exacerbations or flares in individuals with RA, recognizing a disease flare or a potential joint infection and directing the individual to seek further evaluation and treatment is imperative for the comprehensive management of these patients. Although disease flares and joint infections are often difficult to distinguish, both present with warm, red, and painful joints. Given the typically recognizable symptoms, one strategy would be to direct the patient to contact the physician managing their arthritis if they develop fevers, chills, or warmth, redness, or severe pain in a joint and to delay exercise training that loads affected joints until after evaluation and treatment. During the course of a flare, training should be altered to include primarily isometric strengthening and range of motion flexibility exercises.

In addition to recognizing acutely inflamed or infected joints, the patient and practitioner should be aware of the development of regional musculoskeletal problems. While typically the result of overuse or repetitive actions, regional musculoskeletal disorders should prompt an acute adjustment in the training regimen. Persons with arthritis, especially RA, are more prone to the development of compressive neuropathies, especially posterior tibial, median, ulnar, and posterior interosseus nerves. Development of neuropathic pain (usually described as burning, shooting, numbness, or tingling) in these distributions should alert the practitioner to syndromes such as tarsal tunnel or carpal tunnel syndrome. Additionally, awareness of and ability to diagnose other common regional musculoskeletal disorders such as rotator cuff tendonitis, trochanteric bursitis, and iliotibial band syndrome are helpful in the management of persons with arthritis. Once diagnosed, treatment for these conditions usually involves rest, physical therapy, and occasionally steroid injection. During the acute phase of inflammation, inciting activities involved in the patient's training program should be replaced with an alternative activity that does not aggravate the affected area. Nonetheless, maintaining range of motion in the affected area is an essential part of rehabilitation. By minimizing repetitive actions and offering various exercise modes, many regional musculoskeletal problems can be prevented.

Exercise testing in patients with arthritis should be tailored to the patient's arthritis disease status. Submaximal testing may be preferable in individuals with severe disease, and in patients with severe lower extremity involvement, arm ergometry may be necessary for testing. It is worth noting that for standard graded maximal tests without spirometry, $VO_{2\,max}$ estimations are often based on American College of Sports Medicine metabolic equations derived from steady-state exercise (20). These equations have been shown to overestimate $VO_{2\,max}$ in patients with arthritis and those with cardiovascular disease when graded exercise protocols are used (21,22). In order to avoid exercise prescriptions at higher than intended intensity, take care to choose a protocol with well-validated $VO_{2\,max}$ estimation equations. Several equations have been validated for graded exercise protocols (refer Chapter 10), and one equation has been validated using the Modified Naughton protocol in a population with knee OA (21,22). Additionally, if exercise prescriptions are based on maximal heart rate prediction equations, having the patient check their own heart rate during exercise to verify that they are within the targeted range is especially important in this population where heart rate may vary significantly depending on the mode of exercise.

DISEASE-SPECIFIC ADJUSTMENTS FOR EXERCISE PRESCRIPTION

Recently, a work group published recommendations on exercise prescription for individuals with RA and OA. These recommendations are based on available evidence as well as proceedings at the 2002 Exercise and Physical Activity Conference in St. Louis, Missouri. This group recommends that individuals with RA desiring cardiovascular fitness train at an intensity of 60–85% maximal heart rate, a frequency of two to three times per week, and duration of 30–60 min, and using whole body and dynamic modes such as walking, stationary cycling, dancing, and aerobic aquatics (23) (Table 2). For neuromuscular rehabilitation in RA, recommendations include dynamic

Table 2
Guidelines for Aerobic Exercise Prescription in Patients with Arthritis*

	Rheumatoid arthritis	Osteoarthritis – hip and knee
Intensity	60–85% max HR	50–70% max HR
Frequency	Two to three times per week	At least three times per week
Duration	30–60 min	Accumulate 30 min per day
Mode	Walking, stationary cycling, and aerobic aquatics†	Walking, stationary cycling, and aerobic aquatics†

HR, heart rate.

* Based on recommendations for cardiovascular fitness gains (23).

† Specific modes should be tailored to disease severity, accessibility, and patient preference.

resistance training at 50–80% of maximal load, two to three times per week, at a volume of 8–10 exercises, 8–10 repetitions, and 1–2 sets (Table 3).

Recommendations for individuals with hip and knee OA are to perform aerobic exercise at an intensity of 50–70% maximal heart rate, a frequency of at least three times per week, and a cumulative duration of at least 30 min per day while utilizing a mode tailored to the individual patient (23) (Table 2). Additionally, given the prevalence of obesity in patients with OA and the contribution of obesity to OA and cardiovascular disease pathogenesis, a plan for moderate weight loss should be incorporated into the exercise prescription for overweight and obese individuals with OA. Because skeletal muscle weakness appears to correlate with radiographic presence of knee OA, resistance training with a goal for strengthening large muscle groups, especially quadriceps, should be included in a comprehensive rehabilitation plan for those with OA. Recommendations for resistance training in OA suggest that beginning programs at 40% of one repetition maximum (RM), with one set of 4–6 repetitions, 2 days a week, and increasing volume and intensity by 5–10% per week (24) (Table 3). It is worth noting that these recommendations for both RA and OA were not designed to

Table 3
Guidelines for Resistance Training Prescription in Patients with Arthritis*

	Rheumatoid arthritis*	Osteoarthritis – hip and knee†
Intensity	50–85% 1 RM	40–80% 1 RM
Frequency	Two to three times per week	Two to three times per week
Volume	Eight to ten exercises using major muscle groups	Eight to ten exercises using major muscle groups
	Eight to ten repetitions	Four to six repetitions
	One to two sets	One set

RM, repetition maximum.

* Based on recommendations for neuromuscular gains (23).

† Based on recommendations for comprehensive management of older adults with osteoarthritis (24).

address CR-specific goals, and the exercise studies upon which these recommendations were based did not have cardiovascular endpoints. Most important, given the vast range in disease activity for RA and OA, individualized exercise prescription and progression is imperative.

While the CR health professional is often focused on aerobic and resistance training to improve cardiovascular benefit, incorporating flexibility and range of motion exercises into the exercise routine of the patient with arthritis will promote their comprehensive care. Patients with arthritis should be encouraged to perform gentle stretching and flexibility exercise of both large and small joints at least once daily several times a week (24). Also, it is important to emphasize the importance of warm-up and cool-down exercises and consider icing after exercise.

Precautions for exercise training should be similar to those given to all individuals participating in exercise programs but may be tailored for the patient with arthritis to include noting joint or muscle pain with exercise, postexercise pain lasting more than an hour, joint swelling or redness, and fatigue.

COMMON CHRONIC ADAPTATIONS TO EXERCISE TRAINING

In individuals with RA, exercise training appears to improve strength and cardiorespiratory fitness, but effects on function and radiographic progression are less clear [reviewed in (25)]. Several studies have shown no detrimental effects of exercise on radiographic progression (26–30). However, a recent investigation reported that high-intensity weight-bearing exercise (70–90% of predicted maximal heart rate) may hasten progression of radiographic damage in shoulders and ankle (subtalar) joints with pre-existing severe damage (31). Again, although more trials are warranted to validate these results, in individuals with severely damaged joints, conventional wisdom would guide rehabilitation toward exercise modalities, such as aquatics-based programs that minimize loading on severely damaged joints.

In individuals with OA, exercise training can reduce pain and improve strength and function (32), but these studies have primarily been limited to populations with OA of the knee rather than that of the hip or generalized OA. There are recent reports suggesting that a combination of strengthening and aerobic exercise may promote beneficial changes in cartilage glycosaminoglycan content in individuals at risk for OA (33). Unfortunately, there are limited investigations evaluating the impact of chronic aerobic or resistance exercise on the radiographic progression of arthritis or on cardiovascular endpoints. Again, given the lack of evidence-based guidance, conventional wisdom recommends minimizing joint loading of moderately to severely affected joints as much as possible, as would be provided in aquatics-based programs. Although facilities in all programs might not be conducive to aquatic exercise, if that modality is available, CR programs might promote aquatic aerobics for individuals with arthritis.

Many physicians recommend quadriceps-strengthening exercises to patients with symptomatic knee OA. Although a number of investigations suggest that resistance training, specifically quadriceps-strengthening, reduces pain and disability in knee OA, few evaluate the impact of strengthening on radiographic progression. However, in one investigation that evaluated the impact of *baseline* quadriceps strength on disease progression, greater quadriceps strength appeared to promote progression of OA in

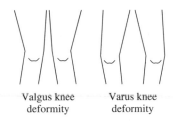

Valgus knee   Varus knee
deformity   deformity

Fig. 1. Graphical depiction of valgus and varus knee deformities.

individuals with valgus and varus knee deformities (Fig. 1) and medial and lateral knee laxity *(34)*. While these findings warrant validation in a training trial, when recommending quadriceps strengthening to patients with OA and malaligned or lax kness, it is reasonable to discuss this as a potential, but not verified, risk. Also, although there is limited clinical trial evidence, orthotic devices, such as valgus-corrective braces for valgus deformities of the knee and lateral heel wedges for varus knee deformities, may counteract these biomechanical factors as well as provide other benefits such as decreasing nonsteroidal usage *(35)*.

OTHER IMPORTANT AREAS OF CONCERN

- RA deformities may require adjustment of machines used in exercise training. In patients with severe deformities, exercise prescription in conjunction with occupational and physical therapists is reasonable. For upper extremity deformities, handgrip adaptive devices may be useful. For foot deformities, referral to a podiatrist may be helpful in providing individualized orthotics or suggesting shoes with a wide toe box for hallux valgus deformities. Similarly, knee bracing and shoe orthotics may be helpful for knee arthritis and assistive devices such as canes and walkers, typically recommended by physical therapists may allow patients with severe hip or knee arthritis to increase cumulative aerobic activity in daily activities.
- Consideration of RA involvement in the cervical spine, typically manifested initially as neck pain radiating to the occiput, is essential. Possible cervical instability is evaluated with flexion and extension radiographs of the cervical spine and, when identified, should be evaluated for need for surgical stabilization. Isometric and minimally dynamic exercises of cervical muscles may improve symptoms in individuals with RA and cervical spine instability who chose not to have surgical stabilization *(36)*, but individuals with cervical instability should not participate in contact sports or typical resistance training involving loading of the cervical spine.
- One means of minimizing joint loading in individuals with moderate-to-severe hip, knee, and ankle arthritis is aquatics therapy. In addition, to reduce joint loads, exercise in water provides some resistance for muscle strengthening and may provide an analgesic benefit for painful joints. In persons with RA, for a given VO_2, heart rate appears to be higher on land than in water, such that to achieve aerobic benefits with aquatics therapy, heart rate targets should be increased by 9 beats/min during aquatics therapy *(24)*.
- More information on arthritis-specific exercise programs, including Arthritis Foundation/YMCA aquatics programs (AFYAP) and People with Arthritis Can Exercise (PACE®) can be found at http://www.arthritis.org and http://www.rheumatology.org. More details regarding arthritis-specific exercise physiology can be found in the excellent reference *(22)*.

- Given the lack of evidence for exercise prescription for primary and secondary prevention of cardiovascular disease in patients with arthritis, future exercise studies should address cardiovascular and radiographic endpoints in individuals with these chronic diseases.

SUMMARY

As the aging population increases, the number of individuals with arthritis presenting for CR is likely to increase dramatically. Recognizing the typical joints involved in RA and OA and signs of disease complications will help in promoting the rehabilitation of these patients. As with all patients, attention to nutrition, risk factor management, and psychosocial assessment are important in the rehabilitative effort. Most important, as with all patients, exercise testing and prescriptions should be individualized to accommodate each patient's disease activity, deformities, and overall functional status.

REFERENCES

1. Lawrence RC, Helmick CG, Arnett FC, Deyo RA, Felson DT, Giannini EH, Heyse SP, Hirsch R, Hochberg MC, Hunder GG, Liang MH, Pillemer SR, Steen VD, Wolfe F. Estimates of the Prevalence of Arthritis and Selected Musculoskeletal Disorders in the United States. *Arthritis Rheum.* 1998;41:778–799.
2. Hootman JM, Helmick CG. Projections of US Prevalence of Arthritis and Associated Activity Limitations. *Arthritis Rheum.* 2006;54:226–229.
3. Centers for Disease Control and Prevention. Prevalence of Disabilities and Associated Health Conditions Among Adults–United States, 1999. *MMWR Morb Mortal Wkly Rep.* 2001;50:120–125.
4. Kvien TK. Epidemiology and Burden of Illness of Rheumatoid Arthritis. *Pharmacoeconomics.* 2004;22:1–12.
5. Gonzalez-Gay MA, Garcia-Porrua C, Hajeer AH. Influence of Human Leukocyte Antigen-DRB1 on the Susceptibility and Severity of Rheumatoid Arthritis. *Semin Arthritis Rheum.* 2002;31:355–360.
6. Padyukov L, Silva C, Stolt P, Alfredsson L, Klareskog L. A Gene-Environment Interaction Between Smoking and Shared Epitope Genes in HLA-DR Provides a High Risk of Seropositive Rheumatoid Arthritis. *Arthritis Rheum.* 2004;50:3085–3092.
7. Mehraein Y, Lennerz C, Ehlhardt S, Remberger K, Ojak A, Zang KD. Latent Epstein-Barr Virus (EBV) Infection and Cytomegalovirus (CMV) Infection in Synovial Tissue of Autoimmune Chronic Arthritis Determined by RNA- and DNA-In Situ Hybridization. *Mod Pathol.* 2004;17:781–789.
8. Firestein GS. Etiology and Pathogenesis of Rheumatoid Arthritis. In *Kelley's Textbook of Rheumatology.* Philadelphia, PA: W.B. Sanders; 2005:996–1042.
9. Jacobsson LT, Knowler WC, Pillemer S, Hanson RL, Pettitt DJ, Nelson RG, del Puente A, McCance DR, Charles MA, Bennett PH. Rheumatoid Arthritis and Mortality. A Longitudinal Study in Pima Indians. *Arthritis Rheum.* 1993;36:1045–1053.
10. Mutru O, Laakso M, Isomaki H, Koota K. Cardiovascular Mortality in Patients with Rheumatoid Arthritis. *Cardiology.* 1989;76:71–77.
11. Kvalvik AG, Jones MA, Symmons DP. Mortality in a Cohort of Norwegian Patients with Rheumatoid Arthritis Followed from 1977 to 1992. *Scand J Rheumatol.* 2000;29:29–37.
12. Myllykangas-Luosujarvi R, Aho K, Kautiainen H, Isomaki H. Cardiovascular Mortality in Women with Rheumatoid Arthritis. *J Rheumatol.* 1995;22:1065–1067.
13. Solomon DH, Karlson EW, Rimm EB, Cannuscio CC, Mandl LA, Manson JE, Stampfer MJ, Curhan GC. Cardiovascular Morbidity and Mortality in Women Diagnosed with Rheumatoid Arthritis. *Circulation.* 2003;107:1303–1307.
14. Buckwalter JA, Saltzman C, Brown T. The Impact of Osteoarthritis: Implications for Research. *Clin Orthop Relat Res.* 2004:S6–S15.

15. Di Cesare PE, Abramson SB. Pathogenesis of Osteoarthritis. In *Kelley's Textbook of Rheumatology*. Philadelphia, PA: W.B. Sanders; 2005:1493–1500.
16. Towheed TE, Maxwell L, Anastassiades TP, Shea B, Houpt J, Robinson V, Hochberg MC, Wells G. Glucosamine Therapy for Treating Osteoarthritis. *Cochrane Database Syst Rev*. 2005;(2):CD002946.
17. Bellamy N, Campbell J, Robinson V, Gee T, Bourne R, Wells G. Viscosupplementation for the Treatment of Osteoarthritis of the knee. *Cochrane Database Syst Rev* 2005;(2):CD005321.
18. Polsky D, Doshi JA, Marcus S, Oslin D, Rothbard A, Thomas N, Thompson CL. Long-Term Risk for Depressive Symptoms after a Medical Diagnosis. *Arch Intern Med*. 2005;165:1260–1266.
19. Marks R, Allegrante JP, Lorig K. A Review and Synthesis of Research Evidence for Self-Efficacy-Enhancing Interventions for Reducing Chronic Disability: Implications for Health Education Practice (Part II). *Health Promot Pract*. 2005;6:148–156.
20. American College of Sports Medicine. Appendix D-Metabolic Calculations. *Guidelines for Exercise Testing and Prescription*. Media, PA: Williams & Wilkins; 1995:269–287.
21. Berry MJ, Brubaker PH, O'Toole ML, Rejeski WJ, Soberman J, Ribisl PM, Miller HS, Afable RF, Applegate W, Ettinger WH. Estimation of VO2 in Older Individuals with Osteoarthritis of the Knee and Cardiovascular Disease. *Med Sci Sports Exerc*. 1996;28:808–814.
22. Kraus VB, Wiggin D. Arthritis. *Clinical Exercise Physiology*. Champaign, IL: Human Kinetics; 2003:443–464.
23. Minor M, Stenstrom CH, Klepper SE, Hurby M, Ettinger WH. Work Group Recommendations: 2002 Exercise and Physical Activity Conference, St. Louis, Missouri. Session V: Evidence of Benefit of Exercise and Physical Activity in Arthritis. *Arthritis Rheum*. 2003;49:453–454.
24. American Geriatrics Society Panel on Exercise and Osteoarthritis. Exercise Prescription for Older Adults with Osteoarthritis Pain: Consensus Practice Recommendations. A Supplement to the AGS Clinical Practice Guidelines on the Management of Chronic Pain in Older Adults. *J Am Geriatr Soc*. 2001;49:808–823.
25. Van den Ende CH, Vliet Vlieland TP, Munneke M, Hazes JM. Dynamic Exercise Therapy in Rheumatoid Arthritis: A Systematic Review. *Br J Rheumatol*. 1998;37:677–687.
26. Nordemar R, Ekblom B, Zachrisson L, Lundqvist K. Physical Training in Rheumatoid Arthritis: A Controlled Long-Term Study. I. *Scand J Rheumatol*. 1981;10:17–23.
27. Hansen TM, Hansen G, Langgaard AM, Rasmussen JO. Longterm Physical Training in Rheumatoid Arthritis. A Randomized Trial with Different Training Programs and Blinded Observers. *Scand J Rheumatol*. 1993;22:107–112.
28. Stenstrom CH, Lindell B, Swanberg E, Swanberg P, Harms-Ringdahl K, Nordemar R. Intensive Dynamic Training in Water for Rheumatoid Arthritis Functional Class II–A Long-Term Study of Effects. *Scand J Rheumatol*. 1991;20:358–365.
29. Hakkinen A, Sokka T, Kotaniemi A, Hannonen P. A Randomized Two-Year Study of the Effects of Dynamic Strength Training on Muscle Strength, Disease Activity, Functional Capacity, and Bone Mineral Density in Early Rheumatoid Arthritis. *Arthritis Rheum*. 2001;44:515–522.
30. de Jong Z, Munneke M, Zwinderman AH, Kroon HM, Ronday KH, Lems WF, Dijkmans BA, Breedveld FC, Vliet Vlieland TP, Hazes JM, Huizinga TW. Long Term High Intensity Exercise and Damage of Small Joints in Rheumatoid Arthritis. *Ann Rheum Dis*. 2004;63:1399–1405.
31. Munneke M, de Jong Z, Zwinderman AH, Ronday HK, van Schaardenburg D, Dijkmans BA, Kroon HM, Vliet Vlieland TP, Hazes JM. Effect of a High-Intensity Weight-Bearing Exercise Program on Radiologic Damage Progression of the Large Joints in Subgroups of Patients with Rheumatoid Arthritis. *Arthritis Rheum*. 2005;53:410–417.
32. Roddy E, Zhang W, Doherty M, Arden NK, Barlow J, Birrell F, Carr A, Chakravarty K, Dickson J, Hay E, Hosie G, Hurley M, Jordan KM, McCarthy C, McMurdo M, Mockett S, O'Reilly S, Peat G, Pendleton A, Richards S. Evidence-Based Recommendations for the Role of Exercise in the Management of Osteoarthritis of the Hip or Knee–The MOVE Consensus. *Rheumatology (Oxford)*. 2005;44:67–73.

33. Roos EM, Dahlberg L. Positive Effects of Moderate Exercise on Glycosaminoglycan Content in Knee Cartilage: A Four-Month, Randomized, Controlled Trial in Patients at Risk of Osteoarthritis. *Arthritis Rheum.* 2005;52:3507–3514.
34. Sharma L, Dunlop DD, Cahue S, Song J, Hayes KW. Quadriceps Strength and Osteoarthritis Progression in Malaligned and Lax Knees. *Ann Intern Med.* 2003;138:613–619.
35. Brouwer RW, Jakma TS, Verhagen AP, Verhaar JA, Bierma-Zeinstra SM. Braces and Orthoses for Treating Osteoarthritis of the Knee. *Cochrane Database Syst Rev.* 2005;(1):CD004020.
36. Kauppi M, Leppanen L, Heikkila S, Lahtinen T, Kautiainen H. Active Conservative Treatment of Atlantoaxial Subluxation in Rheumatoid Arthritis. *Br J Rheumatol.* 1998;37:417–420.

21 Cardiac Rehabilitation for Elderly Cardiac Patients

Daniel E. Forman, MD

CONTENTS

Age itself is a powerful risk factor for cardiovascular disease. As a result, older adults are inherently prone to incident cardiac events as well as to insidious cardiovascular pathologies that often lead to major disability and frailty. Eighty percent of cardiac deaths, longer hospital stays, and greater subsequent disability all occur among cardiac patients aged ≥ 65 years *(1)*, an age group that is also the fastest growing segment of the population. Given this fundamental vulnerability and these demographic trends, cardiac rehabilitation is an important consideration for elderly. This is especially relevant because an average 60-year-old can expect to live > 23 more years, an average 70-year-old > 15 more years, and an average 80-year-old > 8 more years *(2)*. Cardiac rehabilitation may help improve mortality, morbidity, and quality of living among older cardiac patients.

Ironically, cardiac rehabilitation remains severely underutilized among elderly cardiac patients, particularly among women. Moreover, there are still insufficient data from randomized controlled trials to clearly gauge benefits of cardiac rehabilitation in older adults *(1,3,4)*. Older patients as well as their families, physicians, and insurers often de-prioritize this option, especially because it often entails added logistic and financial challenges to what is already often an arduous convalescence. High incidence of depression, social isolation, and limited socioeconomic status among elderly also likely exacerbate such disinclination.

From: *Contemporary Cardiology: Cardiac Rehabilitation*
Edited by: W. E. Kraus and S. J. Keteyian © Humana Press Inc., Totowa, NJ

CARDIAC REHABILITATION IN HISTORICAL CONTEXT

When cardiac rehabilitation first started in the early 1970s, it was primarily organized as post-myocardial infarction exercise surveillance for middle-aged. Its relevance to the elderly often seemed inherently ambiguious. Subsequently, cardiac rehabilitation has evolved from its earliest into comprehensive risk modification, programming, yet relevance to older adults remains unclear while elderly patients with Elderly coronary artery disease (CAD) are increasingly likely to survive incident cardiac events, they are then prone to cascading disease and infirmity. A context in which broader secondary prevention of cardiac rehabilitation may seem fertile or irrelevant. Comorbidities, such as arthritis, chronic obstructive pulmonary disease (COPD), and dementia, not only curb referral but they fundamentally hamper traditional cardiac rehabilitation goals for the patients who are referred. Whereas Vigorito et al. *(5)* assert that cardiac rehabilitation goals can be individually tailored for each elderly enrollee to identify vital goals even for those who are functionally or cognitively limited, this strategy remains controversial.

The 4th edition of the American Association of Cardiovascular and Pulmonary Rehabilitation (AACVPR) guidelines for cardiac rehabilitation addressed issues of aging and presented a strong case for exercise training and risk factor among the elderly *(6)*. However, in remarkable contrast, the 2005 American Heart Association (AHA) guidelines on Cardiac Rehabilitation and secondary prevention downplayed this critical issue *(7)*. Other than mentioning under-use of cardiac rehabilitation in older adults and urging more study, issues of aging are essentially omitted. This tack seems especially remarkable because the guidelines emphasize broadening candidacy for cardiac rehabilitation to include those with heart failure (HF), peripheral arterial disease, and valvular heart disease. In other words, eligibility to cardiac rehabilitation includes a spectrum of cardiovascular pathologies that soar in relation to age, but the clinical complexities associated with age are not discussed.

MODIFIABLE PHYSIOLOGIC VULNERABILITIES ASSOCIATED WITH AGING

Abundant data show that exercise and risk factor interventions can modify age-related cardiovascular physiological changes that predispose to disease. A hallmark of the aging process is a progressive decline in physical activity, which represents a significant cardiovascular hazard *(8)*. Maximal aerobic capacity, measured as VO_2 peak, declines up to 20% per decade in healthy men and women in their 70s and 80s, accelerating as age increases, especially in the context of concurrent disease. However, regular exercise and physical activity can slow and even reverse functional declines and lead to improved function and longevity. Hakim et al. *(9)* showed that men (aged 61–81 up) who walked < 0.25 mile/day had a twofold increased risk of coronary heart disease compared to those who walked > 1.5 mile/day (5.1 versus 2.5%; $p < .01$).

On a more constitutive level, investigators have demonstrated that specific liabilities of senescence can be modified. Typical aging includes stiffening of the central vasculature, especially as elastin fragments and calcium and collagen deposition increase in the vessel walls *(10)*. Moreover, endothelial capacity to synthesize vital peptides for vasomotor regulation and vascular homeostasis declines, with decreasing coronary flow reserve capacity and increasing vulnerability to unstable atheromatous lesions.

Exercise is one means to modify these vascular aging phenomena; Tanaka et al. *(11)* showed that 3 months of aerobic exercise (primarily walking) reduced a β-stiffness index by 20% ($p < .01$). Taddei et al. *(12)* compared endothelial function in sedentary and athletic elderly adults and showed 25% ($p < .05$) enhanced endothelial-mediated performance among the elderly with greater daily activity.

Exercise and pharmacological interventions can also modify typical aging patterns of the heart. In typical aging, the heart pumps against increased afterload pressures (in part due to vascular stiffening) *(10)* and develops myocyte hypertrophy as a natural compensatory means to modify ventricular wall stresses. Myocyte apoptosis is exacerbated in the process, which in turn induces ventricular mural fibrosis and stiffening of the matrix. Age-associated diastolic filling impairments relate to these mural changes, as well as to age-related changes in myocyte mechanics that extend the timing of calcium uptake into the sarcoplasmic reticulum. However, Levy et al. *(13)* used nuclear techniques to show that 6 months of endurance training leads to 14% increase in resting and exercise peak early left ventricular (LV) filling rates ($p = .02$ and .04, respectively) among older men, along with 19% improvements in VO$_2$ peak. In that study, multivariate analysis showed that changes in peak LV filling correlated significantly to the improved functional capacity.

On an even more basic level, ambient inflammation, catabolism, and oxidative damage also increase with aging and probably underlie age-related frequency of atherosclerosis, hypertension, plaque rupture (supply ischemia), and muscle weakening. Studies demonstrate exercise-training benefits in reducing inflammation, catabolic peptides, and oxidative stress, with associated improvements in anabolic milieu and functional capacity *(14,15)*. Gielen et al. *(14)* showed that 6 months of aerobic training leads to significantly reduced tumour necrosis factor-α (TNF-α), interleukin-1β (IL-1β), IL-6, and iNOS in skeletal muscle of HF patients compared with sedentary controls even while serum levels were unaffected. Statins can similarly modify inflammation *(16)* with theoretical pertinence to managing older cardiac patients.

Therefore, exercise and lifestyle modifications can potentially modify aging phenomena that are otherwise tant amount to the substrate of cardiovascular disease. Furthermore, exercise and lifestyle changes can modify functional limitations that often arise from cardiovascular disease. Studies demonstrate, for example, that after exercise training, tasks that were previously associated with breathless exhaustion for frail elders tend to become more easily tolerated (i.e., below the ventilatory threshold) *(17)*. Although many view frailty as a rationale to omit cardiac rehabilitation, those with limited function may derive the greatest proportional improvements with reduced debility as well as modified disease *(18)* and improved quality of life.

Consistently, pleiotropic benefits from exercise and lifestyle modifications extend beyond cardiovascular effects. Senescence is, for example, associated with a predictable loss of skeletal muscle mass and strength [(i.e., sarcopenia *(19)*] that typically compound cardiovascular limitations. As exercise improves cardiovascular performance, it also stimulates muscle mass, endurance, and strength *(20)* that add to cardiovascular efficiency. Improved mood, stress and metabolism have also been attributed to cardiac rehabilitation in the elderly (21).

Cardiac rehabilitation has unique potential to foster an environment where aerobic and strength training as well as risk factor modification can be safely initiated, supervised, and monitored for elderly despite their innate vulnerabilities and limitations. For most elders, the idea of exercise and risk modifications is often daunting, especially at the onset. Unfortunately, although many community centers tout exercise programs for older adults, enrollment of participants with cardiac conditions is often discouraged and/or a source of excessive anxiety (22). Furthermore, training regimens in some group programs are standardized and simplistic, missing opportunities to develop personalized regimens that have greater potential to achieve exercise training benefits, ensure safety and better integrate exercise with other lifestyle modification goals. Older adults, who have been predominantly sedentary, usually benefit from very modest exercise intensities (and low medication doses) at the outset of rehabilitation, with therapy then advancing in intensity and range to best enhance function and health. For these adults, standardized group programs that are fixed at one intensity may never feel safe or suitable.

UTILITY OF TRADITIONAL RISK FACTOR MODIFICATION AMONG ELDERLY

Although some aspects of risk modification for elderly still remain theoretical, overall rationale for treating traditional cardiac risk factors for elderly is already clear, with compelling reasoning for inclusion in a comprehensive cardiac rehabilitation program.

Hypertension

Among its many attributes, cardiac rehabilitation affords a unique opportunity to monitor blood pressure (BP) at rest and with exertion and to titrate vital antihypertensive therapy. It also facilitates close hemodynamic monitoring, of key value because elderly hypertensives are also prone to orthostatic hypotension, especially when antihypertensive therapy is initiated. Cardiac rehabilitation also provides an opportunity to assess and modify lifestyle contributors to hypertension. Salt sensitivity increases in stiff senescent vasculature, and for most elders, this becomes a liability when they are enticed by restaurants and processed foods that are laden with salt. Alcohol-use also can exacerbate hypertension, with alcoholism being a common geriatric problem. Likewise, nonsteroidal anti-inflammatory drug use has been associated with detrimental renal effects and associated hypertension, a problem for the many elders who rely on these medications for chronic pain relief. Finally, excess weight and inactivity are other well-known contributors to hypertension. Both are also synergistic goals in a cardiac rehabilitation program.

As an exercise program, cardiac rehabilitation also promotes exercise-associated BP-lowering effects. Still, multiple studies demonstrate that exercise alone yields only modest systolic BP changes with persistent vascular stiffening thought to moderate BP-lowering benefits (23). For older adults, medications (24) combined with risk factor modification and exercise provide optimal BP reduction.

Lipids

While importance of lipid disorders as risk factors for cardiovascular disease in the elderly has sometimes been considered controversial, accumulating evidence suggests that treating elevated low-density lipoprotein (LDL)-cholesterol levels is beneficial (25). The PROspective Study of Pravastatin in the Elderly at Risk (PROSPER) was a primary and secondary prevention trial designed to specifically study efficacy of cholesterol reduction with pravastatin 40 mg among older adults aged 70–82 years. At 3.2 years, pravastatin reduced the risk of the primary combined cardiac endpoint by 15%. Furthermore, combining data from PROSPER, Cholesterol and Recurrent Events (CARE), and Long-Term Intervention with Pravastatin in Ischaemic Disease (LIPID) shows that pravastatin 40 mg reduced total strokes by 22% *(26)*.

Given the notorious difficulty in statin compliance, even among younger adults, cardiac rehabilitation is particularly valuable for elderly candidates, especially because dietary modification is additionally complicated by diets lower in sodium and fat. Propensity to depression (especially after a cardiac event or surgery) also often confounds dietary interventions. Cardiac rehabilitation can help manage these difficult issues.

Tobacco

In 1998, 10.4% of men and 11.2% of women 65 years of age or older were current smokers, but the proportion declined to less than 5% among persons over age 85 years *(27)*. Nonetheless, smoking cessation goals for elderly are still highly beneficial. In a population study, 7178 persons aged 65 years or older were studied; current smoking was associated with a relative risk for cardiovascular death of 2.0 in men and 1.6 in women, independent of other risk factors. Although adverse effect of smoking on mortality was greatest in seniors aged 65–74 years, current smoking was associated with a persistent survival disadvantage in both men and women over the age of 75 years *(28)*. Cardiac rehabilitation provides opportunities for exercise training, counseling, support groups, and nicotine replacement all with proven efficacy to achieve smoking cessation.

Diabetes

In the Framingham Heart Study, the relative risk for coronary heart disease in diabetic men over age 65 years was 1.4, whereas, in women, diabetes conferred a relative risk of 2.1. In both men and women, the excess risk for coronary heart disease in diabetics was greater in persons over age 65 years than in those younger than 65 years *(29)*. Therefore, strategies to modify diabetic risk among elderly are prudent.

Whereas unforeseen weight loss among elderly may often indicate underlying disease or depression, excess weight in the elderly is an important cardiovascular risk that can be successfully modified through diet and exercise. Accumulating visceral fat with aging is associated with insulin resistance. Age-related skeletal muscle wasting adds to the proportion of body fat that predisposes to impaired metabolism and cardiovascular risks. Cardiac rehabilitation helps achieve vital weight loss in a population that is also prone to the detrimental issues of malnutrition, depression, and anorexia *(30)*.

DATA DEMONSTRATING FEASIBILITY OF CARDIAC REHABILITATION IN ELDERLY

In a 2001 review, Pasquali et al. *(3)* identify the lack of robust data regarding cardiac rehabilitation in older adults and criticize the few elderly-specific trials for being predominantly observational (nonrandomized) with only one including a nonexercise control group. They assert that the true benefits of cardiac rehabilitation cannot be determined without randomization and that there is selection bias in studying only those referred to cardiac rehabilitation. Furthermore, although the studies ostensibly compared outcomes in young and old, the investigators did not account for baseline differences in clinical characteristics, diagnoses, or functional capacities, which may have further confounded the results. Nonetheless, they acknowledge that the studies showed consistent improvements in exercise capacity and quality of life, universal safety, and modest improvements in lipids.

Among these studies, Lavie et al. *(31)* reported a 34% improvement in exercise capacity, a 6% reduction in body fat, and a 6% increase in high-density lipoprotein (HDL)-cholesterol among older (> 65 years) adults. In an analogous study, HDL-cholesterol improved 3%, the LDL/HDL ratio decreased 5%, percent fat decreased 7%, and exercise tolerance improved 43% among cardiac rehabilitation participants ≥ 65 years *(32)*. In this particular study, improvements in anxiety, depression, mental health, energy, general health, pain, well being, and quality of life were also observed. Subsequently, Lavie *(33)* showed that lipids, body fat, exercise tolerance, and quality of life were also greater among older adults (age >75 years) in cardiac rehabilitation. Balady et al. *(34)* also studied patients aged >75 years and reported a 36% increase in exercise tolerance in men and a 32% improvement in women. Those with an initial peak metabolic equivalent (MET) level of <5 (34) demonstrated the greatest benefits in exercise tolerance, increasing from 4.1 ± 0.7 to 8.3 ± 3.5 METS ($p < .0001$).

A trial by Stahle et al. *(35)* stands out due to its randomized controlled design. A group of 101 patients aged 65–84 years (mean age 71 years) recovering from an acute coronary event were randomized to a supervised outpatient exercise-training program ($n = 50$) or to a control group ($n = 51$). By 3 months, exercise tolerance as well as self-estimated level of physical activity, fitness, and quality of life were significantly better in the exercise group compared with controls [from 104 ± 24 to 122 ± 27 watts in exercisers ($p < .001$) versus 102 ± 30 to 105 ± 37 watts among controls].

More recently, Marchionni et al. *(36)* studied 270 post-MI patients aged 65–86 years. Ninety patients aged 45–65 years were compared to 90 patients aged 66–75 years and 90 patients aged > 75 years. Patients in each age strata were randomized between hospital-based cardiac rehabilitation, home-based cardiac rehabilitation, and no cardiac rehabilitation (control). Total work capacity increased with hospital- and home-based cardiac rehabilitation but was unchanged in the control group. Although improvements were greatest in the young and middle-aged groups, they were also significant in those > 75 years. Thereafter, total work capacity drifted downward toward baseline among those who completed hospital-based cardiac rehabilitation, whereas gains were preserved among those who originally completed home-based cardiac rehabilitation. Health-related quality of life improved in middle-aged and old cardiac rehabilitation (hospital- and home-based) and control groups but only with cardiac rehabilitation in the very old patients. Complications were similar across treatment and age groups. Costs were lower for home-based cardiac rehabilitation than for hospital-based cardiac rehabilitation.

HOME-BASED VERSUS HOSPITAL-BASED MODELS OF CARDIAC REHABILITATION FOR THE ELDERLY

Marchionni's study highlights a key issue pertaining to the future of cardiac rehabilitation, particularly pertinent for the elderly. Owing to advancing technologies, an opportunity exists to shift program design from a traditional hospital-based cardiac rehabilitation program to a home-based cardiac rehabilitation model. These technologies provide home-based participants a closer link to hospital personnel, and even other patients, as they progress through cardiac rehabilitation programming.

Many proponents of home-based cardiac rehabilitation laud the fact that it affords greater cost efficacy (37). Carlson et al. (38) showed that a modified cardiac rehabilitation program, oriented to home training, cost $738 less per patient than tradition formats and required 30% less staff. Furthermore, home-based training also affords unique advantages in providing better access to older adults for whom travel to the hospital and/or spousal care obligations make hospital-based cardiac rehabilitation especially difficult.

Nevertheless, the curricula of home-based programs lack the same standardization as those in hospital formats. Most emphasize only exercise and lack comprehensive risk factor modification. Furthermore, the very technical communication links that make home-based options safer and more effective may seem overwhelming to some elderly.

Recently, a comprehensive Cochrane review of home- versus center-based physical activity programs studied older adults without any cardiac disease (39). This review was limited to training studies and did not evaluate efficacy of risk factor modification. Six trials including 224 participants who completed home-based training were compared to 148 participants who received center-based training. Despite significant heterogeneity of trials and data, in the short-term, center-based programs tended to demonstrate better functional gains (e.g., 207% versus 70% improvements in walking time, $p < 0.001$), but the home-based programs were better in terms of long-term exercise adherence [e.g., 75.1–78.7% of home-based participants in one trial were still adhering to their exercise program compared with 52.6% of the center-based participants ($p < 0.0005$)].

Although this review supports home-based training, it does not fully explore the complexities of achieving comprehensive risk reductions and/or achieving safe exercise training for cardiac patients. Likewise, training regimens were also extremely simple, omitting considerations such as strength training, which would likely afford disproportionate value to some elders.

SUMMARY

The benefits of cardiac rehabilitation for elderly remain more conceptual than proven. Although cardiac rehabilitation originated primarily as a mechanism to mobilize patients after an MI, it has grown in scope and sophistication that seem well suited to modify cardiovascular disease as well as the vulnerabilities associated with aging that particularly predispose elderly adults to cardiovascular disease. Although seminal research demonstrates that exercise and risk factor modifications are important considerations for elderly, study of cardiac rehabilitation programs themselves has not yet fully substantiated programmatic efficacy. Critical research is still needed, and such inquiry will likely reinforce rationale among patients and their doctors to consider this therapy. It seems likely that cardiac rehabilitation constitutes a key opportunity to achieve cost-effective healthcare and a higher quality of life for our elderly patients.

REFERENCES

1. Oldridge, N. Cardiac Rehabilitation in the Elderly. *Aging (Milano)*. 1998;10, 273–283.
2. Social Security tables. http://www.ssa.gov/OACT/STATS/table4c6.html
3. Pasquali SK, Alexander KP, Petersen ED. Cardiac Rehabilitation in the Elderly. *Am Heart J.* 2001;142:748–755.
4. Ades P. Cardiac Rehabilitation and Secondary Prevention of Coronary Heart Disease. *N Engl J Med.* 2001;345(12):892–902.
5. Vigorito C, Incalzi RA, Acanfora D, et al. Recommendations for Cardiac Rehabilitation in the Very Elderly. *Monaldi Arch Chest Dis*, 2003;60:25–39.
6. American Association of Cardiovascular and Pulmonary Rehabilitation. Special Considerations. In *Guidelines for Cardiac Rehabilitation and Secondary Prevention Programs*, MA Williams (ed.). Champaign, IL: Human Kinetics; 2004:135–176.
7. Leon AS, Franklin BA, Costa F, et al. Cardiac Rehabilitation and Secondary Prevention of Coronary Heart Disease. *Circulation*. 2005;111:369–376.
8. Fleg JL, Morrell CH, Bos AG, et al. Accelerated Longitudinal Decline of Aerobic Capacity in Healthy Older Adults. *Circulation*. 2005;112(5):674–682.
9. Hakim AA, Curb JD, Petrovitch H, et al. Effects of Walking on Coronary Heart Disease in Elderly Men: The Honolulu Heart Program. *Circulation*. 1999;100(1):9–13.
10. Wei JY. Age and the Cardiovascular System. *N Engl J Med*. 1992;327:1735–1739.
11. Tanaka H, Dinenno FA, Monahan KD, et al. Aging, Habitual Exercise, and Dynamic Arterial Compliance. *Circulation*. 2000;102(11):1270–1275.
12. Taddei S, Galetta F, Virdis A, et al. Physical Activity Prevents Age-Related Impairment in Nitric Oxide Availability in Elderly Athletes. *Circulation*. 2000;101:2896.
13. Levy WC, Cerqueira MD, Abrass IB, et al. Endurance Exercise Training Augments Diastolic Filling at Rest and During Exercise in Healthy Young and Older Men. *Circulation*. 1993;88(1):116–126.
14. Gielen S, Adams V, Mobius-Winkler S, et al. Anti-Inflammatory Effects of Exercise Training in the Skeletal Muscle of Patients with Chronic Heart Failure. *J Am Coll Cardiol*. 2003;42(5):861–868.
15. Kasapis C, Thompson PD. The Effects of Physical Activity on Serum C-Reactive Protein and Inflammatory Markers: A Systematic Review. *J Am Coll Cardiol*. 2005;45(10):1563–1569.
16. Jain MK, Ridker PM. Anti-Inflammatory Effects of Statins: Clinical Evidence and Basic Mechanisms. *Nat Rev Drug Discov*. 2005;4(12):977–987.
17. Yerg JE, Seals DR, Hagberg JM, Holloszy JO. Effect of Endurance Exercise Training on Ventilatory Function in Older Individuals. *J Appl Physiol*. 1985;58:791–794.
18. Ades PA, Savage PD, Cress ME, et al. Resistance Training on Physical Performance in Disabled Older Female Cardiac Patients. *Med Sci Sports Exerc*. 2003;35(8):1265–1270.
19. Short KR, Nair KS. Mechanisms of Sarcopenia of Aging. *J Endocrinol Invest*. 1999;22:95–105.
20. Bunce S, Schroeder K. Interventions for Sarcopenia and Muscle Weakness in Older People. *Age Ageing*. 2005;34(4):414–415.
21. Ades PA. Cardiac Rehabilitation in Older Coronary Patients. J AM Geriatr Soc. 1999;47:98–105.
22. Heath JM, Stuart MR. Prescribing Exercise for Frail Elders. *J Am Board Fam Pract*. 2002;15:218–228.
23. Stewart KJ, Bacher AC, Turner KL, et al. Effect of Exercise on Blood Pressure in Older Persons: A Randomized Controlled Trial. *Arch Intern Med*. 2005;165(7):756–762.
24. Staessen JA, Gasowski J, Wang JG, et al. Risks of Untreated and Treated Isolated Systolic Hypertension in the Elderly: Meta-Analysis of Outcome Trials. *Lancet*. 2000;355:865–872.
25. Shepard J. Blauwh GJ, Murphy MB, et al. Pravastatin in Elderly Individuals at Risk of Vascular Disease (PROSPER): A Randomized Controlled Trial. *Lancet*. 2002;360:1623–1630.
26. Byington RP, Davis BR, Plehn JF, et al. Reduction of Stroke Events with Pravastatin: The Prospective Pravastatin Pooling Project. *Circulation*. 2001;103:387–392.

27. Reducing Tobacco Use: A Report of the Surgeon General. *MMWR*. 2000;49:797–801.
28. LaCroiz AZ, Lang J, Scherr P, et al. Smoking and Mortality Among Older Men and Women in Three Communities. *N Engl J Med*. 1991;324:1619–1625.
29. Fox CS, Sullivan L, D'Agostino RB Sr, Wilson PW; Framingham Heart Study. The Significant Effect of Diabetes Duration on Coronary Heart Disease Mortality: The Framingham Heart Study. *Diabetes Care*. 2004;27(3):704–708.
30. Savage PD, Brochu M, Poehlman ET, Ades PA. Reduction in Obesity and Coronary Risk Factors after High Caloric Exercise Training in Overweight Coronary Patients. *Am Heart J*. 2003;146(2):317–323.
31. Lavie CJ, Milani RV, Littman AB. Benefits of Cardiac Rehabilitation and Exercise Training in Secondary Coronary Prevention in the Elderly. *J Am Coll Cardiol*. 1993;22:678–683.
32. Lavie CJ, Milani RV. Effects of Cardiac Rehabilitation Programs on Exercise Capacity, Coronary Risk Factors, Behavioral Characteristics, and Quality of Life in a Large Elderly Cohort. *Am J Cardiol*. 1995;76:177–179.
33. Lavie CJ, Milani RV. Effects of Cardiac Rehabilitation and Exercise Training Programs in Patients > or = 75 Years of Age. *Am J Cardiol*. 1996;78:675–677.
34. Balady GJ, Jette D, Scheer J, Downing J. Changes in Exercise Capacity Following Cardiac Rehabilitation in Patients Stratified According to Age and Gender. Results of the Massachusetts Association of Cardiovascular and Pulmonary Rehabilitation Multicenter Database. *J Cardiopulm Rehabil*. 1996;16:38–46.
35. Stahle A, Mattsson E, Ryden L, Unden A, Nordlander R. Improved Physical Fitness and Quality of Life Following Training of Elderly Patients after Acute Coronary Events. A 1 Year Follow-up Randomized Controlled Study. *Eur Heart J*. 1999;20:1475–1484.
36. Marchionni N, Fattirolli F, Fumagalli S, et al. Improved Exercise Tolerance and Quality of Life with Cardiac Rehabilitation of Older Patients after Myocardial Infarction: Results of a Randomized, Controlled Trial. *Circulation*. 2003;107:2201–2206.
37. King AC, Pruitt LA, Phillips W, et al. Comparative Effects of Two Physical Activity Programs on Measured and Perceived Physical Functioning and Other Health-Related Quality of Life Outcomes in Older Adults. *J Gerontol A Biol Sci Med Sci*. 2000;55(2):M74–M83.
38. Carlson JJ, Johnson JA, Franklin BA, VanderLaan RL. Program Participation, Exercise Adherence, Cardiovascular Outcomes, and Program Cost of Traditional Versus Modified Cardiac Rehabilitation. *Am J Cardiol*. 2000;86:17.
39. Ashworth NL, Chad KE, Harrison EL, Reeder BA, Marshall SC. Home Versus Center Based Physical Activity Programs in Older Adults. *Cochrane Database Syst Rev*. 2005;(1):CD004017. doi:10.1002/14651858.CD004017.pub2.

22

Expanding Your Model: Optimizing Referrals and Introducing Disease Management

Linda K. Hall, PhD

CONTENTS

INTRODUCTION

Cardiac and pulmonary rehabilitation programs require personnel from a myriad of professional backgrounds and training. Because this group has such broad professional expertise and diversity, there is the potential for expanding the impact that cardiac rehabilitation (CR) programs may have within the hospital and in the community. In fact, the American Association of Cardiovascular and Pulmonary Rehabilitation is currently exploring interactive relationships with other organizations that will foster the changing nature of cardiac and pulmonary rehabilitation into a disease management (DM) forum. This will necessitate a restructuring of current programs, expanding the roles of staff and the way in which the needs of patients and clients are met. This chapter has two sections: the first addresses the roles of the program management in facilitating and enhancing program effectiveness relative to current regulations, and the second section establishes a platform for program growth and development toward a DM delivery model.

From: *Contemporary Cardiology: Cardiac Rehabilitation*
Edited by: W. E. Kraus and S. J. Keteyian © Humana Press Inc., Totowa, NJ

MAXIMIZING CURRENT MANAGEMENT

Health Care Finance

"We face a demographic tsunami" according to David Walker, comptroller general of the United States *(1)*. An aging population, health care inflation, and advanced medical technology will create a perfect storm is the admonition of Douglas Holtz-Eakin, Director of the Congressional Budget Office *(1)*. Additionally, health care chief financial officers, business and industry leaders, and human resource executives are cogently aware of the criticality of rising health care costs. The year 2004 brought forth a 12.6% increase as a national average for health care spending and served as a warning for these leaders that there is not an end in sight for the next 5 years. This increase foretells that business and industry's contribution to employee health benefits will rise 54%, and as a result, employee contributions may triple by 2010 *(2)*. According to the Centers for Medicare and Medicaid Services (CMS), health expenditures in the United States will reach $2.6 trillion by 2010 and $3.6 trillion by 2014 *(3,4)*.

Tight labor markets (nursing and pharmacist shortages), lower payments from public insurers, and the growing cost of pharmaceuticals and technology are causing a decline in operating margins for America's hospitals from 3.7% in 2002 to 3.3% in 2003. Because of this, hospitals face huge strains in maintaining adequate net profits with reimbursement levels dropping, revenues declining, and costs increasing *(5)*. The cuts in Medicare and Medicaid in 2005 and 2006 brought an additional cause for concern *(6)*. And the increasing amount of uncompensated care that is brought about when the uninsured seek medical care adds to the burden that hospitals face *(7)*.

As health care organizations face shrinking revenues, they look for marginal services to remove from the operating budget. Often CR program's financial status is marginal. It is important for the program manager or director to be a strong advocate for the CR program he/she serves. He/she must be a student of the research that delineates the benefits of these programs and create a case for cost savings related to reduced emergency room visits and hospitalizations, as well as track side-stream revenue derived from program-identified interventions such as coronary re-vascularizations and implants of automatic implantable coronary defibrillators (AICD) and pacemakers.

Insurance Reimbursement for Outpatient Education and Exercise

In March 2006, CMS determined that the evidence supported expansion of the covered diagnoses for CR to include heart valve repair or replacement, percutaneous transluminal coronary angioplasty (PTCA) or coronary stenting, and heart or heart–lung transplant *(8)*. This supersedes the original Medicare coverage, Section 3525 published in September 1982 in the Intermediary Manual part 3 *(9)*.

At the time of this writing, CMS is reimbursing $31.03 for each session of CR, an amount that is then adjusted by the wage index for the specific region where the program is located *(10)*. This may reduce the payment depending on the cost of living index of the geographical area.

Pulmonary Rehabilitation (PR) is remunerated according to a Local Coverage Determination (LCD) that is regionally based. Currently there is no National Coverage Determination (NCD) by CMS. Local coverage is according to the specific personnel providing the service, e.g. physical therapy is paid in 15 minute increments, a nurse or respiratory therapist or other health professional is paid by the session. With PR there is additional remuneration for each 15 minutes of education appropriately documented in the patients medical record *(11)*. Diabetes self-management education (DSME) is a service that is paid for by insurance, as are services for physical, occupational, and speech therapies. Additionally, medical nutrition therapy (MNT) has been added to the coverage arena for patients requiring nutrition re-education and counseling. In all of these cases, the patient must be referred by a physician and have the appropriate diagnostic code *(12)*. For an extensive review of reimbursement issues, read chapter 28.

Program management must make every effort to have primary physicians refer their patients for all of the areas and services covered under National and Local Coverage Determinations. For example, more than 40% of patients referred to CR programs have diabetes. It is important to recognize that many of these patients would be appropriate candidates for MNT, and this would increase revenue as well as insure excellent education outcomes for patients.

Evidence Supports the Efficacy and Potential Profitability of Cardiac Rehabilitation

There is much research that has established the benefits of CR programs without additional risks to the patient. Well established are the following:

- Meta-analyses of clinical trials consistently demonstrate a 25–30% reduction in total and cardiovascular mortality *(13,14)*.
- Health-related quality of life is significantly improved *(15,16)*.
- Improved endothelium-dependent vasodilatation leading to a marked reduction of myocardial ischemia and coronary events *(17–19)*.
- Reduction in re-hospitalization and health care expenditures and prolongation of life *(20,21)*.
- Improvement of exercise capacity is a consistent and strong beneficial result distancing the older participant from disability *(23)*.
- Reduction in fatigue and dyspnea in patients with heart failure and in patients with valve replacement/repair *(17,18)*.

These are but a few of the many, however, most salient results of CR on the referred patient population. Unfortunately, despite the above evidence, a treatment gap occurs relative to ensuring that appropriate patients undergo CR. Although many reasons contribute to this treatment gap, an initial issue is securing program referral, especially in the female, elderly, and minority groups with approximately 20–30% of all clinically appropriate patients being referred *(21,22)*.

Utilizing all of the documented benefits of CR and inpatient care paths, it is essential to work to obtain consensus with physicians for blanket referral and/or standing orders to refer appropriate in-hospital patients to CR and education. Extend the standing orders to referral to outpatient rehabilitation and DM to improve patient outcomes and reduce re-hospitalizations, emergency room visits, morbidity, and mortality.

Patient Satisfaction as a Driver for Program Implementation

Health care is becoming extremely competitive with hospitals competing against one another for occupied beds and physicians looking for increased income streams taking screening tests and procedures out of the hospital and doing them in their offices. Market share is determined by the reputation that is perceived by the public and future users of the health care system. The paying customer includes employers determining health care contracts, health plans, and provider groups determining compensation formulas and consumers who select their health plan based on whether it is a point of service or preferred provider plan *(22)*. Patient's satisfaction is a measure of the patient's perception of their health and quality-of-life outcomes and the satisfaction they have with the quality of care and services including physician interaction. Often this is as important as clinical measures such as reduced blood pressure or lipid profiles as a result of care.

It is the experience at Press Ganey, the health care industry's leading patient satisfaction consultant, that services such as CR score high on the patient satisfaction grid of most health care organizations because of the personal attention and care offered in such a program. In fact, programs such as CR are often viewed as going the extra mile to ensure that the hospital and staff does all of the right things to help the patient get well *(24)*. Because these are outpatient services, they may be viewed as the exit program from the hospital, which often leaves the patient with the perception of excellent service.

Management of CR programs should extend "this positive identity" of the hospital, which was brought about because of patient satisfaction with CR. Opportunities to promote and advance CR and the hospital include providing community education sessions, lunch and learn programs, television appearances and interviews, and newspaper articles on the benefits of CR.

DISEASE MANAGEMENT – THE MODEL OF THE FUTURE

Over the past 15 years, a new process for managing chronic conditions called DM has developed. DM evolved as a mechanism to manage increasing health care costs. The results have been encouraging to business and industry as a way of slowing the current escalating trends. Ultimately, the process was defined by the Disease Management Association of America. "Disease Management is a system of coordinated healthcare interventions and communications for populations with conditions in which patient self-care efforts are significant. Disease management

- Supports the physician or practitioner/patient relationship and plan of care
- Emphasizes prevention of exacerbations and complications utilizing evidenced based guidelines and patient empowerment strategies, and
- Evaluates clinical, humanistic, and economic outcomes on an on going basis with the goal of improving overall health" *(25)*.

CMS has initiated The Chronic Care Improvement Program providing the opportunity for health care institutions to apply for grants to work with Medicare and Medicaid to help beneficiaries to manage their health, adhere to physician plans of care, and obtain the medical care they need to reduce their health risks *(26)*. The difficulty with all of these programs is that they have not been operational for a period of time long enough to give health and dollar-saving outcomes.

Janet Wright, MD, in testimony before the House Committee on Ways and Means made the following observations: "As an example of highly effective DM, I call your attention to a mature and profoundly valuable program which has provided education in self-management and health preservation, linked patients and doctors through frequent progress reports, and not just satisfied, but indeed, life changed its participants. That program is one of the original disease management approaches known as Cardiac Rehabilitation"*(27)*. Thus, we have as a basic approach for intervening with all of the chronic diseases promulgated in this book, the utilization of a tried and true DM program, the principles of intervention promoted by the example of CR.

Approximately two-thirds of all deaths in the US are directly related to five chronic diseases – heart [coronary artery disease (CAD)], chronic obstructive pulmonary disease (COPD), cancer, stroke, and diabetes. Chronic disease accounts for 75% of the nation's total health care costs. Because chronic disease, once diagnosed, is constant, continuing, and prolonged, the resulting pain and suffering decreases the quality of life of millions of Americans *(28)*. Chronic disease is so costly because of increasing technology, improvements in environmental and social conditions, and the increase in life expectancy. The improvements in environment and social conditions have led to an increase in sedentary living, poor eating habits, and tobacco use as leisure time increases because of time-saving technology *(29)*.

Three modifiable health-damaging behaviors, smoking, sedentary living, and obesity, are directly related to the five leading causes of death and suffering brought on by chronic diseases. Because smoking is the risk factor attributed as the leading cause of death, Medicare is considering paying for two smoking cessation opportunities per year as an effort to reducing morbidity *(30)*. Smoking produces long-term chronic diseases that are resource intensive. In essence, death is the least expensive end point in chronic diseases related to smoking.

Overweight and obesity are current epidemics in the United States and the world for that matter. Predictions are that it will surpass smoking as a health-related and chronic disease producing risk factor within the next 10 years. The total cost for obesity equals $117 billion tied up in caring for the diseases associated with obesity summarized in Table 1. Obesity is costly to business and industry because of loss of 39.3 million workdays and 239.0 million restricted activity days that have a huge impact on productivity. This is a health risk that occupies the minds and efforts of many consumers as is evidenced by the expenditure of over $33 billion annually on weight-loss products and services *(31)*.

The direct and indirect costs of sedentary living, as it is related to chronic disease, was in excess of $150 billion in 2000 and occupies approximately 15% of the total health care budget *(32–34)*. The costs of cardiovascular disease and diabetes combine to $396 billion a year. A 30% reduction in these two diseases would save $119 billion a year. Is this feasible? Yes, Hu *(35,36)* found that 2.5 h of brisk walking per week brought about a 30% reduction in cardiovascular disease, stroke, and type 2 diabetes. All-cause mortality rates would be similarly affected, with as much as a 30% reduction, by physical activity expending an average of 1000 kcal/week (approximately 2 miles/day, 5 days/week) *(34)*. Reviewing Table 1 demonstrates the enormous effect that these three lifestyle choices or risk factors have on the development or exacerbation of chronic disease in the United States today. The costs, morbidity, and mortality consequences of these account for more than 75% of health care dollars and premature deaths annually.

It is important to recognize that many of the diseases listed in Table 1 are ones that are primary focuses of CR and Pulmonary Rehabilitation (PR) or comorbidities for patients referred to CR and PR. Essentially, the majority of efforts to correct these major health risk factors occur as secondary prevention, after the patient has incurred the disease and is now in the process of rehabilitating and managing the disease and its exigencies. Managing the disease will stem the increasing exacerbations of these

Table 1
Chronic Diseases Caused or Enhanced by Three Risk Factors: Smoking, Obesity,
and Sedentary Lifestyle

Smoking (28–30)	Obesity (31)	Sedentary Lifestyle (32,33)
Chronic lung disease	Heart disease	Angina
Emphysema	Diabetes	Heart attack
Asthma	Congestive heart failure	Coronary artery disease
Heart disease	Angina	Breast cancer
Stroke	Gout	Colon cancer
Cancer of the lung	Stroke	Congestive heart failure
Cancer of the larynx	Hypertension	Depression
Cancer of the esophagus	Gall bladder disease	Gallstone disease
Cancer of the mouth	Osteoarthritis	High blood triglycerides
Cancer of the bladder	Asthma	High blood cholesterol
Cancer of the cervix	Sleep apnea	Hypertension
Cancer of the pancreas	Uterine cancer	Poor cognitive function
Cancer of the kidneys	Breast cancer	Low- and high-density lipoproteins
Increased blood pressure	Colorectal cancer	Low quality of life
Peripheral vascular disease	Kidney cancer	Obesity
Sudden cardiac death	Gallbladder cancer	Osteoporosis
Osteoporosis	Dyslipidemia	Pancreatic cancer
Peptic ulcer disease	Complications of pregnancy	Peripheral vascular disease
Impotence	Menstrual irregularities	Physical frailty
Dental disease	Hirsutism	Premature mortality
	Stress incontinence	Prostate cancer
	Psychological disorders	Sleep apnea
	Surgical risk	Stiff joints
		Stroke
		Type 2 diabetes

chronic diseases that would occur if the disease progressed unchecked and as a result decrease the cost.

Using the above information and lessons from the past such as managed care and of the future, DM, hospital administration, and program managers and directors should become driving forces for CR programs in the following ways:

- focus on prevention, early diagnosis, and monitoring of patients using specific clinical pathways,
- become an integrated partner in employee health management efforts,
- provide comprehensive outpatient care in one centralized setting,
- create a community presence outside of the hospital facilities, for example, churches, clubs, schools (Fig. 2),
- pay close attention to patient's psychosocial needs,
- identify and aggressively manage other chronic diseases and comorbidities, and
- look for creative cost saving opportunities (37).

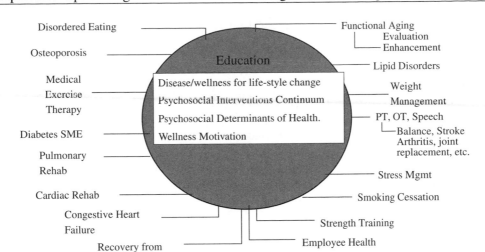

Fig. 1. Disease management integration *38*.

Using these guidelines, it is appropriate to call together all of the services that work with patients in an outpatient setting to discuss how as an integrated service center, your hospital may better service the patients you serve. Use as a model the services depicted in Fig. 2. The ideal would be to have all of these services located within one physical setting with designated drive up and parking areas to facilitate patient assess. When that is not feasible, it is essential that the coordination between services be fluid and supportive of patient care and needs. Additionally, electronic patient records, a call system for follow-up, and a data management system that tracks patient outcomes over time and is interactive between each service so that patient data and care is integrated are essential.

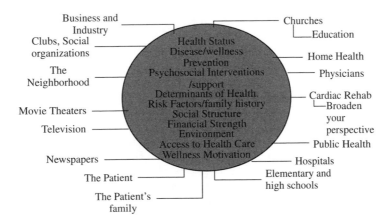

Fig. 2. Community integrated disease management *38*.

CONCLUSION

The objectives outlined in this chapter will assist program management in being a comprehensive advocate for their CR program. The focal points of the chapter epitomize the comprehensive outpatient cardiac programs that Dr Wright described to the House Ways and Means Committee and have been in operation since the late 1960s. It is appropriate to take this model and apply it, because few patients enter CR program free of another chronic disease such as diabetes, osteoporosis, cystic fibrosis, arthritis, congestive heart failure, peripheral vascular disease, obesity, pulmonary disorders such as COPD, and many cancers, to name a few. Each of these diseases may be significantly impacted in their health outcomes by exercise, lifestyle, and nutrition intervention (Table 1) as epitomized by the CR model.

REFERENCES

1. Wolf R. As Social Security Surges and Medicare Takes Off, the Deficit will Soar, The Result: Fiscal Hurricane. *USA Today*, November 15, 2005:1.
2. Weatherly LA. The Rising Cost of Health Care: Strategic and Societal Considerations for Employers, SHRMOnline, *Research Quarterly*. 2004. Available at http://www.shrm.org/.
3. Bush GW, Carter J, Ford GR, Rogers PG, Ray RD, Simmons HE, Schoeni PQ, Goldberg MA. *Building a Better Health Care System: Specifications for Reform*. Washington, DC: National Coalition on Health Care; 2004.
4. Appleby J. Health Care Tab Ready to Explode. *USA Today*, February 24, 2005:1.
5. HPK Group, LLC. The Hospital Financial Dilemma. Available at http://www.hpkgroupllc.com/hospitalcosts.htm, retrieved 24 February 2005.
6. Evans M. Good News, Bad News; Hospital's Net Profit Margin Up, Operating Margin Down. Modern Healthcare, November 1, 2004. Available at http://www.Kellogg.norhtwestern.edu/news/hits041101mh.htm, retrieved 7 March 2005.
7. National Coalition on Health Care, Facts on Health Insurance Coverage. Available at http://www.hchc.org, retrieved 2 March 2005.
8. Centers for Medicare and Medicaid Services. Coverage Decision Memorandum for Cardiac Rehabilitation Programs, March 22, 2006. Available at http://www.CMS.gov, retrieved 22 March 2006.
9. Health and Human Services, Health Care Finance Administration: Payment for Services Furnished to Patients in Hospital Based and Free Standing Cardiac Rehabilitation Clinics. *Fed Regist*. 1982;41:934.
10. AACVPR. *Guidelines for Cardiac Rehabilitation and Secondary Prevention Programs: Reimbursement*, 4th ed. Champaign, IL: Human Kinetics Publishers; 2004:192–193.
11. TriSpan Health Services Intermediary. Outpatient pulmonary rehabilitation services local coverage determination (LCD). Bulletin 2005–75, February 17, 2005, pp. 1–17.
12. Hart AC, Hopkins CA (eds.). *ICD-9-CM Professional*. Salt Lake City, UT: Ingenix; 2004.
13. Jolliffe JA, et al. Exercise-Based Rehabilitation for Coronary Heart Disease. *Cochrane Database Syst Rev*. 2001;(1):CD001800.
14. Stewart KJ, et al. Cardiac Rehabilitation Following Percutaneous Revascularization, Heart Transplant, Heart Valve Surgery and Chronic Heart Failure. *Chest*. 2003;123:2104–2111.
15. Ades PA. Cardiac Rehabilitation and Secondary Prevention of Coronary Heart Disease. *N Eng J Med*. 2001;345:892–902.
16. Wenger NK, et al. Cardiac Rehabilitation as Secondary Prevention. Agency for Health Care Policy and Research and National Heart, Lung and Blood Institute. *Clin Pract Guidel Quick Ref Guide Clin*. 1995;17:1–23.
17. Afzal A, et al. Exercise Training in Heart Failure. *Prog Cardiovasc Dis*. 1998;4:175–190.

18. Carstens V, et al. Exercise Capacity Before and After Cardiac Valve Surgery. *Cardiology*. 1983;70: 41–49.

19. Hambrecht R, et al. Regular Physical Activity Improves Endothelial Function in Patients with Coronary Artery Disease by Increasing Phosphorylation of Endothelial Nitric Oxide Synthase. *Circulation*. 2003;107:3152–3158.

20. Hambrecht R, et al. Effect of Exercise on Coronary Endothelial Function in Patients with Coronary Artery Disease. *N Engl J Med*. 2000;342:454–460.

21. Ades P, et al. Cost Effectiveness of Cardiac Rehabilitation After Myocardial Infarction. *J Cardiopulm Rehabil*. 1997;17:222–231.

22. Bonderstam E, et al. Effects of Early Rehabilitation on Consumption of Medical Care During the First Year After Myocardial Infarction in Patients Greater Than or Equal to 65 Years of Age. *Am J Cardiol*. 1995;75:767–771.

23. Bolus R, Pitts J. Patient Satisfaction: The Indispensable Outcome. *Managed Care Magazine*. April 1999. Available at http://www.managedcaremag.com/archives/9904,9904.patsais.html, retrieved February 24, 2005.

24. Press Ganey Client Forum. Best Inpatient/Outpatient Practices. Available at http://www.pressganey.com.

25. DMAA. Disease Management Association of America. Available at http://www.dmaa.org.

26. Centers for Medicare & Medicaid Services. The Chronic Care Improvement Program. May 25, 2004. Available at http://www.cms.hhs.gov/medicarereform/ccip/.

27. House Committee on Ways and Means. Statement of Janet S. Wright, M.D., Testimony Before the Subcommittee on Health of the House Committee on Ways and Means. May 11, 2004.

28. CDC. Chronic disease overview. *Chronic Disease Overview*. Available at http://cdc.gov/nccdphp/overview.htm, retrieved March 18, 2005.

29. CDC. *CDC Chronic Disease Prevention. The Power of Prevention*. Atlanta, GA: U.S. Department of Health and Human Services; 2003.

30. Centers for Medicare & Medicaid Services. Proposed Decision Memo for Smoking & Tobacco Use Cessation Counseling (CAG-00241N), December 2004. Available at http://www.cms.hhs.gov/mcd/viewdraftdecisionmemo.asp?id=130, retrieved March 22, 2005.

31. Flegal KM, Carroll, MD, Ogden CL, Johnson CL. Prevalence and Trends in Obesity Among US Adults, 1999–2000. *JAMA*. 2002;288(14):1723–1727.

32. Booth FW, Gordon SE, Carlson CJ, Hamilton MT. Invited Review: Waging the War on Modern Chronic Diseases: Primary Prevention Through Exercise Biology. *J Appl Physiol*. 2000;88:774–787.

33. Booth, FW, Chakravarthy MV, Corbin CB, Pangrazi RP, Franks D. Cost and Consequence of Sedentary Living: New Battleground for an Old Enemy. *Res Dig*. 2002;3(16):1–8.

34. Pate RR, Pratt M, Blair SN Haskell WL, Macera CA, Bouchard C, Buchner D, Ettinger W, Heath GW, King AC, et al. Physical Activity and Public Health. A Recommendation from the Centers for Disease Control and Prevention and the American College of Sports Medicine. *JAMA*. 1995;273:402–407.

35. Hu FB, Sigal RJ, Rich-Edwards JW, Colditz GA, Solomon CG, Willett WC, Speizer FE, Manson JE. Walking Compared with Vigorous Physical Activity and Risk of Type 2 Diabetes in Women: A Prospective Study. *JAMA*. 1999;282:1433–1439.

36. Hu FB, Stampfer MJ, Colditz GA, Ascherio A, Rexrode KM, Willett WC, Manson JE. Physical Activity and Risk of Stroke in Women. *JAMA*. 2000;283:2961–1967.

37. Hall LK. Creating a Discharge Destination. AACVPR National Meeting, Charlotte, NC; 2002.

23   The Role of the Physician-Medical Director in Cardiac Rehabilitation

Philip A. Ades, MD

CONTENTS

INTRODUCTION

Cardiac rehabilitation (CR) services are physician-directed and implemented by an interdisciplinary team of healthcare professionals that include nurses, exercise physiologists, physical therapists, dieticians, and behavioral specialists *(1–3)* (Fig. 1). While day-to-day care issues in CR are coordinated by the interdisciplinary team, the overall plan of care, formal progress assessments, and backup plans for emergency management and medical management are coordinated by the Medical Director. The Medical Director should have a strong background and interest in clinical and preventive cardiology, exercise physiology, human behavior, and psychology and should be a team leader *(4)*. The roles and duties of the Medical Director are summarized in Table 1 and discussed below.

From: *Contemporary Cardiology: Cardiac Rehabilitation*
Edited by: W. E. Kraus and S. J. Keteyian © Humana Press Inc., Totowa, NJ

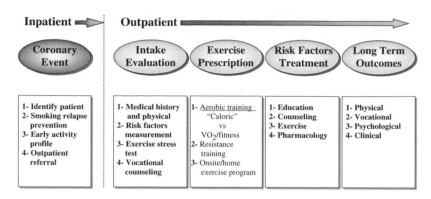

Fig. 1. Elements of cardiac rehabilitation [Adapted from reference *(3)*].

Table 1
Roles of the Medical Director

1. Design and coordinate policies and procedures
2. Design and perform intake evaluation
3. Monitor patient progress and adjust treatment plan
4. Coordinate program safety parameters and emergency management
5. Communicate and interface with referring physicians
6. Coordinate regulatory and reimbursement issues

DESIGN AND COORDINATE POLICIES AND PROCEDURES

Every CR program should have a Policies and Procedures Manual that defines the clinical and therapeutic activities of the CR service. The Medical Director should act as a team leader to establish and keep current the Policies and Procedures Manual and should be a primary teacher of medical management issues to the CR staff. The Medical Director is also the primary person to assure that policies and procedures are compliant with medico-legal parameters such that CR treatment guidelines are standard of care for the community in which the program is based. The hospitals' legal advisor and Medicare Compliance Officer should review the Policies and Procedures Manual. The Policies and Procedures Manual should address the following issues:

- Diagnostic eligibility criteria for patient participation.
- Identification of systematic processes to facilitate patient referrals.
- Components of the intake evaluation.
- Description of exercise training modalities and risk factor treatment modules.
- Description of patient education and behavioral treatment modules.
- Identification of clinical outcome measures.
- Processes for emergency management.
- Processes for documentation of daily treatment routines, medical management issues and communication of results and patient progress to referring physicians.

- Components of the exit evaluation.
- Planning for long-term exercise and lifestyle therapy.

DESIGN AND PERFORM INTAKE EVALUATION

The Medical Director as team leader should design the CR intake evaluation. The goals of the CR intake evaluation are several. First, and foremost, is the task of ascertaining that the patient has an appropriate diagnosis for participation in CR and that exercise training as prescribed by the Medical Director will be safe and effective. Second, the clinical stability of the patient is assessed, and pharmacologic therapy is optimized, both to prevent exertional coronary ischemia and to utilize agents that have been proven to prolong life and/or prevent major cardiac events *(5)*. Third, cardiac risk factors are measured or extracted from the medical record, including measures of lipid profiles, serum glucose, blood pressure, body mass index, waist circumference, and peak aerobic capacity at exercise stress testing. Fourth, appropriate dietary and pharmacologic therapies are instituted to treat cardiac risk factors to established goals *(5,6)*. Finally, the Medical Director, with the input of program staff, should design an exercise training prescription that is oriented toward attaining improved physical function and risk factor goals for each individual patient (see Chapters 2, 13, 14, 16 and 17). Exercise training protocols will differ greatly by patient characteristics. For example, an older women struggling with poor physical function and a need to maintain physical independence in the home setting will often need an exercise program that focuses on increasing strength and endurance; so, it is often important to include a component of resistance training *(7,8)*. On the contrary, a younger male with multiple components of the metabolic syndrome will need an exercise prescription that focuses on maximization of exercise-related caloric expenditure, using longer bouts of walking and other aerobic exercises, to maximize weight loss *(9)*.

MONITOR PATIENT PROGRESS AND ADJUST TREATMENT PLAN

The Medical Director should outline the plan by which progress of the individual patient is monitored and communicated to the primary care physician. Different models exist for patients enrolled in CR relative to whether it is the referring physician or the Medical Director of the CR program that is monitoring patient progress and adjusting the care plan as needed. In the case where the Medical Director is monitoring patient progress, it is clear that any changes in the treatment plan should be clearly communicated with the referring physician, and certainly, no changes in pharmacologic therapy should be made without the input of the referring physician. On the contrary, in some programs, the Medical Director is only available for medical emergencies, with the referring physician performing the intake evaluation and monitoring of patient progress. In this model, closer contact is needed between the referring physician and program staff.

COORDINATE PROGRAM SAFETY PARAMETERS AND EMERGENCY MANAGEMENT

The singular most important role of the Medical Director is to design and maintain a CR program that is medically safe for participants. Safety protocols include guidelines for excluding highest risk patients, provisions for the closer monitoring of high-risk patients, and establishing protocols for emergency management for the rare but predictable emergencies that include sustained arrhythmias, acute coronary events, and cardiac arrest. Patients with any of the following conditions or measures should not enter CR before the condition is stabilized, and if they are already participating, they should be seen by the Medical Director before continuing in the program *(10)*. These include but are not limited to

- unstable angina.
- severe aortic stenosis.
- hypertrophic obstructive cardiomyopathy.
- class IV heart failure.
- resting systolic hypertension (≥ 200 mmHg).
- resting diastolic hypertension (≥ 110 mmHg).
- uncontrolled ventricular or supraventricular arrhythmias.
- random blood glucose < 80 or > 300 mg/dl until corrected.

As determined by the Medical Director, patients with more severe heart disease may require closer than usual monitoring which may include extended electrocardiographic monitoring, more individualized staff contact, more frequent than usual checking of vital signs, and/or a limitation of exercise intensity. Finally, processes need to be in place for the care of cardiac emergencies such as myocardial infarction, cardiac arrhythmias with hemodynamic collapse, or cardiac arrest. The Medical Director or a designated physician needs to be able to respond to these emergencies within seconds, and appropriate support staff need to be available. Each day that CR is being performed, there needs to be written evidence of who is designated as the responsible physician during an emergency. Intermittent "mock" codes should be performed, and all CR staff need to be certified in basic cardiac life support while advanced cardiac life support for some staff is preferred.

COMMUNICATION AND INTERFACING WITH REFERRING PHYSICIANS

The individual patient appropriately looks to his/her primary care physician for guidance in making health care decisions. From the point of view of the primary care physician, CR is part of the overall care plan for the patient with heart disease, and it needs to be coordinated with other aspects of patient care. Without timely, high-quality written communication from the CR program to the referring physician, the lifestyles and behaviors learned while in CR will not be supported or perpetuated long-term. At a minimum, communication between the CR program and the referring physician should include the following:

- Baseline evaluation and plan of care.
- A progress report half-way through the CR program.
- A final summary of participation with plans for long-term exercise and preventive care.

Supplemental communications may include updates on clinical events requiring medical intervention such as changes in anti-anginal medications or the need for intensification of pharmacologic therapy for improved blood pressure or lipid control. The Medical Director needs to be available to CR staff in an ongoing fashion to evaluate patients when needed and to communicate assessments and possible changes in therapies to the referring physician when appropriate.

COORDINATE REGULATORY AND REIMBURSEMENT ISSUES

Physician involvement is a major component of obtaining reimbursement for Phase II CR services because these services are provided "incident to" physicians' services. The Centers for Medicare and Medicaid Services (CMS) coordinates the care of more than 50% of CR participants nationwide; thus, their reimbursement guidelines and policies are closely monitored and are often adapted for CR coverage for private insurance carriers. Until recently, CMS covered Phase II CR only for services relating to the following diagnostic categories:

- Acute myocardial infarction.
- Coronary artery bypass surgery.
- Chronic stable angina with a positive exercise electrocardiogram or imaging stress test.

However, in the new CMS coverage policy for coverage of CR of March 2006, it has been decided that Phase II CR services be expanded to include patients after a percutaneous coronary intervention such as placement of a coronary stent, in the absence of an acute myocardial infarction, patients after heart valve replacement, and patients after cardiac transplantation but not patients with chronic heart failure *(11)*. It should be noted that many commercial insurance companies already do provide coverage for these diagnoses, but these need to be verified on a company-by-company basis. Because CR coverage remains "incident to" physicians' professional services, the patient still needs to be referred to CR by their personal physician and their progress in CR needs to be followed and documented in the CR chart either by the Medical Director of the CR program or by the primary physician. This progress report needs to be done at least once during a 3-month CR program and is in addition to the baseline and summary reports described above. This same physician will make adjustments to the plan of care as necessary to maintain patient safety and/or to attain patient outcome goals. A second issue important to CMS and other health insurance companies is that a physician be designated to be available to manage medical emergencies in the CR program. This physician can be the Medical Director of the CR program or, alternatively, can be the hospital emergency "code" team that is specially trained to deal with such emergencies in a timely fashion. Finally, CMS requires what is called "direct physician supervision" of the exercise area during Phase II CR. Technically, this is similar to what is provided for trained Registered Nurses or Exercise Physiologists to perform diagnostic exercise stress testing. The physician does not have to be physically present in the room but must be in the area of the exercise program and thus available for urgent situations. For example, this might include seeing clinic patients in a room down the hall if it does not preclude a prompt response, but it would not include performing medical procedures that cannot be interrupted or being in an adjacent building. Whereas Nurse Practitioners or Physicians Assistants may perform several of the roles of the Medical Director such as the intake or exit evaluation of the patient, the physician supervision aspect of CR must be performed by a Medical Doctor. It is not clear if a Nurse Practitioner can refer a patient to Phase II CR or if this needs to be done by an MD.

SUMMARY

Medical directors of CR programs are optimally situated to assure that systematic application of behavioral lifestyle treatments and pharmacologic therapies are applied to attain favorable clinical outcomes in patients with coronary heart disease. As the leader of the CR team, the role of the Medical Director is pivotal to define program policies, to perform patient assessments, to communicate in an effective and timely fashion with the referring physician, to assure patient safety, and to ascertain that the plan of care is effectively attaining favorable patient outcomes for participants.

THE FUTURE

Currently, many CR programs have a nurse or Exercise Physiologist functioning effectively as the program director to design policies and procedures. They cover medical emergencies with a hospital "code" team. If an urgent clinical issue arises for a given patient, they need to navigate many barriers to interrupt the personal physician for clinical direction. However, the personal physician is rarely able to physically come and examine the patient. Furthermore, the personal physician is rarely trained in the necessary concepts important to function as a CR staff physician, such as knowledge of exercise physiology, cardiology, or behavioral change techniques. Optimally, both the American Association of Cardiovascular and Pulmonary Rehabilitation and the American Heart Association support the concept that the Medical director for each CR program be the person responsible to assure that systems are in place to attain favorable clinical outcomes for participating patients (4). A physician-Medical Director is also well situated to best communicate with referring physicians.

One shortcoming of the current CR model is that patients at high risk for the development of coronary heart disease must suffer an acute coronary event before they "qualify" for a preventive program that is covered by their medical insurance. A challenge to Medical Directors of CR prevention programs is to develop innovative preventive services that are affordable within the current reimbursement model. Such a model might include a baseline risk factor analysis and a symptom-limited stress test for patients deemed at high risk, an evaluation that is covered by most insurers. Subsequently, patients can participate in health-club-style prevention programs that can include exercise, behavioral weight-loss programs, diabetic weight-loss and nutrition programs, or programs for individuals with relatively asymptomatic coronary heart disease in the absence of a recent coronary event. Follow-up evaluations would measure the response of cardiovascular risk factors such as hypertension, hyperlipidemia, and obesity. Such programs can be made available at reasonable costs, often well below the equivalent cost of a pack of cigarettes per day. Engaging patients at increased risk of heart disease calls for an expansion of the current model of what is often termed Phase III CR. In certain settings, this can also be expanded to include other chronic disease states where exercise is felt to be beneficial such as rheumatoid and osteoarthritis, chronic pulmonary disease, mental depression, and the dynamic process of healthy aging where two overriding goals are to maintain independence and prevent physical disability.

REFERENCES

1. Wenger NK, Froelicher ES, Smith LK, et al. Cardiac Rehabilitation. *Clinical Practice Guideline No.17.* Rockville, MD: US Dept of Health and Human Services, Public Health Service, Agency for Health Care Policy and Research and the National Heart, Lung and Blood Institute, AHCPR Publication No.96-0672; 1995.
2. Balady GJ, Ades PA, Comoss P, Limacher M, Pina I, Southard D, Williams MA, Bazzaare T. Core Component of Cardiac Rehabilitation/Secondary Prevention Programs. *Circulation.* 2000;102: 1069–1073.
3. Ades PA. Cardiac Rehabilitation and the Secondary Prevention of Coronary Heart Disease. *New Engl J Med.* 2001;345:892–902.
4. King ML, Williams MA, Fletcher GF, et al. Medical Director Responsibilities for Outpatient Cardiac Rehabilitation/Secondary Prevention Programs: A Scientific Statement from the American Heart Association/American Association for Cardiovascular and Pulmonary Rehabilitation. *Circulation.* 2005;112:3354–3360.
5. Smith SC Jr, Blair SN, Bonow RO, et al. AHA/ACC Guidelines for Preventing Heart Attack and Death in Patients With Atherosclerotic Cardiovascular Disease: 2001 Update. A Statement for Healthcare Professionals from the American Heart Association and the American College of Cardiology. *J Am Coll Cardiol.* 2001;38;1581–1583.
6. Expert Panel on Detection, Evaluation, and Treatment of High Blood Cholesterol in Adults. Executive Summary of the Third Report of National Cholesterol Education Program (NCEP), Expert Panel on Detection, Evaluation, and Treatment of High Blood Cholesterol in Adults (Adult Treatment Panel III), *JAMA.* 2001;285:2486–2497.
7. Brochu M, Savage P, Lee M, Dee J, Cress ME, Poehlman ET, Tischler M, Ades PA. Effects of Resistance Training on Physical Function in Older Disabled Women with Coronary Heart Disease. *J. Appl. Physiol.* 2002;92:672–678.
8. Ades PA, Savage PD, Cress ME, Brochu M, Lee NM, Poehlman ET. Resistance Training Improves Performance of Daily Activities in Disabled Older Women with Coronary Heart Disease. *Med Sci Sports Exerc.* 2003;35(8):1265–1270.
9. Savage P, Brochu M, Poehlman E, Ades PA. Reduction in Obesity and Coronary Risk Factors after High Caloric Exercise Training in Overweight Coronary Patients. *Am Heart J.* 2003;146:317–323.
10. American Association of Cardiovascular and Pulmonary Rehabilitation. *Guidelines for Cardiac Rehabilitation and Secondary Prevention Programs,* 4th ed. Champaign, IL: Human Kinetics; 2004.
11. CMS. Available at http://www.cms.hhs.gov/mcd/viewdraftdecisionmemo.asp?id=164 and http://www.cms.hhs.gov/mcd/viewdraftdecisionmemo.asp?id=164.

24 Assessment and Treatment of Risk in the Clinic Setting

William E. Kraus, MD

CONTENTS

The assessment of global cardiovascular risk at baseline and in response to therapy is an important component in both cardiac rehabilitation (CR) and the clinic setting that accompanies it. At our institution, we assess risk before and following a period of CR using established modifiable markers of cardiovascular risk, including status of lipids, blood pressure, metabolic syndrome, diabetes mellitus, central adiposity, depression, social support, and others. The goal is then to modify the risk to prevent downstream cardiovascular morbidity and mortality. Although much is accomplished in the setting of the CR program itself, much can be accomplished in the clinic-based visits with physicians and physician extenders to reinforce messages from the CR program, to titrate and optimize medical therapy, as addressed in previous chapters, and to further refine risk modification strategies when CR is completed. For lifestyle modification to be successful in the clinic setting, the provider must base the approach on a behavioral construct that to the clinician makes sense and can readily be employed. We have found the standard Stages of Change construct *(1)* to be the most useful in our clinics.

ASSESSMENT OF RISK IN THE CARDIAC REHABILITATION SETTING

It is useful to assess modifiable cardiovascular risk using established markers prior to and following a period of CR. First, such an assessment can focus the attention of the individual participant and the CR staff on targeted areas of particular interest

From: *Contemporary Cardiology: Cardiac Rehabilitation*
Edited by: W. E. Kraus and S. J. Keteyian © Humana Press Inc., Totowa, NJ

during the rehabilitation period. In addition, such information can be shared as a report of the program success to referring providers, thus becoming a reinforcing strategy for participant recruitment. Such assessments also can be added to the medical record for individual CR participants. Second, the staff can use these data to assess the effectiveness of the program in general, as well as the effectiveness of particular strategies to modify risk for particular risk markers [e.g., blood pressure, low-density lipoprotein (LDL) cholesterol, weight, and waist circumference]. Ineffective strategies can be modified and adapted to be more effective or abandoned if found to have no utility. Third, such longitudinal data can be extremely useful in research projects, conducted under the supervision of qualified personnel and the institutional Review Board, to address outstanding and untested hypotheses regarding CR programs in general. By adding to the general literature in this area, the entire field will be advanced.

We have used the format illustrated in Fig. 1 to collect relevant data on individual participants. Such data are shared with the referring health care provider and can become

DUKE CARDIAC REHABILITATION

PATIENT'S NAME:
MD:

INITIAL SUMMARY

HISTORY NUMBER:

Thank you for referring your patient to the Duke Cardiac Rehabilitation Program. Here is a plan of care for your patient aimed at helping him/her reach optimal health. It will be expected that each patient attend two nutritional classes, two educational lectures each week, stress management sessions and regularly attend exercise sessions three times per week. Our medical staff will monitor each patient and will be available to assist you in risk factor management, including screening for behavioral risk factors. A final report will be sent to you regarding the patient's participation and progress at discharge. If you have any questions or concerns, please contact any member of the cardiac rehabilitation team at (919) 660-6724.

Your patient's modifiable risk factors include:

	Initial	Comments
Metabolic Syndrome		
Smoking		
Hypertension		Average of first 3 BP readings
systolic		
diastolic		
Hyperlipidemia		
Total		
LDL		Goal for LDL is <70
HDL		Goal for HDL is >40
TRG		Goal for TG is <150
Diabetes		
HBA1C		Goal is between 4.3-6
Fasting glucose		Average of first 3 fasting glucoses
Framingham Risk		
Exercise METS		
6 Minute Walk (meters)		
Waist Circumference (cm)		Goal for
Educational score		20 total questions
Behavior Modification		
Nutrition component		

MEDICATIONS AT ENTRY:

LIFESTYLE PLAN with GOALS:

VOCATIONAL REHABILITATION: ☐ VR services requested ☐ VR services waived
EXERCISE HISTORY:
EXERCISE THERAPY PLAN - Target Ranges
FREQUENCY: 3 times/week   MODE: ☐WALK ☐BIKE ☐NUSTEP ☐POOL ☐UBE ☐EFX ☐ROWER
INTENSITY: Training HR Range: RHR + 20-30 RPE: 11-13 CALORIC EXPENDITURE GOAL: 1000 kcals/week
DURATION: Warm-up: 5-10 min/session   Aerobic Conditioning: Cool Down: 5-10 min/session
STR/FLEX: Weight Training recommended? ☐ Yes ☐ No   Stretching recommended? ☐ Yes ☐ No
DISCHARGE PLANNING:
ADDITIONAL COMMENTS:

_____ Date _____   _____ Date_____
Exercise Physiologist   Medical Director

Fig. 1. (*Contd.*)

DUKE CARDIAC REHABILITATION

PATIENT'S NAME:
MD:
HISTORY NUMBER:

EXIT SUMMARY

Program dates: Number of sessions:

	Initial	Exit	%Change	Comments
Metabolic Syndrome				
Smoking				
Hypertension				Average of first and last 3 BP readings
systolic				
diastolic				
Hyperlipidemia				
Total				
LDL				Goal for LDL is <70mg/dL
HDL				Goal for HDL is >50mg/dL
TRG				Goal for TG is <150 mg/dL
Diabetes				
HBA1C				
Fasting glucose				Average of first and last 3 fasting glucoses
Framingham 10 yr. CHD Risk				
Exercise METS				
6 Minute Walk (meters)				
Waist Circumference (cm)				Goal for
Educational score				20 total questions

MEDICATIONS AT DISCHARGE:

PROGRESSION TOWARD GOALS: .

BEHAVIOR MODIFICATION:

NUTRITION COMPONENT:

OTHER SERVICES ATTENDED: Regular lecture attendance ☐   Stress Management series ☐   Relaxation/Meditation class ☐
Strength training ☐   Flexibility program ☐   Consistent exercise outside of cardiac rehab ☐

RECOMMENDED EXERCISE PLAN

	AEROBIC EXERCISE	STRENGTH	FLEXIBILITY
FREQUENCY			After each exercise session
INTENSITY		10-15 reps, 1-3 sets	
TYPE			
TIME	20-60minutes		
ENERGY EXPENDITURE	1000 calories/week		

———————————————
EXERCISE PHYSIOLOGIST

———————————————
MEDICAL DIRECTOR
If you have any concerns, please call our team at 660-6724.

Cardiac Rehab Plan
☐ Join the Fred Cobb Healing HEARTS program
☐ Join the Duke Health and Fitness Center
☐ Home exercise program
☐ Discharge to exercise facility of choice

Fig. 1. Initial and Exit Summaries for Use in Cardiac Rehabilitation. Such summaries can be useful in communication to referring caregivers about the course and response to the treatment program. Also the collected data can be useful in program efficacy assessments and research.

part of the medical record of the individual patient. In addition, data are collected in a longitudinal database for subsequent program-wide assessments, as previously discussed.

ASSESSMENT AND MODIFICATION OF RISK IN THE CLINIC SETTING

As noted, the clinic visit, either by a member of the CR team or the referring physician, is an important ancillary component of the CR experience for the individual. The potential effectiveness of such visits to the successful institution of prevention strategies cannot and should not be underestimated. There is an evolving body of literature supporting the concept that attention of the physician and/or physician extender to particular behaviors (e.g., smoking, inactivity, and poor eating habits) is likely the most important component of a behavior-change strategy. We have found that there are at least four steps to a successful intervention with an individual in the behavioral change arena: (i) bringing attention to the behavior, (ii) discussion of the behavior with the individual, (iii) developing an effective strategy for changing behavior, and (iv) following up with the progress of the strategy at the next encounter. It is clear, however, that such approaches take time and the pressures of current medical practice require that strategies to address behavior change in the medical clinic require strategies that are at once effective and time-efficient. I will discuss some methods that we have found effective in our clinics for accomplishing each of these ends.

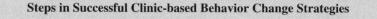

Steps in Successful Clinic-based Behavior Change Strategies

➢ Bring Attention to the Behavior – Surveying

➢ Discussion of Importance of Changing the Behavior

➢ Agreeing on Plan and Contracting

➢ Follow-up

Bringing Attention to the Behavior

There are several conceivable methods whereby one might bring a particular behavior to the attention of the individual. When this comes from the physician, the individual becomes aware that the physician believes that it is important. For example, taking weight or waist circumference or asking about eating and physical activity behaviors are important components of drawing the individual's attention to the issue and stressing that the health care provider believes that the issue is important enough to seek and record this information. We have found that short surveys administered about eating and physical activity behaviors, administered in the waiting room while the individual is waiting to see the caregiver, also provide an effective strategy for collecting the information. It is essential, however, in order for this strategy to be effective that the information subsequently be addressed and referenced during the clinic encounter with the physician and reinforced by other health care team members. Such data should also become part of the clinic record, preferably in the clinic note.

Discussion of the Behavior in the Clinic with the Individual

As noted, it is important, once the data are collected on a given behavior, to discuss the behavior with the individual during the clinic encounter. That being said, it is clear, given the time pressures on practitioners in the clinic, that not all behaviors of interest can be effectively addressed in each clinic visit. That is, we have found it particularly ineffective to mention, as a parting comment during a clinic encounter that the individual "should lose weight, eat better and get more regular exercise." Although better than nothing, the absence of a detailed, if brief, encounter on important behavioral issues will rarely lead to significant or long-term behavior change. Rather, the care provider must spend some time, even if short, explaining the importance of the behavior under issue. We have found that addressing one of the four potentially important behaviors in each visit is an efficient and effective means to promote behavior change. In the prevention cardiovascular clinic, the important behaviors that should be addressed are smoking, poor nutrition choices, lack of sufficient physical activity, and type A behavior. How does one chose which behavior to address in a given clinic visit?

CHOOSING WHICH RISK FACTOR TO ADDRESS: THE TRANSTHEORETICAL MODEL OF BEHAVIORAL CHANGE

In chapter 7, Dr Collins and colleagues discuss the background and use of the Transtheoretical Model of Behavior Change in assisting in developing a program for an individual. This model can also be used in the clinic setting to decide which behavior, of several that could be chosen, should be addressed in any given encounter. For example, should an individual be a smoker, have a poor diet, excessive job-related stress, and be physically inactive, one might ask which behavior might be best to address first. One approach might be to assess in which stage of precontemplation, contemplation, or planning the individual is, by prompting with questions such as "Have you considered stopping smoking?" and "Have you made plans to stop smoking within the next several months?" Depending upon this survey of prospective behaviors, it might make sense first to address those behaviors to which the individual is willing or even eager to direct their attention. For example, in an individual that responds to such queries with "I enjoy smoking and do not wish to consider stopping at the present but I do want to consider changing my diet and getting more exercise," it does not make sense to address first the smoking issue in preference to the diet and exercise issues.

A SERIES OF CLINIC VISITS BECOMES A PROGRAM FOR BEHAVIOR CHANGE

Given constraints on time that a practitioner can spend in any one clinic visit and limitations on the ability of any one individual can absorb in one visit, and given the other potential issues to address (e.g., medication changes), it is our habit to address only one behavior in each visit and attempt to move the behavior change along the spectrum of the Transtheoretical Model spectrum (precontemplation to contemplation to planning to action to maintenance and reinforcement) in each clinic encounter. This typically may take from 5 to 15 min. Thus, in reality, *a series of clinic visits becomes a program of behavior change*, and, for example, it may take up to sixteen sequential clinic visits to address and promote effective behavior change in each of four distinct behaviors.

DEVELOPING A BEHAVIOR-CHANGE PLAN

As noted, developing a behavior-change plan is an essential step in the process of promoting lifestyle changes in the clinic setting. This may take as little as 5 min and as much as 15 min in the clinic setting. Let us use increasing physical activity as an example. One should probe the individual's lifestyle and where, within the normal routine, a dedicated period of physical activity and exercise might fit. As it does not require large changes in physical activity to make a significant difference in health parameters *(2–4)*, and modest changes in physical activity are relatively easy to make, formulating a plan with an individual in the clinic setting is facile. Often, for example, to promote daily moderate level activity of about 30-min duration, we often suggest that the individual walk the dog daily – whether he has one or not! Once a plan is made, it is important to document it in the clinic record for later reference.

Follow-Up at the Next Encounter – the Importance of Contracting

The final essential step in a clinic-based process promoting behavior change is follow-up and reinforcement. By recording the plan in the clinic note, the clinician is prepared to query progress at the next visit. In addition, we find contracting to be a useful exercise, as well. For example, if weight loss is a goal, one might agree on a target of a given amount of weight loss in the interim until the next visit (e.g., agreeing on a 10-lb weight loss in 5 months). One useful strategy to reinforce the understanding is to contract on the behavior (looking the individual in the eyes, shaking hands on the agreement, and recording it in the chart). This can be particularly effective in helping the individual recall the contract. The contract and progress in achieving the agreement is then reviewed at the next encounter and a new contract formed. Often, when it is important to reinforce behavior and when change is actively taking place, more as opposed to less frequent, clinic visits should be arranged.

SUMMARY AND OUTSTANDING QUESTIONS

In summary, assessing global cardiovascular risk is important in both the CR setting and the cardiovascular prevention clinic that works in parallel. Assessing risk permits one to assess the effectiveness and make necessary adaptation of procedures and tactics for promoting lifestyle changes in these settings. In the clinic setting, promotion of lifestyle change is a progressive process, often based on behavioral change strategies, such as the Transtheoretical Model, where a series of stepwise counseling can be considered a program. Although many of the suggestions presented in this summary are seemingly rational and self-evident, many questions are in need of scientific testing for efficacy in randomized trials. For example, an important question might be that, when multiple behaviors need to be addressed, whether it is better to address a behavior that the individual is open to change (i.e., contemplative) or one that potentially presents the greatest risk (e.g., smoking). Scientific studies addressing such questions will greatly assist those that promote lifestyle change strategies in the clinic setting.

REFERENCES

1. Prochaska J, DiClemente C. Stages and Processes of Self-Change for Smoking: Toward an Integrative Model of Change. *J Consult Clin Psycho*. 1983;51:390–395.
2. Kraus WE, Houmard JA, Duscha BD, et al. Effects of the Amount and Intensity of Exercise on Plasma Lipoproteins. *N Engl J Med*. 2002;347:1483–1492.
3. Houmard JA, Tanner CJ, Slentz CA, Duscha BD, McCartney JS, Kraus WE. Effect of the Volume and Intensity of Exercise Training on Insulin Sensitivity. *J Appl Physiol*. 2004;96:101–106.
4. Slentz CA, Duscha BD, Johnson JL, et al. Effects of the Amount of Exercise on Body Weight, Body Composition, and Measures of Central Obesity: STRRIDE–A Randomized Controlled Study. *Arch Intern Med*. 2004;164:31–39.

25 Cardiac Rehabilitation Staffing

Gregory J. Lawson, MS, RCEP, FAACVPR

CONTENTS

Appropriate staffing for contemporary cardiac rehabilitation programs demands a multidisciplinary approach. Even if budgetary constraints and/or small patient census justify only a few staff, these professionals must have competencies across various disciplines: medicine, nursing, exercise physiology, physical and occupational therapy, psychology, sociology, pharmacology, and education. Cardiac rehabilitation includes baseline patient assessments, nutritional counseling, aggressive risk factor management (lipids, hypertension, weight, diabetes, and smoking), psychosocial and vocational counseling, and physical activity counseling and exercise training, and the use of appropriate cardio-protective drugs (1). Staff must be able to perform assessments, teach, and provide effective interventions in the following realms: cardiopulmonary and musculoskeletal anatomy, physiology, and pathology; cardiovascular disease risk factors; nutrition; physical functioning and exercise therapy; psychosocial; health behavior; vocational; and pharmacy.

INPATIENT CARDIAC REHABILITATION STAFFING

Once stable after a cardiovascular event or procedure, most patients are good candidates for inpatient cardiac rehabilitation. Treatment involves early mobilization, identification and education of cardiovascular risk factors, medication instruction, and discharge planning that includes referral to outpatient cardiac rehabilitation. After documented physician referral, the inpatient cardiac rehabilitation staff must conduct baseline cardiovascular, pulmonary, musculoskeletal, and psychosocial assessments. On the basis of these, an individualized program of physical activity and education should be administered to the patient by the cardiac rehabilitation staff. This team includes, at minimum, each nurse who is responsible for the patient on each

From: *Contemporary Cardiology: Cardiac Rehabilitation*
Edited by: W. E. Kraus and S. J. Keteyian © Humana Press Inc., Totowa, NJ

nursing shift. Specific staff duties necessary to meet the goals of inpatient cardiac rehabilitation may be and are often delegated to a multidisciplinary team including certified nursing assistants; registered dieticians; physical and occupational therapists, exercise specialists, and exercise physiologists; pharmacists; social workers; and discharge planners. Some programs, usually those with large patient populations, may have a Cardiac Rehabilitation Coordinator or Cardiac Rehabilitation Educator (usually a nurse) who coordinates the above team of providers, assumes their respective roles, and/or is responsible for special patient populations (e.g., higher-risk patients). For smaller programs, and for patients experiencing a short length of stay, the patient's nurse or any one of the above providers may be cross-trained to take on multiple roles (Table 1). Regardless of which professional staff is doing the work of inpatient cardiac rehabilitation, everyone in this team should be familiar with and competent (within their respective job descriptions) relative to clinical indications and contraindications

Table 1
Summary of Staff Assignments Designed to Meet Typical Inpatient Cardiac Rehabilitation Patient Goals

Goal	Job function	Job title
Initial assessment and explanation of event or procedures	Basic cardiovascular nursing	Patient's RN or CRE/Coord.
Early physical activity including ambulation	Leads patient with transfers, bedside exercises, and ambulation	RN, PT, OT, CNA, ExSp, or CRE/Coord.
Heart healthy diet	Nutrition assessment and instruction	RN, RD, or CRE/Coord.
Smoking cessation	Smoking assessment, advice, and intervention	RN or CRE/Coord.
Effective emotional management	Psychosocial assessment and stress management intervention	RN, SW, Behavioral Specialist, Psychologist, or CRE/Coord.
Medication management	Medication instruction	RN, Pharmacist, or CRE/Coord.
Effective diabetes management	Medication and lifestyle instruction	RN, RD, CDE, or CRE/Coord.
Effective discharge planning (for first few weeks at home)	Planning for transitional care if necessary; instruction on home activities and emergency preparedness; medication prescriptions; follow-up appointments; referral to outpatient cardiac rehabilitation	SW, DP, RN, or CRE/Coord.

CNA, Certified Nursing Assistant; CDE, Certified Diabetes Educator; CRE/Coord., Cardiac Rehabilitation Educator/Coordinator; DP, Discharge Planner; ExSp, Exercise Specialist; OT, Occupational Therapist; PT, Physical Therapist; RD, Registered Dietician; RN, Registered Nurse; SW, Social Worker.

for cardiac rehabilitation *(2)*. Moreover, staff who are responsible for early mobilization and physical activity of patients must be familiar with the adverse responses to physical activity which require discontinuation of activity *(2)*.

OUTPATIENT CARDIAC REHABILITATION STAFFING

After discharge from the hospital, most patients with cardiovascular disease are good candidates for outpatient cardiac rehabilitation, including those recovering from a myocardial infarction, coronary revascularization, cardiac transplant, or valve surgery and patients with stable angina or heart failure. Historically, the cornerstone of outpatient cardiac rehabilitation has been appropriately prescribed and medically monitored/supervised exercise therapy in a clinical setting. This requires personnel who have the following competencies: basic cardiovascular, pulmonary, and musculoskeletal assessment; electrocardiogram (ECG) interpretation; medical emergency management; and exercise therapy theory and practice. Moreover, because contemporary outpatient cardiac rehabilitation programs are more focused toward disease management and have, by necessity, adopted a case management approach to patient care *(3)*, core staff must also have competencies in cardiovascular risk factor management, basic psychosocial assessment and intervention, and behavioral counseling. Core staff must be able to perform individual patient assessments of basic cardiovascular and behavioral issues, help patients to set realistic goals regarding these, and evaluate progress toward these goals (Table 2) *(4)*. As with inpatient programs, various disciplines can be employed to meet program goals.

Typically, core outpatient staff consists of nurses and exercise physiologists in some combination, depending on program philosophy, goals, and census (see Fig. 1 for a flexible staffing model). Additional staff from other disciplines may be employed on a part-time basis to provide specific patient education and instruction. For example, a registered dietician who works primarily in an outpatient nutrition clinic may spend several hours per week teaching patients in the outpatient cardiac rehabilitation clinic. In programs that employ a nontraditional cardiac rehabilitation model, whereby the patients attend fewer clinic visits, and the exercise is primarily or all home-based *(5)*, staff (primarily nurses) interact with patients via telephone and periodic office visits. Regardless, program staff still must have competency in the areas of exercise assessment, prescription, and evaluation.

Some programs call their staff "Cardiac Rehabilitation Case Managers" or "Cardiac Rehabilitation Specialists" rather than by their original disciplinary training ("Cardiac Rehabilitation Nurse" or "Cardiac Rehabilitation Exercise Specialist"). This demonstrates that clinical personnel are cross-trained and are accountable for various responsibilities (see Table 3 for sample generic job description).

To demonstrate competency and expertise, it is highly recommended that clinical cardiac rehabilitation staff obtain certification(s) in their respective fields (Table 4) *(6)*. Clinical staff should demonstrate the knowledge, skills, and abilities (KSAs) necessary to provide safe and effective services to their patients, many of which are delineated by the American College of Sports Medicine (ACSM) *(2)*. Any clinical staff person who is responsible for conducting cardiac rehabilitation supervised exercise should possess the KSAs for either the ACSM Exercise Specialist® or the ACSM Registered Clinical Exercise Physiologist® (Table 5). Additional training in Preventive

Table 2
Staff Competencies for Individual Patient Assessments, Goal Setting, Treatment Strategies (Patient Behaviors), and Outcome Evaluation

Core component	Assessment, goal setting, treatment strategies, and outcome evaluation
Patient assessment	*Review medical history* *Assess*: Vital signs, current clinical status, administer a battery of standardized measurement tools to assess status in each component of care. *Goal*: Develop a goal-directed treatment plan with short- and long-term goals for cardiovascular risk reduction and improvement in health-related quality of life. *Evaluate outcomes*: Reinforce/revise goals and/or treatment strategies if necessary.
Lipid management	*Assess*: Lipid profile, current treatment, and compliance. *Goal*: Assist patient to improve lipid profile. *Strategies (behaviors)*: See Nutritional and Physical Activity Counseling. *Evaluate outcomes*: Reinforce/revise goals and/or treatment strategies if necessary.
Hypertension management	*Assess*: Resting blood pressure (BP), current treatment strategies, and patient's adherence. *Goal*: Assist patient to improve blood pressure. *Strategies (behaviors)*: See Nutritional and Physical Activity Counseling. *Evaluate outcomes*: Reinforce/revise goals and/or treatment strategies if necessary.
Diabetes management	*Assess*: Diabetes present; HbA1C and fasting blood glucose (FBG); current treatment strategies and patient's adherence. *Goal*: Assist patient to improve blood glucose control. *Strategies (behaviors)*: See Nutritional and Physical Activity Counseling. *Evaluate outcomes*: Reinforce/revise goals and/or treatment strategies if necessary.
Weight management	*Assess*: Weight, height, body mass index (BMI) – determine risk. *Goal*: Assist patient to reduce weight by at least 10% (1–2 lb/week). *Strategies (behaviors)*: Create energy deficit of 500–1000 kcal/day with diet and exercise. See Nutritional and Physical Activity Counseling. *Evaluate outcomes*: Reinforce/revise goals and/or treatment strategies if necessary.
Psychosocial management	*Assess*: Psychological distress (depression, anxiety, hostility, etc.); refer patients with clinically significant distress to appropriate behavioral health specialists. *Goal*: Assist patient to reduce psychological distress. *Strategies (behaviors)*: Teach coping and stress management skills. Promote adherence. *Evaluate Outcomes*: Reinforce/revise goals and/or treatment strategies if necessary.

(Continued)

Table 2 (Continued)

Exercise training and counseling	*Assess*: Functional capacity; physiological responses to exercise; current (past 7 days) physical activity behavior – include leisure and usual activities (occupational, domestic, etc.). Specify time (min/day) frequency (days/week), and intensity (e.g., moderate or vigorous). *Goal*: Individualized exercise prescription defining frequency (times/week), intensity [target heart rate (THR), rated perceived exertion (RPE), metabolic equivalent (MET) level], duration (min), and modality to achieve aerobic, muscular, flexibility, and energy expenditure goals. Example: 30 min a day on most (at least 5) days/week at moderate (3–5 MET) intensity level. *Strategies (behaviors)*: Assist patient to implement exercise prescription in Cardiac Rehabilitation and/or Home Program; promote adherence. *Evaluate outcomes*: Reinforce/revise goals and/or treatment strategies if necessary.
Nutritional counseling	*Assess*: Current dietary behavior – dietary content of fat, cholesterol, sodium, calories; eating/drinking habits. *Goal*: Individualized prescribed diet based on needs assessed. *Strategies (behaviors)*: Teach nutritional information and dietary skills; provide instructional resources; promote adherence. *Evaluate outcomes*: Reinforce/revise goals and/or treatment strategies if necessary.
Smoking cessation	*Assess*: Smoking status – current, recent, former, never. If current or recent, stage of change, amount of tobacco/day (or other nicotine). *Goal*: Abstinence from smoking and use of all tobacco products. *Strategies (behaviors)*: Teach smoking cessation information and skills; provide instructional resources; promote adherence. *Evaluate outcomes*: Reinforce/revise goals and/or treatment strategies if necessary.

Cardiology, Motivational Interviewing, and use of the Stages of Change Model should be encouraged. All cardiac rehabilitation staff should have current training in basic life support skills and participate regularly in emergency drills *(6)*. During supervised exercise sessions, the recommended patient to staff ratio is 5:1 for early outpatient (Phase II) programs and 15:1 for intermediate to long-term programs *(7)*. A second staff person should be available in case of emergencies. In rare instances, the acuity of individual patients may demand a very low (even 1:1) patient to staff ratio.

Cardiac rehabilitation programs can benefit immensely from volunteer staff, such as graduate or undergraduate students working to fulfill academic requirements for clinical experience *(8)*. Student interns can provide a source of positive motivation and encouragement to current patients. They can assist with orientations and act as a resource to current patients regarding protocols and procedures. They can assist with supervision of current client activities, data collection, and outcome tracking. Student interns must have a written job description and be supervised by department staff.

Also, it would be a tremendous oversight to discount the importance of a good clerical/secretarial component. Too often, for perceived financial limitations, clinical personnel are left spending a disproportionate amount of time with clerical and secretarial

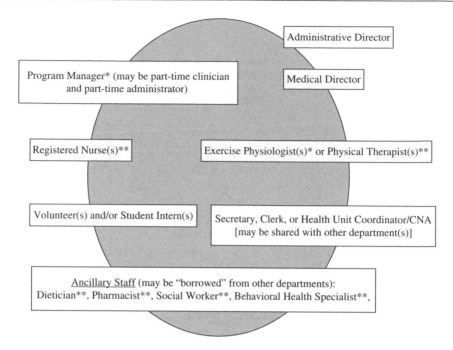

Fig. 1. Flexible Staffing Model for outpatient cardiac rehabilitation. *May have alternative job title and may oversee other services such as inpatient cardiac rehabilitation and/or other outpatient primary or secondary prevention services. **These may have alternative job titles, for example, "Cardiac Rehab Specialist," and/or may also perform functions within inpatient cardiac rehabilitation and/or other outpatient primary or secondary prevention services.

duties. In reality, having a competent secretary or health unit coordinator, even if shared with other departments, allows clinical staff to focus on and improve patient outcomes and program delivery, which often results in higher departmental productivity.

MEDICAL DIRECTOR

Provision of cardiac rehabilitation services, both inpatient and outpatient, should be led by a Medical Director. The Medical Director is ultimately responsible for ensuring that systems are in place to facilitate the process by which cardiac rehabilitation staff, in conjunction with referring physicians, assist patients to reach cardiac rehabilitation specific goals most effectively (9). In addition to providing general medical oversight of the program (medical policies, procedures, and regulations), the Medical Director, who is often trained in cardiology, internal medicine, or family medicine, must ensure that the program is safe, comprehensive, cost-effective, and medically appropriate for individual patients. The Medical Director must also maintain effective communication with community physicians who care for patients eligible for program participation.

PROGRAM ADMINISTRATION

Cardiac rehabilitation staff are accountable to the institution providing the services they deliver and so must have a program administrator. This person may be the director of all cardiovascular services or nursing services or may be the director of

Table 3
Generic Job Description for Cardiac Rehabilitation Clinical Personnel

1. Provides cardiac and pulmonary rehabilitation and prevention services to a diagnostically and developmentally diverse population that is commensurate with the client's age, cognitive ability, and developmental needs.

2. Works collaboratively with cardiac rehabilitation staff, physicians, and other departments to enhance the continuum of care and productive working relationships.

3. Develops and implements patient exercise and education care plans and programs according to prescribed treatment and clinical pathways.

4. Assesses and evaluates patient's physical, functional, and psychosocial status to assist patient in the design of an exercise, education, and lifestyle modification program to meet activities of daily living (ADL), recreational, and vocational needs.

5. Evaluates patient progress and creates or modifies goals and objectives, discharges with appropriate program to maintain and continue optimal lifestyle function and follows up with patient to determine adherence and success.

6. Documents patient assessments and progress according to departmental guidelines. Maintains accurate patient attendance and charge records for the charging and billing process.

7. Assists with set up, storing, inventory, and maintenance of program equipment and supplies.

8. Provides and presents formal and informal exercise and risk factor topics to patients and families.

9. Maintains confidentiality of patient, employee, or medical center information at all times. Ensures all information, and conversations regarding patients are secured from general public access.

10. Participates in unit/department performance-improvement activities to ensure the development and implementation of processes, which support quality patient care and effective work performance.

11. Participates in all staff meetings and mandatory in services and training programs to ensure continued understanding of all departmental policies, procedures, and performance-improvement processes.

12. Maintains/develops competencies associated with this job description (see examples in Table 2 list).

the clinic or groups of services in which cardiac rehabilitation operates. The immediate supervisor of the inpatient cardiac rehabilitation program is often the nurse manager of the inpatient cardiac care unit; however, in larger programs, the supervisor may be a person who directs both the inpatient and the outpatient cardiac rehabilitation services. The outpatient cardiac rehabilitation supervisor (or manager, coordinator, or director) often has dual responsibilities as both administrator and clinician *(10)*. This person must possess qualities and skills that ensure the best patient care and also must understand and implement effective business strategies for customer service, department operations, human resources, and financial management *(11)*.

Table 4

Example of ACSM Exercise Specialist Knowledge, Skills, and Abilities *(9)*

Exercise physiology and related exercise science

- Describe activities that are primarily aerobic and anaerobic.

Pathophysiology and risk factors

- Examine the role of diet on cardiovascular risk factors such as hypertension, blood lipids, and body weight.

Health appraisal, fitness, and clinical exercise testing

- Describe the importance of relative and absolute contraindications of an exercise test.

Electrocardiography and diagnostic techniques

- Define the electrocardiogram (ECG) criteria for initiating and/or terminating exercise testing/training.

Patient management and medications

- Describe mechanisms and actions of medications that may affect exercise testing and prescription.

Medical and surgical management

- Describe indications and limitations for medical management and interventional techniques in different subsets of individuals with coronary artery disease (CAD) and peripheral arterial disease (PAD).

Exercise prescription and programming

- Design a supervised exercise program beginning at hospital discharge and continuing for up to 6 months for the following conditions: myocardial infarction (MI); angina; left ventricular assist device (LVAD); congestive heart failure; percutaneous coronary intervention (PCI); coronary artery bypass graft (CABG); medical management of CAD; chronic pulmonary disease; weight management; diabetes; and cardiac transplants.

Nutrition and weight management

- Describe and discuss dietary considerations for cardiovascular and pulmonary diseases, chronic heart failure, and diabetes that are recommended to minimize disease progression and optimize disease management.

Human behavior and counseling

- List and apply five behavioral strategies as they apply to lifestyle modifications, such as exercise, diet, stress, and medication management.

Safety, injury prevention, and emergency procedures

- List medications that should be available for emergency situations in exercise testing and training sessions.

Program administration, quality assurance, and outcome assessment

- Discuss the role of outcome measures in chronic disease management programs such as cardiovascular and pulmonary rehabilitation programs.

Core areas are listed with *only one* example of specific knowledge, skills and abilities (KSAs) in each core area.

Table 5
Recommended Certifications for Allied Health Personnel Working in Cardiac
Rehabilitation Programs

For personnel with the following degree, background, or current discipline	Recommended certification(s)
Bachelors, Masters, or Doctorate in Exercise Science, Exercise Physiology, etc.	• *Registered Clinical Exercise Physiologist®* by American College of Sports Medicine (ACSM) http://www.acsm.org • *Exercise Physiologist Certification* by American Society of Exercise Physiologists http://www.asep.org
Associate, Bachelors, Masters, or Doctorate in Nursing	• *Cardiac/Vascular Certification* by American Nurses Credentialing Center http://www.nursingworld.org/ancc/ • *Exercise Specialist®* by ACSM http://www.acsm.org
Physician	• *Exercise Specialist®* by ACSM http://www.acsm.org
Physical Therapist	• *Cardiovascular and Pulmonary Certification* by American Physical Therapy Association http://www.apta.org • *Exercise Specialist®* by ACSM http://www.acsm.org

STRATEGY FOR STAFFING

Considerations for staffing outpatient cardiac rehabilitation include program goals, patient census, budget, facility space, regulatory requirements of state (licensure) and federal (reimbursement) agencies, and availability of qualified and interested personnel. Any one or combination of these factors may hamper the most effective staffing model that a particular institution or clinic may choose. However, this should not dissuade the champion of a particular cardiac rehabilitation service from providing a program. Although it is rare for all of the above considerations to meld together for an ideal staff mix, successful staffing models can be achieved when available resources are effectively matched with well-defined and articulated program goals. Of course, over time, resources and goals will inevitably change, and so must staffing, to maintain program effectiveness and productivity.

Staffing cardiac rehabilitation has evolved from a high degree of medical supervision and monitoring some 35 years ago to various degrees of medical supervision with delegation of most services to allied health care personnel today *(6,12)*. Many of the original cardiac rehabilitation services in the 1950s and 1960s began with physicians providing direct care and working individually with inpatients. As the safety of low-level exercise was established, physicians delegated cardiac rehabilitation (physical activities including bedside exercises and hallway ambulation) to nurses. Many nurses began to take on the dual role of nurse and educator, teaching the patient about cardiovascular risk factors. Larger institutions began to employ physical and occupational therapists to conduct the physical activity component of inpatient cardiac rehabilitation, and registered dieticians were engaged to provide nutrition assessments and instruction. Length of hospital stay from 1960 through even 1980 was long enough such that there was ample time to provide patient education and several days of physical activity. Consequently, many health care providers became involved with inpatient cardiac rehabilitation. However, as length of hospital stay shortened considerably throughout the 1980s and 1990s, the amount of education and activity that could be done with patients was truncated significantly. This provided the impetus for a tremendous increase in outpatient cardiac rehabilitation services.

Formal outpatient cardiac rehabilitation was introduced in the mid- to late 1960s, and as with inpatient programs, staffing consisted primarily of physicians and nurses. Through the 1970s, physicians delegated most of the work to nurses. As these programs grew and became more prevalent throughout North America, and with the development of the exercise science profession *(7)*, programs began to employ exercise physiologists.

Contemporary cardiac rehabilitation staffing models are successful when they deal creatively with fiscal limitations and ensure delivery of comprehensive, cost-effective, and individualized care and do so by respecting the contributions of various professional disciplines and cross-training staff for necessary competencies.

REFERENCES

1. Cardiac Rehabilitation and Secondary Prevention of Coronary Heart Disease: An American Heart Association Scientific Statement. *Circulation.* 2005;111:369–376.
2. American College of Sports Medicine. *Guidelines for Exercise Testing and Prescription*, 7th ed. Baltimore, MD: Lippincott Williams & Wilkins; 2006:176–177, 332–337.
3. Ades PA, Balady GJ, Berra K. Transforming Exercise-Based Cardiac Rehabilitation Programs into Secondary Prevention Centers: A National Imperative. *J Cardiopulm Rehabil.* 2001;21:263–272.
4. Sanderson, BK, Southard, D, Oldridge, N. Outcomes Evaluation in Cardiac Rehabilitation/Secondary Prevention Programs. *J Cardiopulm Rehabil.* 2004;24:68–79.
5. Ratchford AM, Hamman RF, Regensteiner JG, Magid DJ, Gallagher SB, Mernich JA. Attendance and Graduation Patterns in a Group-Model Health Maintenance Organization Alternative Cardiac Rehabilitation Program. *J Cardiopulm Rehabil.* 2004;24:150–156.
6. American Association of Cardiovascular and Pulmonary Rehabilitation. *Guidelines for Cardiac Rehabilitation and Secondary Prevention Programs*, 4th ed. Champaign, IL: Human Kinetics; 2004:6, 45–46, 194–196, 203.
7. American College of Sports Medicine. *Resource Manual for Guidelines for Exercise Testing and Prescription*, 5th ed. Baltimore, MD: Lippincott Williams & Wilkins; 2006:602–605, 629.
8. Heggestad J. *Cardiac Health & Rehabilitation and Graded Exercise Testing: Policy and Procedure Manual*, 3rd ed. Los Angeles, CA: Academy Medical Systems; 1998:92–95.
9. Medical Director Responsibilities for Outpatient Cardiac Rehabilitation/Secondary Prevention Programs: An American Heart Association/American Association of Cardiovascular and Pulmonary Rehabilitation Scientific Statement. *Circulation.* 2005;112:3354–3360.

10. Sharratt MT, Squires RW, Pescatello LS. A North American Survey of Educational Background and Job Responsibilities of Cardiopulmonary Rehabilitation Program Directors. *J Cardiopulm Rehabil.* 1997;17:9–15.

11. Segrest W, Castillo A, Adams J, Tolentino R, Hartman J. Quality Patient Care in a Successful Business Model. *J Cardiopulm Rehabil.* 2003;23:426–429.

12. Bennett SB, Pescatello LS. A Regional Comparison of Cardiac Rehabilitation Personnel: Adherence to the 1995 American Association of Cardiovascular and Pulmonary Rehabilitation Guidelines by Staff Position. *J Cardiopulm Rehabil.* 1997;17:92–102.

26 Reimbursement Issues

Patricia McCall Comoss RN, BS, FAACVPR

CONTENTS

INTRODUCTION

In its half-century history, two parallel developments have formed a firm and lasting foundation for the contemporary practice of cardiac rehabilitation. First and foremost was decades of research to build the evidence base that defines the safety and effectiveness of cardiac rehabilitation. Other chapters in this book summarize much of that science and suggest related practical applications. The concurrent effort contributed to a business model that would make the operation of cardiac rehabilitation programs sustainable. Knowledge of reimbursement issues is the cornerstone of that model. Therefore, the purpose of this chapter is to

- identify the latest rules/regulations that govern public payment of cardiac rehabilitation services and
- provide recommendations for how programs and practitioners can meet those requirements and secure payment for services rendered.

REIMBURSEMENT FOR PROGRAMS

Both public agencies and private health insurance companies pay for cardiac rehabilitation services in the United States. Medicare is the largest payer by far. Most cardiac rehabilitation programs report that 50–80% of their patient mix is covered under Medicare. It is for this reason, as well as the fact that a number of private payers take their lead from Medicare, that programs work hard to identify and comply with Medicare requirements. Failure to do so would not only deprive a program of adequate reimbursement, it could also result in legal and financial penalties.

From: *Contemporary Cardiology: Cardiac Rehabilitation*
Edited by: W. E. Kraus and S. J. Keteyian © Humana Press Inc., Totowa, NJ

Rules and Regulations

The Health Care Financing Administration (HCFA) first approved coverage of cardiac rehabilitation in 1980 *(1)*. As the preceding Medicare statute written in 1965 neither identified cardiac rehabilitation nor provided a benefit category for its coverage *(2)*, payment could only be made to the then new program through an existing benefit category. Therefore, in its *Coverage Issues Manual (CIM), Section 35-25*, HCFA directed that cardiac rehabilitation could only be reimbursed if it was provided "incident to physician services" *(3)*. The terms of that document governed the delivery and payment of cardiac rehabilitation services until early 2006. In March of that year, more than 25 years after Medicare coverage was originally granted, the Centers for Medicare/Medicaid Services (CMS, formerly known as HCFA) totally revised its coverage guidelines *(4)*.

As is the current trend in the development of practice guidelines in all areas of medicine, the new guidelines are largely evidence-based. However, the old payment mechanism, "incident to physician services," remains intact. Only an amendment to the Medicare statute can cause that to change. To facilitate that change, legislation has been introduced in both houses of Congress *(5,6)*. Table 1 summarizes major requirements in the new Medicare guidelines.

Billing and Coding

Once a program is organized and operated according to Medicare requirements, a process must be established to bill for and collect allowed reimbursement. Use of the correct diagnostic and procedure codes is key to timely reimbursement.

The 2006 National Coverage Determination (NCD) expands the number of patient groups eligible for cardiac rehabilitation participation under Medicare. Table 2 summarizes those diagnoses along with their respective diagnostic codes (7). Notably absent from the list is congestive heart failure (CHF). In updating its guidelines, CMS determined that "there is insufficient evidence to support coverage at his time" *(8)*. However, many private payers already include CHF as a covered diagnosis. For all payers, medical record proof of the qualifying diagnosis must be contained in each patient's cardiac rehabilitation chart. Examples include

- hospital discharge summary confirming date of myocardial infarction,
- operative report describing surgery/interventional procedure, and
- physician's office visit note explaining patient's angina pattern.

Once qualifying diagnosis is confirmed and a medical evaluation clears the patient as appropriate for cardiac rehabilitation participation, outpatient sessions are scheduled 2–3 times per week for as few as 3–4 or as many as 12–18 weeks. Each session typically consists of a combination of exercise and education/counseling services usually lasting about 1 hour. Although a few initial visits may be performed 1:1, most services are performed in small group sessions with a staff to patient ratio of 1:4 or 1:5 *(9, p. 195)*. Regardless of staff ratio or duration of the visit, each session is billed as a bundled charge versus the itemized or time-based services of other therapies.

Only two codes exist in the Common Procedure Terminology (CPT) system for billing cardiac rehab sessions. The difference between them is whether or not electrocardiogram (ECG) telemetry monitoring is used to display patient responses during

Table 1
Major Requirements for Medicare Reimbursement

Program structure	Program operation
Location • Hospital outpatient department • Physician-directed clinic	Approved diagnoses • See Table 2 for Medicare list • Private payers may cover additional diagnoses including congestive heart failure (CHF)
Emergency plan • Equipment – standard life-saving equipment including defibrillator, oxygen, resuscitation equipment, and medications • Personnel – all trained in basic life support (BLS); added training in advanced cardiac life support (ACLS) for those qualified to provide those services	Comprehensive services • Medical evaluation • Prescribed exercise • Risk factor modification • Education/counseling Appropriate EKG monitoring • Determined by clinicians
Direct physician supervision • Assumed to be met when rehab provided on hospital premises • Arrangements for daily coverage and immediate physician response required in off-site locations	Incident to documentation • See Table 4
Personnel • Emergency capability as above • Special training in exercise therapy for cardiac patients	Timing • Ideally initiated 1–3 weeks after hospital discharge • Extenuating circumstance may delay start • A 12-month look-back period allowed for patients with myocardial infarction (MI)
Length of stay • Maximum of 36 sessions • Frequency – sessions scheduled 2 or 3 times per week • Duration – 12 to 18 weeks	Extensions/Re-admissions • Case-by-case consideration for sessions beyond 18 weeks but not to exceed 72 sessions • No lifetime limit – may repeat rehab for each qualifying cardiac episode

Modified from (4).

Table 2
Medicare Approved Diagnoses and Related Codes

Primary diagnoses	ICD-9 codes	Supporting diagnoses	ICD-9 codes
Post acute myocardial infarction (MI) (< 8 weeks old)	410.0–410.9 (depending on area of MI)		
Old MI (> 8 weeks old)	412		
Stable angina pectoris	413.9		
Post coronary artery bypass (CABG)	V45.81	Coronary artery disease	414.01 (native) 414.05 (bypass)
Post coronary angio-plasty/stent (PTCA)	V45.82	Coronary artery disease	414.01 (native) 414.05 (bypass)
Heart transplant	V42.1	Cardiomyopathy; Congestive heart failure	425.0–425.9 (based on type) 428.0–428.9
Heart valve replacement	V43.3	Specific valve disorder	424.0–424.3

Excerpted from *(7)*.

performance of the exercise portion of the session *(10)*. While the new Medicare coverage guidelines state that extent of monitoring is a clinical decision, most fiscal intermedaries (FI) continue to enforce of continuous telemetry monitoring:

93797 = Physician services for outpatient cardiac rehabilitation, without continuous ECG monitoring (per session)

93798 = Physician services for outpatient cardiac rehabilitation, with continuous ECG monitoring (per session)

No other CPT codes are available to bill for cardiac rehabilitation visits performed by the usual cardiac rehabilitation staff [registered nurses (RN), clinical exercise physiologists (CEP), and physical therapists (PT)]. Supplemental services provided by mental health specialists, PT, or dietitians are subject to established qualifications for those services and are billed separately by those disciplines. They are viewed as an exception, not a routine part of a rehabilitation visit, and rationale for their use must be justified in the patient's medical record.

Charges and Reimbursement

As is the case throughout the healthcare system, there is a substantial difference between what is charged for cardiac rehabilitation sessions and what will ultimately be collected. Charges (the price a provider assigns to a service) vary widely from one program to another. Cost of delivering the CR service is one obvious determinate of charge. But pricing is also influenced by patient demographics, regional wage/price indices, and local competition. No published data are available to document trends in cardiac rehabilitation pricing. However, recent observations by the author identified a range of $75–300 per session in hospital-based cardiac rehabilitation programs located in the mid-Atlantic area. High-end charges are primarily found in the cities (e.g., Philadelphia), whereas a few rural sites still charge under $100 per session.

Depending upon the payer, there may/may not be any relationship between charges and payments. Negotiations between managed care companies and providers typically result in payments near 50% of charge plus a co-pay amount from the patient. In contrast, Medicare has been paying a fixed fee for cardiac rehabilitation sessions since 2000 when Ambulatory Payment Classifications (APCs) went into effect *(11)*. APC 0095 is synonymous with CPT 93798. The approved reimbursement on those codes averages near $35 nationally with Medicare now paying about two-thirds of that allowed amount. The patient or his/her secondary insurance company is obligated to pay the balance. Medicare's contracts with providers prohibit waiving of the patient's portion. Every attempt must be made to collect the two-part total. Bills are submitted to payers at the end of each month for the total number of visits completed during that time period. Hospitals bill on the standard UB-04 form, and physician offices/clinics use form 1500 *(12)*.

PAYMENT TO PHYSICIANS

Chapter 25 discusses physician roles in cardiac rehabilitation in greater detail. In this chapter, major aspects of those roles are related to available payment mechanisms.

Physician involvement in cardiac rehabilitation has been under government scrutiny for the last 5 years. In 2002, the Office of the Inspector General (OIG) began doing site visits to cardiac rehabilitation facilities "to determine whether hospitals had complied with national Medicare outpatient cardiac rehabilitation coverage requirements for direct physician supervision and incident to services" *(13)*. In their final report submitted to CMS in 2005 and summarizing the results of findings from 34 inspections, the OIG charged CMS to clarify coverage requirements for those respective roles. As a result, the 2006 Medicare revisions address the previously confusing physician role expectations. In turn, program sponsors are working hard to assure that payments to physicians are tied directly to the specific medical services they provide to the cardiac rehabilitation program or patients.

Medical Director for Cardiac Rehabilitation

Medicare guidelines do not specifically impose a requirement for a Medical Director to oversee the cardiac rehabilitation program. However, other authoritative statements describe the Medical Director's role as "pivotal" *(14)* and assert that "Each program should have a licensed physician serving as medical director" *(15)*. Most importantly, the legislation recently introduced in Congress (S. 329 & H.R. 552) contains more definitive language stating that the Secretary of Health and Human Services would:

> ...*establish standards to ensure that a physician with expertise in the management of patients with cardiac pathophysiology, who is licensed to practice medicine in the State where the cardiac rehabilitation program is offered, is responsible for such program; and, in consultation with appropriate staff, is involved substantially in directing the progress of individual patients in the program. (16)*

In prior decades, many if not most Medical Directors of cardiac rehabilitation programs served in that position on a voluntary basis. Some were the programs' original founders/champions. Few were paid. That situation has changed dramatically in the last few years because of the increased demands of the position. Table 3 summarizes a list of major role expectations.

Today, Medical Directors of cardiac rehabilitation programs are usually appointed to that position by hospital administration or medical staff. They sign a contract or agreement to serve and are paid a stipend reflecting the prevailing hourly rate for a projected number of service hours. No billing or collecting of insurance is involved. Payment is between the hospital (or other program owner) and the physician.

Supervision of Off-Site Program

Whereas the majority of outpatient cardiac rehabilitation programs are hospital-owned as well as located on hospital premises, some physician practices choose to own/operate their own programs out of their office or an adjacent site. Like physician ownership of other diagnostic or therapeutic entities, physician investment in a cardiac rehabilitation facility is subject to all the conditions of the Stark rules that prohibit self-referral. Depending on the corporate structure of the practice, the exception for in-office ancillary services may/may not apply to office-based cardiac rehabilitation programs *(17)*. Legal advice is recommended before proceeding with program installation in an office setting.

Operationally, the same rules/regulations described previously for hospital-based programs apply equally to cardiac rehabilitation programs located in a medical office or a physician-directed clinic. All structural and operational requirements summarized in Table 1 must be met. And, there is an additional requirement for such off-site facilities:

The program must be under the direct supervision of a physician (18).

The intent of that requirement is to assure immediate availability of a physician at all times the program is operating. Such coverage is assumed to be met when cardiac rehabilitation services are performed on hospital premises, essentially because physicians are always around the building and will respond to rehabilitation in the event of an emergency. However, no such assumption can be made for an off-site facility. Therefore, specific arrangements must be made to provide on-site physician coverage. That means that cardiac rehabilitation operating hours need to be matched to the office hours of the covering physician, which may limit available appointment times especially for patients who need to schedule rehabilitation before/after work. The covering physician may be the program owner, Medical Director, or another physician/group with whom an arrangement has been made to provide daily coverage. As with the Medical Director role, there is no mechanism for billing this super-visory role. Fees for time spent are negotiated between the covering physician and the program owner.

Otherwise in off-site venues, cardiac rehabilitation services are provided and billed essentially the same way as in hospitals. For Medicare patients, CMS form 1500 is completed by office staff and sent to the Medicare Carrier, which covers the physician practice. As in the hospital, the standard ICD-9 and CPT codes for cardiac rehabilitation

Table 3
Synopsis of Medical Director Job Description

Program oversight	Patient care

Review and approve program policies/procedures especially those related to
• Medical necessity and medical appropriateness, such as
   o Acceptable diagnoses for cardiac rehab participation
   o Inclusion/exclusion criteria
• Risk stratification and guidelines for extent of monitoring/surveillance
• Requirements for and content of physician orders/treatment plans
• Outcome measurement and program exit criteria
	Enforce safety measures and emergency preparations, including
	• Personal availability to respond to urgent/emergent developments in cardiac rehab or arrangements for another physician to do so (may be Code Team physician in hospital setting)
	• Development/approval of standing orders for staff to follow in event of emergency
	• Requirement of basic life support training for all staff and advanced cardiac life support for licensed staff members who are authorized to deliver that level of care
	• Participate in periodic emergency drills with cardiac rehab staff

Educate other providers • Inform other physicians about the value and benefit of cardiac rehab participation and encourage patient referrals • Teach/update the CR staff about latest evidence-based strategies for secondary prevention use	Assure that face-to-face patient–physician interactions occur periodically during rehab participation either/or • With the patient's referring or primary physician • By the Medical director personally
Meet with clinical and/or administrative staff on a regular basis to discuss business issues, including • Program utilization • Staffing needs • Regulatory compliance • Performance improvement opportunities	Perform hands-on care to selected patients • Manage rehab care as requested by other physicians • Advise/assist with patient cases as requested by staff, including contacting patient's physician as necessary

Provide visible physician presence through frequent walk-through rounds while cardiac rehabilitation sessions are in action

Table 4
Chart Forms Documenting "Incident to" Interactions

Patient referral with evidence of medical evaluation and qualifying diagnosis
- to provide physician clearance for rehab participation

Physician orders for
- Admission assessment and emergency intervention
- Exercise prescription and risk stratification
- Discharge criteria and follow-up instructions
- to record medical decision making for patient's rehab treatment plan

Office visit reports and/or physician office notes
- to exchange an interim rehab report in connection with a regularly scheduled office visit

Urgent events/change in condition form
- to request medical direction for managing new/different signs/symptoms in rehab

apply. No additional billing opportunity accrues because the program is owned/operated by a medical practice.

Physician–Patient Encounters

Because cardiac rehabilitation functions "incident to physician services," the main source of revenue for physicians connected to the program is through face-to-face patient encounters, either for diagnostic services (e.g., stress test) or for ongoing patient management. The patient's referring physician – cardiologist, surgeon, primary care – and/or the program's Medical Director may have occasion to see the patient before or during rehabilitation participation and to bill accordingly. These encounters may physically occur in the rehabilitation facility or be scheduled in the physician's office. In either case, they are billed as office visits using the appropriate Evaluation & Management (E&M) codes for time spent with either new patients (CPT 99201–99205) or with established patients (CPT 99211–99215) *(19)*. Examples of typical scenarios that prompt such face-to-face encounters include

- initial patient approval for rehabilitation participation,
- regularly scheduled medical follow-up during cardiac rehabilitation participation, and
- a change in patient signs/symptoms during rehabilitation participation that triggers an unscheduled office visit.

Table 4 summarizes common chart forms that provide documentation demonstrating staff–physician–patient interactions that fulfill Medicare's requirement for "incident to" services. Contrary to some past practices, paperwork without a patient encounter – such as physician review of rehabilitation charts, interpretation of normal exercise rhythm strips, or signing of other chart forms – is not a billable activity.

SUMMARY

Understanding that billing codes are few and that insurance payments are controlled, most providers of cardiac rehabilitation services are motivated by other than financial goals *(20)*. At best, cardiac rehabilitation programs may break-even. At least, losses can be minimized through good program management while other nonmonetary goals are achieved. Any/all reimbursement available to cardiac rehabilitation is based on services provided by either the program staff or the physicians providing rehabilitation-related patient care. Although any licensed physician can refer patients to cardiac rehabilitation, only those performing a documented medical work product get paid. Strategies suggested in this chapter should help to optimize those available payments.

REFERENCES

1. Health Care Financing Administration. *Coverage Issues Appendix – Section 35-25: Cardiac Stress Testing and Outpatient Hospital Cardiac Rehabilitation Programs.* Washington, DC: U.S. Department of Health and Human Services; 1980.
2. U.S. Congress. *Title XVIII of the Social Security Act: Health Insurance for the Aged and Disabled*, Washington DC; 1965.
3. Health Care Financing Administration. *Coverage Issues Manual – Section 35-25: Cardiac Rehabilitation Programs, Transmittal No. 41.* Washington, DC: U.S. Department of Health and Human Services; 1989.
4. Phurrough SE, Salive M, Baldwin J, McClain S, Schott L, Chin J. *Decision Memo for Cardiac Rehabilitation Programs (CAG – 00089R).* Baltimore, MD: The Centers for Medicare and Medicaid Services; 2006.
5. Crapo M, Lincoln BL, Snow OJ. *Senate Bill 329: The Pulmonary and Cardiac Rehabilitation Act of 2005.* Washington, DC: U.S. Senate; 2007.
6. Pickering C, Lewis J. *House Bill 552: The Pulmonary and Cardiac Rehabilitation Act of 2006.* Washington, DC: U.S. House of Representatives; 2007.
7. American Medical Association. *Physician ICD-9-CM 2007, 9th Revision*-Clinical Modifications Chicago, IL: American Medical Association Press; 2006:119–121, 308–309.
8. Phurrough SE, Salive M, Baldwin J, Mcclain S, Schott L, Chin J. Decision Memo for Cardiac Rehabilitation Programs (CAG-00089R). Baltimore Centers for Medicare and Medicaid Services: 2006.
9. Williams MA, Balady GJ, Carlson JJ, Comoss P, Humphrey R, Lounsbury PF, Roitman JL, Southard DR. *Guidelines for Cardiac Rehabilitation and Secondary Prevention Programs*, 4th ed. Champaign, IL: Human Kinetics; 2004:195.
10. Beebe M, Dalton J, Espronoada M, Evans DD, Glenn RL, Green G, Hayden D, Majerowicz A, Meggs J, Mindeman ML, O'Hara KE, O'Heron MR, Pavloski D, Rozell D, Stancik L, Thompson P, Tracy S, Trajkocski J, Walker A. *Current Procedural Terminology: 2007 Professional Edition.* Chicago, IL: American Medical Association Press; 2006:398.
11. Federal Register. *Addendum A: List of Outpatient Ambulatory Payment Classes with Status Indicators, Relative Weights, Payment Rates, and Coinsurance Amounts.* Washington, DC; 2000.
12. Nelson J. *Outpatient Cardiac Rehab: Tools and Best Practices for Reimbursement and Compliance.* Marblehead, MA: HCPro Inc.; 2005:75–84.
13. Levinson DR. *Final Report: Review of Medicare Outpatient Cardiac Rehabilitation Provided by Hospitals*, Washington, DC: U.S. Department of Health and Human Services, Office of the Inspector General; 2005.

14. King ML, Williams MA, Fletcher GF, Gordon NF, Gulanick M, King C, Leon AS, Levine BD, Costa F, Wenger NK. Medical Director Responsibilities for Outpatient Cardiac Rehabilitation/Secondary Prevention Programs. *J Cardiopulm Rehabil.* 2005;25:315–320.

15. Williams MA, Balady GJ, Carlson JJ, Comoss P, Humphrey R, Lounsbury PF, Roitman JL, Southard DR. *Guidelines for Cardiac Rehabilitation and Secondary Prevention Programs*, 4th ed. Champaign, IL: Human Kinetics; 2004:193–196.

16. Lewis J, Pickering C. *House Bill 552: The Pulmonary and Cardiac Rehabilitation Act of 2007.* Washington, DC: U.S. House of Representatives; 2007:3.

17. Torras H. *Health Care Fraud and Abuse – A Physician's Guide to Compliance*, 2nd ed. Chicago, IL: American Medical Association Press; 2003:119–172.

18. Phurrough SE, Salive M, Baldwin J, McClain S, Schott L, Chin J. *Decision Memo for Cardiac Rehabilitation Programs (CAG – 00089R).* Baltimore, MD: The Centers for Medicare and Medicaid Services; 2006:4.

19. Beebe M, Dalton J, Espronoada M, Evans DD, Glenn RL, Green G, Hayden D, Majerowicz A, Meggs J, Mindeman ML, O'Hara KE, O'Heron MR, Pavloski D, Rozell D, Stancik L, Thompson P, Tracy S, Trajkocski J, Walker A. *Current Procedural Terminology: 2007 Professional Edition.* Chicago, IL: American Medical Association Press; 2006:9–11.

20. Comoss P. Frequently Asked Questions...Action Packed Answers. *J Cardiopulm Rehabil.* 2005;25:67–70.

INDEX

A

Abdominal obesity, 29
Acromegaly, 198
ACSM Exercise Specialist®, 279, 285
  knowledge, skills and abilities, 284
ACSM Registered Clinical Exercise Physiologist®,
  279, 285
Adults
  blood pressure for, 162–163, 171 (*See also*
    Hypertension)
  classification and management, 162–163
  exercise responses to, 171
Adult Treatment Panel III (ATP III) guidelines
  ability to achieve new LDL-C goals, 148–149
  newer clinical trials, 145–146
  newer statin trials, 146–147
  optimal and optional LDL-C level, 147–148
Aerobic exercise, *See also* Exercise program
  blood pressure response to, 185–188
Aging, 87, 142, 190, 200, 231, 240, 243–247, 249, 254,
  259, 268, 298
  physiological vulnerabilities associated with, 244–246
Air displacement method, 27
Air Force/Texas Coronary Atherosclerosis Prevention
  Study (AFCAPS/TexCAPS), 144
Aldosteronoma, 198
Alpha-interferon, 199
Ambulatory Payment Classifications (APCs), 293
American Association of Cardiovascular and Pulmonary
  Rehabilitation (AACVPR), 1–2, 15, 28, 30, 45–46,
  135–136, 244, 253, 268
American College of Cardiology (ACC), 1–2, 103, 121,
  148, 150, 175, 178
American College of Physicians, 30
American College of Sports Medicine (ACSM), 1–2, 34,
  137, 169, 179, 236, 279, 285
American Diabetes Association (ADA), 157, 159, 200
American Heart Association (AHA), 1–2, 15, 27–28, 32,
  103, 118–119, 121, 142–143, 148, 150, 164, 175,
  178, 244, 268
American Hospital Association, 2
American Nurses Credentialing Center, 285
American Physical Therapy Association, 285
Anger, 53–54, 95–96
Angina patients
  exercise program for, 173, 176–178
  exercise training for, 107–108
  risk reduction, 142
Angiotensin-converting enzyme (ACE)-inhibitor
  therapy, 142

Anglo-Scandinavian Cardiac Outcomes Trial–Lipid
  Lowering Arm (ASCOT-LLA) trials, 144–145
Ankle to brachial systolic pressure ratio (ABI), 222, 226
Antihypertensive and Lipid-Lowering Treatment to
  Prevent Heart Attack Trial–Lipid-Lowering Trial
  (ALLHAT-LLT), 145
Anti-insulin receptor antibodies, 199
Antiplatelet therapy, 142, 202
Anxiety, 47, 53–54, 56, 59–60, 95–96, 112–113, 203,
  212, 214, 217, 235, 246, 248, 280
Arthritis, 61, 115, 244, 259–260
  adaptations to exercise training, 238–239
  adjustments for
    acute exercise and exercise testing, 235–236
    disease-specific exercise prescription, 236–238
  aerobic exercise prescription in, 237
  as comorbidity in CR, 231–240
  concern areas, 239–240
  diagnosis and treatment of, 233–234
  osteoarthritis, 231–239
  rehabilitation and exercise management implications,
    234–235
  resistance training prescription in, 237
  rheumatoid arthritis, 231–239
  self-efficacy in patient with, 235
Arthritis Foundation/YMCA aquatics programs
  (AFYAP), 239
Aspirin therapy, 142, 161, 166
  for diabetes mellitus, 161
Atherosclerosis, 28–30, 55, 78, 80, 143, 166, 174, 179,
  201, 221–222, 226, 245
Atherosclerotic vascular disease patients, secondary
  prevention in, 1–2
A to Z trial, 145

B

Balke protocol, 115
Beck Depression Inventory (BDI), 47
Behavioral change
  bringing attention to behavior, 274
  clinic-based strategies, 273–275
  clinic visits and, 275
  developing plan for, 275–276
  importance of, 274–275
  transtheoretical model of, 275–276
Behavioral profile, and hostility, 54–55
Benson's respiratory one meditation, 60
Beta-adrenergic agonists, 198
Beta-blocker therapy, 142

299

Progressive overload exercise training program
  frequency and duration, 10–11
  intensity, 8–10
PROspective Study of Pravastatin in the Elderly at Risk
    (PROSPER), 144–145, 246–247
Prothrombotic status, and obesity, 29
Psychological distress, and cardiovascular disease,
    55, 280
Psychosocial risk factors, 48, 53–55, 62
Pulmonary disease patients, *See* Chronic lung disease
Pulmonary exercise assessments, of chronic lung disease,
    213–214
Pulmonary rehabilitation (PR), 254, 257

Q

Quality Assurance Program, 142

R

Rabson–Mendenhall syndrome, 198
Randomized clinical trial (RCT), 48–49, 173
Recurrent Coronary Prevention Project, 61
Reimbursement for CR programs, 289–297
  billing and coding, 290, 292
  charges and reimbursement, 292–293
  Medicare approved diagnoses and related codes, 292
  payments to physicians, 293–296
  rules and regulations, 290
Relaxation response techniques, for stress management,
    59–61
Resistance exercise, 38–39, 174, 238
  training program, 11–13
    effectiveness of, 12
    flexibility in, 12–13
Responding to resistance, principle in MI, 69
Resting metabolic rate (RMR), 33–34, 37
Retinopathy, 159, 162, 200–202
  and nephropathy, 207
Revascularization, 56, 104, 175, 178, 279
Rheumatoid arthritis (RA), 231–239
Risk assessment, 26–27, 136–137
  cardiac rehabilitation setting, 271–273, 276
  clinical setting, 273–276

S

Saturated fat, 17–18, 21–22, 72, 149, 160, 164
Scandinavian Simvastatin Survival Study (4S), 145
Sedentary lifestyle, 135, 161, 207, 258
Self-hypnosis, for stress management, 59–61
Senior Hypertension and Physical Exercise (SHAPE)
    study, 190
Shifting perceptions and beliefs, for stress management,
    61–62
Six-minute walk test, 71, 115, 226, 228
  in cardiac rehabilitation, 131–139
  ceiling effect, 138
  data uses, 136–137
  determinants of, 134–136
  for exercise prescription, 137

future research directions, 138–139
learning effect, 138
protocol, 132–134
Skin-fold thickness method, 27
Smokers, 77–81, 83, 85–87, 90–92, 94, 96–97, 100, 159,
    164, 214, 226, 247, *See also* Smoking
Smoking, 1–3, 36, 55, 67–68, 70–71, 73, 142–143, 159,
    161, 164, 172, 175, 202, 214, 221, 223, 226–227,
    232, 235, 247, 257–259, 264, 273, 275–278, 281,
    See also Smoking cessation
  cardiovascular disease in, 78–79
  chronic diseases caused by, 258
  coronary disease and, 97
  depression and, 97
  epidemiology of, 78
  pathophysiology of, 78, 80–81
  prevalence, 78–79
Smoking cessation, 142
  assessment of
    smoking and tobacco dependence, 82
    willing and readiness to stop smoking, 82
  behavioral approaches, 89, 91, 94
  benefits of, 81
  brandswitching approach, 91
  cleaning house approach, 94
  clinical tobacco intervention, 83
  cold turkey approach, 89, 91, 94
  cutting back approach, 94
  in future, 100
  and heart disease risk reduction, 80–81
  issues during action stages, 94–100
    challenging destructive thinking, 95–97
    creating reward system, 97–98
    dealing with psychological addiction, 95
    delivery method, 98
    depression, coronary disease and smoking, 97
    effects of smoking rate, 94
    establishing and maintaining support, 97
    increasing awareness of triggers to recidivism, 95
    managing withdrawal symptoms, 98
    planning for withdrawal symptoms, 95
    psychological factors, 96
    relapse prevention, 98–100
    using health locus of control, 96
  motivation to, 87–88
  pharmaceutical agents for, 92–93
  pharmacotherapy, 88–94
  physical addiction to tobacco, 88
  plan, 81, 86, 88
  recognizing tobacco dependence as chronic disease, 86
  strategies when patient
    unwilling to quit, 86–88
    willing to quit, 83–86
  treatment interventions, 81–94
  warm chicken approach, 91
Social isolation, 53–55, 214, 243
Somatostatinoma, 198
Stanford Coronary Risk Intervention Project (SCRIP)
    trials, 143